AGING ISSUES, HEALTH AND FINANCIAL ALTERNATIVES

ARE CHRONIC DEGENERATIVE DISEASES PART OF THE AGEING PROCESS?

INSIGHTS FROM COMPARATIVE BIOLOGY

AGING ISSUES, HEALTH AND FINANCIAL ALTERNATIVES

Additional books in this series can be found on Nova's website under the Series tab.

Additional e-books in this series can be found on Nova's website under the e-book tab.

AGING ISSUES, HEALTH AND FINANCIAL ALTERNATIVES

ARE CHRONIC DEGENERATIVE DISEASES PART OF THE AGEING PROCESS?

INSIGHTS FROM COMPARATIVE BIOLOGY

MICHAEL A. SINGER

New York

For permission to use material from this book please contact us:
Telephone 631-231-7269; Fax 631-231-8175
Web Site: http://www.novapublishers.com

Library of Congress Cataloging-in-Publication Data

ISBN: 978-1-62618-013-0

Library of Congress Control Number: 2013930634

Published by Nova Science Publishers, Inc. † New York

Contents

Preface

Most of the DNA in the human genome does not encode proteins but is involved in regulatory functions. In addition, the human genome is characterized by an extensive array of structural DNA variants arising from de novo mutations plus accumulated structural variants transmitted through an individual's lineage. The result is that each person has a unique genome which is expressed as that person's unique phenotype. Ageing can be understood on both the species and individual level. Each species has a programmed ageing and mortality pattern, but within those broad species-specific boundaries there is considerable individual variation. At the individual level, ageing reflects the integrated effects of that individual's unique mix of DNA structural variants, unique experience-specific epigenetic marks and imperfectly repaired genomic and cellular damage. The extensive genomic and phenotypic variation across individuals makes it very difficult to define what is normal without setting arbitrary limits. This difficulty in establishing normal morphological and behavioral ranges makes the disease construct very problematical. Giving an individual a disease label carries the implication that all individuals with that label share a similar underlying disease molecular phenotype. The current genomic and epigenomic data are not consistent with this implication. Human "chronic degenerative" diseases are not diseases, but rather variations of the ageing process across individuals.

Keywords: Aldosterone; bimodal distribution; chaperone; circadian rhythm; cis-regulatory element; copy number variant (CNV); cortisol; corticosterone; dendrite; disease concept; dopamine; epidemiological studies; epigenetics; epistasis; eusocial; evo-devo; genome wide association study (GWAS); glycated hemoglobin; histone; hyperinsulinemia; immediate early gene (IEG); intimal arterial thickening; mechanosensor; microbiota; micro RNA (miRNA); natural selection; neovascularization; non-coding DNA; Notch signaling; nuclear receptor; pressure mechanosensor; pressure-natriuresis mechanism; personalized medicine; salt intake; single nucleotide polymorphism (SNP); quantitative trait; quantitative trait locus; social environment; stress response; telomere; mTOR pathway; trade-off; transcription factor; transposon; tyrosine kinase receptor; vascular remodeling

Introduction

Collecting information relevant to the pathogenesis of human biomedical conditions as well as designing management strategies for these conditions, have generally relied upon a combination of inputs from clinical studies and experimental studies using traditional laboratory animal models. However, as amply documented (Singer, 2007; 2011), the physiological features of natural animal models can also give valuable insights into human biomedical disorders. Animals have evolved adaptations under the pressure of unusual environmental conditions and these adaptations often represent biological solutions to states similar to those of human biomedical disorders. For example, the American black bear has learned how to avoid disuse osteoporosis and disuse muscle atrophy during a prolonged period of inactivity while hibernating. In addition, the physiological characteristics of natural animal models often challenge concepts held by the biomedical scientific community. As a case in point, humans with an elevated arterial pressure develop cardiac hypertrophy as a consequence of the increased (hemodynamic) pressure load. This state of cardiac hypertrophy is considered pathologic since it can lead to significant systolic and diastolic dysfunction with resulting heart failure. On the other hand, the giraffe has a mean arterial pressure of about 200 mmHg, yet only develops physiological cardiac hypertrophy as a result of this increased pressure load. Why does an increased pressure load lead to apparent pathological cardiac hypertrophy in the human but only physiological cardiac hypertrophy in the giraffe? Regardless, the physiological features of natural animal models can give important insights into human biomedical disorders.

Ageing is generally defined as a progressive decline in "fitness" with advancing chronological age. Within the evolutionary context, this decline in fitness is specifically measured in terms of a decrease in the age-specific probability of survival and the age-specific rate of reproduction. However, the process of ageing can be conceptualized within a much broader context to encompass more generally an age-dependent decline in the physiological functioning of organs (e.g. heart, kidney, brain) and systems (e.g. neuroendocrine system). In humans, ageing is a well-accepted phenomenon, although the boundary separating what biomedical researchers term ageing and what is considered a "disease" has not been clearly defined. In this monograph, natural animal models will be used to examine both the features of ageing and to provide a different perspective on the genesis of human biomedical disorders. This approach should help clarify the boundary between what constitutes ageing (senescence) and what constitutes "disease". This distinction has been further blurred by the concept that ageing per se is now considered a "risk" factor for certain diseases. Defining this boundary is in fact, the central question posed in this monograph; are so- called "chronic degenerative diseases" actually diseases or really manifestations of senescence. It is my contention that "chronic degenerative diseases" are just variants of the ageing process.

A skeptic would argue that the design features of humans and for example black bears and giraffes are so different that one cannot extrapolate from a bear or giraffe to a human. The vasculature of the giraffe is "made" to withstand a high mean arterial pressure and as such the design features of the giraffe do not apply to the hypertensive state observed in the human. Clearly this must be the predominant view since arterial blood pressure measurements in the giraffe were first obtained more than fifty years ago but yet the giraffe has never been embraced as a suitable animal model of human hypertension by those engaged in cardiovascular research.

However, this view is inconsistent with the observation that in general, evolution proceeds by "tinkering" with morphological features that are already in existence and with successful animal design characteristics rather than proceeding discontinuously via the development of completely unique adaptations. As noted by Brakefield (2011), the process of evolution is highly opportunistic and if a particular feature or property is available, evolution will exploit its potential and run with it. Protein coding genes are generally highly conserved and evolutionary change is largely relegated to the regulatory machinery (Brakefield, 2011; Fernald, 2006). In fact, evolution is a very economical process and one example is the observation that blood vessels and nerve fibers often course throughout the body alongside one another and their "wiring" into networks is accomplished by a number of mechanisms common to both systems (Carmeliet and Tessier-Lavigne, 2005). Animal design features form a continuum and as such, for example, the cardiovascular physiology of the giraffe has direct relevance to the cardiovascular physiology of the human.

Part of the motivation in writing this monograph is to counter what I perceive to be two implicit assumptions in the biomedical research field. The first assumption is that somehow the physiology of the human is unique and that there is not a continuum across animals; a "gap" exists between human physiological features and those of "lower animals". Such an assumption presumably underlies why the cardiovascular physiology of the "hypertensive " giraffe or the chronic hyperglycemic state of birds are not considered appropriate models for study by biomedical researchers in the fields of cardiovascular medicine and endocrinology respectively. In addition, this assumption is "supported" by the fact that almost all biomedical experimental research uses rodents which have been genetically simplified by either inbreeding or by being genetically engineered. This assumption has been particularly applied to the "non- morphological" aspects of animal biology; for example, are language, music and the mind unique to humans? In answer to this question, there is now a growing consensus that animal communication systems including human language represent a continuum of complexity and that even the state of the human mind is an evolved entity. This issue is discussed more fully in the Background; Evolution section. A second implicit assumption is that presumed altered physiological functions in the human are considered to be a disease. For example, cognitive decline associated with brain amyloid plaques is called a disease in humans whereas such features are found in other animals and are considered part of senescence. Classifying a decrease in physiological functions as a disease carries the additional assumption that this decrease in physiological functions (disease) can be cured. Such a "disease" can be managed but in most cases not cured. The complexities in genetic/epigenetic mechanisms that have been revealed since completion of the human genome project more than a decade ago (Background; genetics) underscore the simplistic nature of this "disease-cure" assumption.

Since Western medicine has constructed an elaborate house of diseases, what then is a disease? Duffin (2005) has examined the disease concept from an historical perspective. There are a number of components comprising the disease concept and their descriptive features vary according to the prevailing cultural norms and scientific knowledge of that era. Duffin (2005) breaks down the disease concept into illness (symptoms and signs experienced by the sufferer), causation, and prognostic and treatment aspects. On an individual basis, the disease is considered to reside within the person, to be "bad" and hopefully to be discontinuous. I would add to these components, one of "sameness" since this component represents the basis underlying the design feature of current epidemiological studies. By "sameness" I refer to the implicit assumption that individuals suffering from a given disease state all have the same underlying molecular phenotype and that the results of a specific treatment can be generalized to all individuals classified as having that disease state. However, as is evident throughout this monograph, this assumption is not valid. Individual genomes and epigenomes are unique and the statistically mean individual does not exist. Across individuals labeled as having for example insulin resistance or cognitive impairment, there will be a great variation in the underlying molecular phenotypes.

The disease concept also implies a dichotomy between normal and abnormal. Defining the normal state in humans for a given behavioral or physiological trait is problematical. In humans, a "normal" range for quantitative traits such as arterial blood pressure, weight, height and blood glucose concentrations is defined statistically and abnormal values are arbitrarily classified as being more than two standard deviations from the mean (Cochrane, 1972). For behavioral traits such as cognitive functioning defining what is a normal range is much more difficult.

In essence as discussed throughout this book, diseases are really not diseases but just variations (perhaps extreme in some cases) in physiological and metabolic traits that occur naturally across individual animals.

The organization of this monograph is as follows. In the background section, salient details concerning evolution, genetics, phenotypic plasticity and ageing will be presented. Four subsequent sections will review specific chronic degenerative diseases; atherosclerotic vascular disease, hypertension, diabetes and dementia. Each section will explore the characteristics of relevant natural animal models that furnish insights into the interplay between the various biological mechanisms underlying these four "disease" states. In a concluding section, the evidence relating to the question of whether chronic degenerative diseases are actually diseases or part of the ageing process will be reviewed. It is important to remember that each of these four "disease" states (atherosclerotic vascular disease, hypertension, diabetes and dementia) has been extensively studied and there is a large body of experimental studies for each of them. Hence, only a limited number of these studies can be reviewed in this monograph. I have attempted to choose studies that highlight the complex interplay between the multiple biological processes that characterize the underpinnings of each of these "disease" states.

Chapter I

Background

In this Background section, general features of evolution, genetics, phenotypic plasticity and ageing relevant to the subsequent discussion of "chronic degenerative diseases" will be presented. This material is not meant to be comprehensive, but I have tried to highlight in these areas, specific information that I believe will make the sections describing "chronic degenerative diseases" more understandable.

Evolution

The course of evolution has been shaped by the interplay between genetic variation across individual organisms and external factors; environmental pressures including limited resources, competition between individuals and chance and contingency. As pointed out by Gould (1980), gene mutation is the source of genetic variation but natural selection only "sees" the phenotypic expression of these mutations in individuals. Hence individuals are the unit of selection but individual organisms do not evolve. Individuals can only grow, reproduce and die. Evolutionary change occurs in groups of interacting organisms; species are the unit of evolution. In his popular writings, Gould (1989; 1996) has also discussed the role of chance and contingency in the evolutionary process. He argued that evolution cannot be characterized as a process with a directional trajectory of increasingly complex organisms. Quoting from Gould (1996); "We (humans) are glorious accidents of an unpredictable process with no drive to complexity, not the expected results of evolutionary principles that yearn to produce a creature capable of understanding the mode of its own necessary construction".

Over the past two decades, a better understanding of the genetic mechanisms underlying the evolution of animal morphological diversity among species has emerged. This understanding has resulted from the merging of developmental genetics (i.e. the genetic mechanisms underlying embryogenesis) and evolutionary biology into the discipline of evolutionary development biology, dubbed evo-devo. Previously, biologists had generally focused on the role of mutations in protein coding genes as the underlying source of genetic variation central to evolutionary change. Most mutations were eliminated through negative selection while mutations beneficial to the "fitness" state of the organism were spread through the evolving population by positive selection. However, several important observations have confounded this model and have helped shape current views on the evolution of animal form.

One of these observations was the discovery of a suite of interacting (Hox) genes which are critical for the embryonic development of arthropods and tetrapods (Carroll, 2005). Hox genes function to regulate form in the head-tail axis of developing animal embryos. Hox genes contain a DNA sequence known as the homeobox which encodes a protein domain, the homeodomain. Hox genes are arranged in clusters; for example, the fruit fly has a single cluster of hox genes while mammals have four clusters (Veraksa et al., 2000). The protein products of Hox genes (Hox proteins) are a large family of closely related transcription factors with similar DNA binding profiles. The homeodomain is the part of the Hox protein conferring DNA binding. However, the action of Hox proteins on target genes requires the co-binding of multiple cofactors and modulator proteins to the DNA of the target gene (Veraksa et al., 2000). The differential spatial and temporal expression of Hox genes directs different fates to head-tail axis morphological domains (Lemons and McGinnis, 2006). As development proceeds, "head" Hox proteins specify the cell arrangements and structures that result in, for example, chewing organs, "thoracic" Hox proteins specify, for example, loco motor organs, and "abdominal" Hox proteins specify, for example, genital and excretory organs (Lemons and McGinnis, 2006). Hox genes act at multiple levels within developmental gene hierarchies; their protein products (transcription factors) regulate vast numbers of individual target genes (gene regulatory network). Hox proteins regulate other transcription factors which act at very early stages in target pathways and as well regulate genes involved in various signaling cascades. Within this scheme, the number of targets of Hox proteins is extremely numerous. At the downstream end of this hierarchical scheme are the so called realizator genes. The products of these genes are involved in cellular functions such as migration, adhesion, and differentiation. Their unique combinations determine the structural anatomy of a large field of cells (Veraksa et al., 2000).Hence, the result of this multilayered hierarchal scheme is a distinct morphological region linked to a given Hox protein (Veraksa et al., 2000). As pointed out by Carroll (2008), Hox proteins have been evolutionarily conserved; mice and humans share the same set of 39 Hox genes. There is no evidence for any new Hox gene duplications in the mammalian lineage.

How are Hox genes themselves regulated? The cis-regulatory elements of these genes are larger and more complex than those of loci encoding proteins involved in cell-type-specific physiological processes. Upstream steps involved in initiation of Hox gene expression patterns have not been clearly defined, but the maintenance of Hox gene expression patterns requires the action of proteins from the Polycomb and Trithorax group of genes. Polycomb and Trithorax proteins form large multimolecular complexes which modify chromatin structure around Hox genes (epigenetic mechanism) and in this way alter expression profiles of the Hox genes (Veraksa et al., 2000). Many of the Hox gene clusters encode micro RNAs (miRNA) at intergenic regions. Such miRNAs appear to have a regulatory function on the expression of neighboring Hox genes (Lemons and McGinnis, 2006).

Hox gene clusters are only one class of morphological patterning genes; in this case determining form along the anterior-posterior axis. In a similar fashion, other suites of interacting genes direct specific organogenesis. For example, eye development proceeds via morphological transformations of newly generated tissue that are regulated by multiple genes with expression patterns that overlap spatially and temporally. In fruit flies, seven genes collaborate (Fernald, 2006). One of these genes, the homologs eyeless in fruit flies and Pax6 in mammals, is sufficient to induce eye formation even in ectopic sites (Veraksa et al., 2000) and hence Pax6 (eyeless) has been considered a master control gene for eye development. However, Pax6 (eyeless) is also required for patterning part of the developing brain and central nervous system (Carroll, 2008). As with the Hox genes, the protein encoded by Pax6 functions as a transcription factor. Similar to the Hox genes, Pax6 (eyeless) has a large cis-regulating complex which in this particular gene contains six distinct cis-regulatory elements (Carroll, 2008).

In summary, Hox genes and the Pax6 (eyeless) gene are members of the so-called toolkit family of genes. The genetic toolkit consists of a relatively small number of genes which encode protein products (transcription factors) that direct organismal morphological development. Toolkit genes are highly conserved and serve multiple functions in different cell types, body parts and developmental stages.

A second observation that has helped shape current views on the evolution of animal form is related to the role of non- coding DNA. Non- coding DNA refers to DNA that does not code for proteins or structural RNA e.g. ribosomal and transfer RNA. Andolfatto (2005) has examined the evolution of non- coding DNA in two species of Drosophila; D. melanogaster and D. simulans. He compared non- coding nucleotide sites (introns, intergenic regions, 5' and 3' untranslated transcribed regions) with synonymous sites; protein coding sites where, because of the redundancies in nucleotide triplet code, a substitution would not alter the encoded amino acid. The synonymous sites were used as a metric of neutral evolutionary change. Within a species, Andolfatto (2005) found that both polymorphism and evolutionary divergence were significantly reduced in non- coding DNA compared to synonymous sites. This observation implied that within a species, mutations in non- coding DNA were subject to stronger negative selection than synonymous sites. Between species, there was considerable evolutionary divergence for non- coding DNA relative to synonymous sites; this divergence was driven by positive selection. Based on the data, Andolfatto (2005) estimated that changes in non- coding DNA regions contributed much more to adaptive divergence between species (speciation) than did changes in protein coding DNA regions.

Carroll (2005; 2008) has used these observations to explore the genetic mechanisms underlying the evolution of morphological diversity. Toolkit genes such as the Hox genes encode transcription factors which serve multiple roles in that they function independently in different cell types, body parts and developmental stages. Mutations in the coding region of a given Hox gene would alter its protein product (transcription factor) and hence alter all of the genes regulated by that transcription factor. Such a mutation would have widespread effects and be deleterious to organismal fitness. There are modes of gene evolution which increase genetic diversity, but avoid the widespread deleterious effects of the coding region mutation just described (Carroll, 2005). Three such mechanisms are; gene duplication with mutations in only one of the paralogs, expansion of the number of cis regulatory elements for that gene with mutations in some, but not all, of these cis regulatory elements and evolution of a new exon and splicing sites which allows for alternative forms of a protein. Carroll (2008) argues that the absence of new Hox gene duplications in arthropods and tetrapods, the extreme conservation of homeodomains and the potential for mutations in one cis regulatory element to selectively alter just one feature of gene expression favor the proposal that mutations in the cis regulating elements of existing genes is a more likely source of morphological diversity compared with the evolution of new genes. Carroll proposed that cis regulatory element evolution was an essential component of gene regulatory network evolution and was the chief mechanism underlying the diversity of development and form. How do cis regulatory elements evolve? Carroll (2008) proposed several possible mechanisms; mutations in existing cis regulatory elements that create new binding sites for transcription factors, insertion of transposable elements (possessing an array of transcription factor binding sites) into the genome which then function as new cis regulatory elements and direct modification of the properties of the transcription factor binding sites within a cis regulatory element.

In a more recent publication, Wagner and Lynch (2010) discussed another possibility in the evolution of body plans of multicellular organisms. They pointed out that the binding of transcription factors to the appropriate DNA site often requires the cooperative binding of other transcription factors or cofactors such as non- coding RNA. The formation of these transcription factor complexes allows for the integration of converging signals into a signal transcriptional response. Hence the evolution of transcription factor proteins (through modification of the encoding gene) may play an important role in the evolution of body form.

Carroll (2008) has summarized his genetic theory of morphological evolution as follows. Form evolves by altering the expression of functionally conserved proteins and such changes occur chiefly through mutations in cis regulatory elements of pleiotropic developmental regulatory genes (toolkit genes) and of target genes within the vast regulatory networks they control. These principles underlie the evolution of morphological diversity as would be seen for example between species. However, the genesis of adaptations resulting from the action of natural selection on individual organisms, involves individual variation due to many types of structural and nonstructural (epigenetic) modifications of DNA (discussed in the next section on genetics).

The proposals of Carroll are supported by the observed relationship between amounts of genomic non- protein coding DNA and eukaryotic complexity (Taft et al., 2007). Since quantifying a parameter encompassing biological complexity is difficult, Taft et al. used a more general definition comprising the number and different types of cells in the organism and the degree of cellular organization. The number of protein- coding DNA sequences in animals varying from nematodes to humans varies by only 50% whereas the total genomic size across this same range of animals varies by a factor of about one thousand. Across this animal range of increasing biological complexity, there was a good correlation between increasing complexity and the value of the ratio of non- protein coding DNA to total genomic size. Most of this non- (protein) coding DNA transcribed non- (protein) coding RNA and this non- coding RNA has regulatory functions; e.g. modification of chromatin structure, genomic imprinting. As summarized by Taft et al., (2007), the evolution of more developmentally complex organisms has been possible not only via the evolution of suites of highly conserved toolkit proteins, but also through the evolution of an expanded regulatory architecture which is largely transacted by non- (protein) coding RNA. This observation indicates that evolution proceeds primarily through the less costly process of modifying the gene regulatory mechanisms acting on existing protein coding genes rather than the more costly process of creating a host of new protein coding genes. A recent paper comparing the genomes of humans and non-human primates underscores the importance of regulatory DNA in species differences (McLean et al., 2011).

Clearly, we are learning more about the genetic mechanisms underlying the evolution of morphological diversity. However, what about the genetic mechanisms underlying the evolution of behavioral diversity particularly complex behaviors? This is a more difficult issue since morphological diversity is more easily measured and quantified than behavioral diversity. One behavior that has been studied is vocal learning; the ability to modify vocal signals as a result of experiencing the vocal signals of other individuals. Vocal learning is considered to be an important step in language acquisition and has been documented in all songbird species studied, various species of parrots, Anna hummingbirds, sack-winged bats, a harbor seal, elephants, whales and dolphins (Webb and Zhang, 2005; Scharff and Petri, 2011). A genetic basis to language development was found with the discovery of the gene FOXP2. The link between language and FOXP2 was established by analysis of a large family (KE) in which affected members with a speech and language disorder were found to have a point mutation in the gene FOXP2. However, the full phenotype of affected members included features other than a speech and grammar disorder; defects in the ability to move the face and mouth not related to speech and a reduction in nonverbal IQ.

The transcription factor encoded by the gene FOXP2 is characterized by a highly conserved Forkhead domain. This protein domain binds to distinct DNA sequences in its target gene's regulatory regions and this protein domain can be considered as analogous to the homeodomain of the Hox proteins. FOXP2 shows extreme sequence conservation and in fact the exon 7 amino acid sequences for six bird species, the American alligator and the mouse are all identical. Humans have one unique amino acid substitution on exon 7 and share a second amino acid substitution with carnivores such as cat, dog, fox and wolf (Webb and Zhang, 2005). Apparently the Fox P2 protein under appropriate conditions (e.g. dimerization or in complexes with other Fox proteins) can function as either a transcriptional repressor or activator (Scharff and Petri, 2011). The FOXP2 gene in mammals is expressed in multiple sites other than the brain; lung, heart and gut. In addition, as already noted, a mutation in this gene as uncovered in the KE family is associated with multiple neural deficits, not just language and speech abnormalities. In humans, FoxP2 protein appears to be important in embryonic neurodevelopment since downstream target genes are involved in neural functions related to cell communication and signal transduction. The importance of FOXP2 as a toolkit gene is supported by the observation that this gene is expressed during embryonic development in homologous brain regions of monkeys, various rodent species, different bird species, frogs and fish (Scharff and Petri, 2011). In addition, continued expression of FOXP2 in postnatal brains suggests functions beyond those of neural development. As concluded by Haesler et al., (2004), the highly conserved FOXP2 gene sequence and the overall brain expression pattern in avian, reptilian and mammalian brains confirm that FOXP2 has a more general neurodevelopmental role in addition to enabling vocal learning.

In a recent paper, Konopka et al., (2009) compared the transcriptional regulation properties of human and chimpanzee FOXP2. Apparently when chimpanzees and humans diverged from a common ancestor, the human FOXP2 protein acquired two different amino acids not shared with other primates. These two human- specific amino acid changes altered FOXP2 function by conferring differential gene transcriptional regulation. The genes that are differentially regulated by human FOXP2 include those involved in cerebellar motor function, craniofacial formation and cartilage and connective tissue formation suggesting an important role for human FOXP2 in establishing the neural circuitry and physical structure needed for spoken language. However, it is becoming apparent that the differences in language skills between non-human primates and humans are becoming smaller (Grainger et al., 2012).

There are also experimental observations that the development and evolution of vocal learning in song birds is related to changes in the regulation of FOXP2 temporal/spatial expression and not to changes in the coding sequence of the gene itself (Carroll, 2005). A comparative analysis of the FOXP2 coding sequences of humans and song learning and non-learning birds did not reveal any amino acid substitutions that were shared between humans and song learning birds, or any fixed differences between song learning and non-learning birds. However, a much different picture was painted when the expression of the FOXP2 gene was examined. A striking increase in FOXP2 expression was observed in Area X of the brain, a center necessary for vocal learning that is absent from non-learners. This increase in FOXP2 expression occurred in zebra finches over the developmental period when vocal learning occurs. In adult canaries, seasonal changes in FOXP2 expression were observed in Area X associated with changes in the stability of the bird's song. During the breeding season, male canaries sing highly regular and stereotyped song and FOXP2 expression in Area X is low. After the breeding season, song becomes more variable and new syllables are incorporated, and concomitantly FOXP2 in Area X is up regulated. Hence changes in the regulation of the temporal/spatial expression of FOXP2, but not changes in its coding sequence are correlated with the development and evolution of vocal learning in birds. However, the upstream regulation of FOXP2 is largely unknown and although FOXP2 in turn regulates a large number of target genes, only a few have been delineated. Finally, it is important to emphasize that the FOXP2 gene acts in a number of brain areas and is involved in a variety of behaviors in addition to vocal learning and language. In summary, as reviewed by Bolhuis et al., (2010) recent experimental observations suggest that analogous mechanisms underlie vocal learning in birds and humans at the behavioral , neural, genetic and cognitive levels.

Another complex behavior that has been studied is gesturing and in particular pointing. As reviewed by Kaplan (2011), gesturing behaviors (including pointing) are intertwined with speech and language development as well as other cognitive functions. Most research in this area has been done in primates and quoting from Kaplan; "The impression that such research on human and non-human primates gives, however, is misleading because it still infers evolutionary uniqueness of pointing in the primate line, with its link to human symbolic communication and theory of mind." Kaplan (2011) studied pointing gesture in the Australian magpie (Gymnorhina tibicen). The magpie is one of the foremost song birds in Australia and is very territorial as well as being exclusively social. The experimental design was as follows. A taxidermy model of a local eagle predator was hidden under a shrub on the ground in a known magpie territorial site. The investigator recorded the behaviors of the magpies when this predator model was detected. The behaviors observed included; alarm vocalizations and swooping flights; beak pointing at the predator by magpies; other magpies, after initially landing, engaging in eye gaze following at the pointing magpies. Kaplan observed that each pointing magpie's role was to change the state of knowledge of another magpie and it immediately stopped its pointing behavior once the watching magpie had also started viewing the eagle and had issued alarm vocalizations i.e. the pointing act ceased because of another magpie's changed behavior not because the arousal stimulus had diminished. Kaplan proposes that this pointing behavior can be considered a pre-speech behavior and evidence of complex cognitive capacity. Kaplan made this judgment in conjunction with two other previously documented observations; the discovery of mirror-like neurons in the avian brain involved in song learning and the evidence that the brain areas specialized for vocal learning in vocal learners evolved as a specialization of a pre-existing motor pathway that controls movement.

In summary, the prevailing evolutionary model is that morphological and behavioral diversity between species has arisen from modifications in the regulatory elements and factors that act upon suites of highly conserved so called toolkit genes. Diversity occurs predominately through the differential spatial and temporal expression of these genes. Within this context humans are not unique. Our form and our repertoire of behaviors have directly evolved from other animals. However, as individuals we do differ from one another. There are differences in the genome between individuals and in the next section; genetics, we will examine the genetic features underlying phenotypic variation within species e.g. variations between individual humans.

Genetics

The human genome project, completed about a decade ago, raised a number of unexpected questions and as a result new complexities within the genetic machinery have become appreciated. As noted by Mattick (2011), the number of conventional protein coding genes does not scale with development and biological complexity; humans and other vertebrates have about 20,000 protein coding genes in the haploid genome. In contrast the extent of non-coding intronic and intergenic sequences increases markedly with complexity; only 1.5% of the human genome encodes proteins (Mattick, 2003; 2011). As noted in the section; evolution, there is a strong positive correlation between the amount of non- protein-coding sequence and biological complexity across animals from nematodes to mammals. It is also apparent that the non- protein- coding sequences of DNA express large numbers of non - coding RNA, many of which have regulatory functions (Taft et al., 2007).

Although not always stated, studies of the human genome are generally referring to the haploid genome. Prior to discussing the genome project in more detail, a very brief description of chromosome structure is in order. The basic building block is a long strand of DNA wound around numerous protein cores, each formed from a complex of eight histones. The resulting structure is much like a necklace wound around numerous beads. A complex core of eight histones with wrapped around DNA is referred to as a nucleosome. The long chain of nucleosomes comprises chromatin which is compacted into the shape of a chromosome.

Another aspect of (previously unsuspected) complexity relates to the genetic underpinnings of heritability. For example, height has a heritability of 80-90%, yet the more than 40 genetic variants associated with height differences account for only about 5% of height's heritability (Maher, 2008). In fact, the genome project did not solve the question as to the genetic basis of phenotypic variability among (generally healthy) humans (Olson, 2011).

Although the human genome is a distinct entity when compared to the genomes of other species, the human genome itself does not exist in a single structural form; numerous structural variations make each individual human genome unique. In fact, recent data has revealed that about 10% of the human genome is structurally polymorphic at the submicroscopic scale (Li et al., 2012).In the early days of DNA sequencing, the structural genetic variants measured included single nucleotide polymorphisms (SNPs), and small insertions, deletions, inversions and duplications. More recently, larger structural mutations (copy-number variants, CNVs) have been described in the human genome (Feuk et al., 2006; Mills et al., 2011). A CNV is a large segment of DNA that is present at a variable copy number in comparison with a reference genome. Classes of CNVs include insertions, deletions and duplications. In fact, CNVs might help explain "missing" heritability (Maher, 2008). CNVs have also been linked to various human disorders (Cohen, 2007). However, currently mapped SNPs and CNVs account for only a small fraction of genome structural polymorphism (Li et al., 2012; Conrad et al., 2010). Transposons, mobile sequences of DNA, represent another mechanism for producing genetic variation. By moving into new positions within the genome, transposons can create phenotypically significant mutations. Hence a spectrum of structural genetic variants are now known to occur in the human genome varying in size from single nucleotide substitutions and other small changes to large structural genetic variants such as CNVs that can encompass tens or hundreds of base pairs (Feuk et al., 2006). As Olson (2011) points out the accumulation of mutations (SNPs, other small structural changes and large structural variants i.e. CNVs) which are "deleterious" by standard evolutionary criteria probably explains the genetic basis for phenotypic variability among humans.

Phenotypic variation can also be due to variability in the methylation of DNA regions within the same tissue across different individuals (demonstrated in mice and humans by Feinberg and Irizarry, 2010). Interestingly, these variably methylated regions were found particularly in the vicinity of genes with ontogenic functions (development and morphogenesis). Feinberg and Irizarry (2010) also reported that variably methylated DNA regions were associated with variability in the expression of genes nearby to that region. Hence phenotypic variability is due, at least in part, to a combination of structural genetic sequence variants and the variable methylation of DNA sequences, a potentially reversible epigenetic process.

A spin off of the genome project is the ENCODE (encyclopedia of DNA elements) project (Greally, 2007; Check, 2007; ENCODE Project Consortium, 2007; Pennisi , 2007). The pilot project used multiple methods to collect and analyze data on just 1% of the human genome. One part of the project examined what portions of the genome might be involved in the regulation of gene expression; so called non coding DNA. The genome is pervasively transcribed such that 93% of bases are represented in primary transcripts. Most of these transcripts are neither traditional protein-coding transcripts, since protein coding DNA makes up barely 2% of the overall genome, nor easily explained as well defined structural non-coding RNAs (transfer RNA, ribosomal RNA, small nuclear RNA).The transcripts are primarily other types of non-protein coding RNAs which are probably important regulators of gene expression. In the late 2000, a new type of RNA called micro RNA (miRNA) was identified (Lander, 2011). Micro RNAs bind to the 3' UTRs of target mRNAs usually resulting in translational repression or target mRNA degradation and gene silencing (Liu et al., 2012).The human genome may encode over 1000 miRNAs.

The ENCODE investigators also looked at the regulation of transcription. They found evidence of regulatory functions for sequences at transcription start sites but also at other sites in the DNA. About one quarter of promoters (cis regulatory elements that facilitate gene transcription) were at the ends of the genes instead of at the beginning. They described almost tenfold more transcription start sites than the number of established (protein coding) genes consistent with the extensive primary transcript activity of the genome. Many of these novel start sites were located hundreds of thousands of bases away from known start sites. Gingeras (2006) has discussed the complexities of the mammalian transcriptome and the implication that most genomic regions serve multiple functions. Some other surprises were also noted.

The 1% of genomic DNA studied in the ENCODE project contained 400 protein coding genes. Additional exons were identified for more than 80% of these genes, but many of these exons were located thousands of bases away from the gene's previously known exons, sometimes hidden in another gene. Some mRNAs were derived from exons belonging to two genes. The ENCODE pilot data have forced a re-evaluation of what constitutes a gene and suggest that a multidimensional network regulates gene expression (Pennisi, 2007).

Lander (2011) has summarized many of the important discoveries that have emerged from the human genome project and its spin offs over the last decade. The relatively low number (about 21,000) of protein coding genes was one of the early surprising observations. Alternative splicing occurs at more than 90% of protein coding genes so that more proteins exist than protein coding genes. Protein coding DNA sequences comprise only about 1.5 -2% of the genome. Non protein coding DNA sequences appear to evolve and turn over faster than protein coding sequences; hence the evolution of species depends more on innovation in regulatory sequences than changes in proteins. As already noted, a new form of RNA has been defined, micro RNA which has important regulatory functions with respect to mRNA translation. Although only a small fraction of DNA codes for proteins, most if not all of the DNA is actively engaged in RNA transcription; a large fraction of this RNA is so-called long non- (protein) coding RNAs. These RNAs have a variety of functional roles including regulation of gene expression (e.g. HOX genes). Hundreds of thousands of epigenetic marks (histone acetylation and methylation, DNA methylation) are layered atop the genome sequence. These epigenetic marks play key roles in gene expression patterns during development and in response to environmental cues. In addition, the genome contains much structural polymorphism including SNPs and copy number variants.

Recently the ENCODE investigators (2012) reported additional results based upon a larger data set; 1640 genome wide data sets prepared from 147 cell types. The results confirmed and extended previous observations. The latest gene count is 20,687 protein coding genes and 18, 400 RNA coding genes (Pennisi, 2012). In the original pilot report, 93% of bases were transcribed (2007) whereas in the full genome the fraction is 76% (Pennisi, 2012 b). Again the presence of extensive regulatory DNA elements (enhancers) and transcription sites (promoters) were found. Genes are highly interlaced with overlapping transcripts that are synthesized from both DNA strands complicating the definition of a "gene" (Ecker, 2012). Some argue that the basic unit of heredity should be considered the RNA transcript decoded from DNA and not the gene (Pennisi, 2012 b). Genes can be regulated by long range elements (enhancers and promoters) in addition to closely situated regulatory elements (Ecker, 2012). The ENCODE investigators described many genomic enhancer regions, more than 200,000 per cell type. A small fraction of these have been linked to target genes but most have no known targets (Bickmore, 2012). The transcriptional picture is one in which the DNA binding of a few high affinity transcription factors displaces nucleosomes thus exposing genomic regions to the binding of lower affinity transcription factors (Bickmore, 2012). Also transcription factor binding can block DNA methylation rather than the other way around. The ENCODE project data underscore the extensive and sophisticated regulatory elements in the human genome.

An additional layer of complexity is added through epigenetic mechanisms. Although the term epigenetics was coined many years ago, the definition has changed as our understanding of genetic mechanisms has grown. Epigenetics refers to changes in gene expression (function) that occur without a change in DNA sequence and that are stable between cell divisions and sometimes between generations (Carnero and LLeonart, 2011). The two principal mechanisms involved in epigenetic regulation of gene expression are methylation/ demethylation of DNA and post translational modification of histone proteins (acetylation/ deacetylation, methylation/demethylation). With respect to DNA methylation, the prevailing assumption is that in mammals the methylation occurs almost exclusively in the CpG dinucleotide context; cytosine methylation. Histone modifications appear to provide a more labile type of gene transcriptional repression whereas DNA methylation has a more stable silencing effect that is not easily reversed (Cedar and Bergman, 2009). These two principal mechanisms do not function separately but are closely intertwined. The central unit of chromatin is the nucleosome which consists of short strands of DNA wound around an octet of histone proteins. Structural changes in chromatin structure influence DNA transcription (Cedar and Bergman, 2009; Baylin and Schuebel, 2007). An open chromatin structure (less tightly packed) is associated with greater distances between nucleosomes and favors DNA transcription. The opposite is true of a closed chromatin structure. The balance between open and closed parts of the genome facilitates proper gene expression patterns in given cell types and also prevents unwanted gene transcription (Baylin and Schuebel, 2007).

The cells in an individual multicellular organism have identical DNA sequences (hence the same genetic instructional sets), yet maintain different terminal phenotypes i.e. neurons, cardiomyocytes, endothelial cells etc. Epigenetic mechanisms are important regulators of development and cell differentiation (Cedar and Bergman, 2009). The basic methylation of the animal genome is bimodal with almost all CpG dinucleotides methylated except those located in CpG islands. CpG islands are enriched in CpG dinucleotides, under methylated and found upstream of many mammalian genes. The developmental sequence of DNA methylation in mammals has become clarified (Lister et al., 2009). Prior to implantation, most CpGs in the embryonic genome are unmethylated. At the time of implantation, developmental cues induce a complex interaction between histones and DNA methylation which results in the aforementioned bimodal DNA methylation pattern. Post implantation as cellular differentiation occurs, pluripotency genes in embryonic stem cells are silenced through a cooperative interplay of DNA methylation and histone modifications. In addition, during cell division the DNA methylation patterns and the chromatin structure of the parent cell are faithfully reproduced in the daughter cells. Gene functional repression is due to a combination of DNA methylation and histone modifications. These two processes also alter the packing arrangement of nucleosomes (DNA- histone complexes) in the chromatin structure. Open chromatin which is usually formed from acetylated histones and unmethylated DNA contains actively transcribing genes whereas compact chromatin formed from methylated DNA and non-acetylated histones contains transcriptionally repressed genes. Compacted chromatin restricts access of transcriptional machinery to the DNA. Long term repression plays an important role in the programming of gene expression profiles in the developing animal. This long term repression is maintained by a closed chromatin structure as a result of DNA methylation and histone modifications. Developmental cues can activate genes in these regions by altering histone modifications and demethylating DNA, with the result that chromatin assumes an open configuration.

In a recent study, Lister et al., (2009) mapped the DNA methylome of two human cell lines; human embryonic stem cells and fetal lung fibroblasts. In the differentiated fibroblast, essentially all of the DNA methyl cytosines detected were in the CpG context, whereas in the embryonic stem cells about 25% of methylated DNA cytosines were in non CpG contexts.

This observation suggests that embryonic stem cells may use different DNA methylation mechanisms than differentiated cells to regulate gene expression patterns. Particularly in the non CpG context, DNA methylation density was reduced at sites of protein - DNA binding in stem cells. These sites are regions where proteins that regulate gene expression in the pluripotent state can bind to DNA. Non CpG methylation disappeared when embryonic cells were induced to differentiate. The data of Lister et al., (2009) confirm that different methylation patterns are observed in embryonic stem cells and differentiated cells, that these different patterns correlate with differences in transcriptional activity between these two cell lines and that epigenetic mechanisms are important gene regulators in the process of cellular differentiation.

Some of the early steps in the regulation of cell differentiation by epigenetic mechanisms have been described by Tran et al., (2012). These investigators used Drosophila male germ line stem cells as a test system. This cell line undergoes asymmetric division into self-renewed germ line stem cells and sibling (daughter) cells that subsequently undergoes differentiation. Histone proteins are a major carrier of epigenetic information and the investigators measured the cellular distribution of "old" pre-existing histones versus newly synthesized histones. Following cell division and DNA replication, pre-existing "old" histones selectively segregated into the germ line cells whereas newly synthesized histones were enriched in the differentiating sibling daughter cells. This data indicate that the asymmetric cellular distribution of pre-existing versus newly synthesized histones is one of the early steps by which existing epigenetic information can be maintained in stem cells and new epigenetic information can be reset in sibling cells that undergo differentiation.

In addition to developmental cues, environmental cues can also induce epigenetic modifications in gene expression patterns. For example, the quality/nature of the maternal-infant interaction during a critical time window in the early post natal period can modify the intensity of the stress response in the offspring even as adults. This example is discussed in the section Atherosclerotic Vascular Disease; Stress hormones. A second example is exemplified by the observation that the differential feeding of female honeybee larvae by nurse bees can determine caste development; queen bee versus worker bee. Finally, there has been documented a correlation between early life socioeconomic status and the methylation pattern of gene promoter regions in later adult life. These last two examples are discussed in the section; Phenotypic plasticity. In these examples environmental cues induce long lasting changes in gene expression patterns through epigenetic mechanisms.

Mandrioli (2004) has discussed the evolutionary role of DNA methylation. In vertebrates, actively transcribing genes are non-methylated whereas silenced genes are methylated. Also, methylation of cytosine residues can silence the expression of transposon-encoded genes, prevent transposon- mediated DNA rearrangements and silence the read through transcription from transposon promoters into neighboring host genes. In contrast, in insects DNA methylation is associated with active gene transcription rather than the silencing of genes. It is speculated that in insects, DNA methylation acts to guarantee the expression of specific and important genes susceptible to transcriptional interference. None the less, the differences between the function of methylation in vertebrates and invertebrates underscore the tinkering that characterizes evolution whereby the same mechanism can be used for different purposes.

Recently, Li et al., (2012) examined the correlation between genomic methylation status and structural mutability in the human genome. Not all regions of the genome are equally susceptible to the occurrence of mutations. These investigators found a strong association between male germ line (human sperm samples) DNA hypo methylation and genomic instability. Methylation deserts (i.e. the approximately 1% of the genome in the male germ line with the lowest occurrence of DNA methylation) had about ten times the amount of structural mutations compared to the genome wide average. These methylation deserts were also highly enriched for fast evolving loci that regulate tissue specific gene expression. These data point to connections between the epigenome, genomic "hot spots" of mutability and evolution.

DNA methylated states are propagated through mitosis but the evidence is not so clear that post translational histone modifications are transmitted across cell division. Some epigenetic information can also be transmitted through meiosis and gamete formation in multicellular organisms. The evidence for trans generational transfer of epigenetic effects has been discussed by Youngson and Whitelaw (2008) and Rando (2012).

Another source of genetic variation is through the creation of new protein coding genes. Several mechanisms have been described (Carvunis et al., 2012). One process, which has been well documented, is through the re-organization of pre-existing genes notably after gene duplication. A second mechanism involves de novo gene "birth" and a possible mechanism for such new gene "birth has been proposed by Carvunis et al., 2012). The mechanism has an intermediary step involving proto-genes. The frequency of de novo gene birth is unknown but is probably more common than previously believed. Recently, a new gene was "created" in an experimental situation with a bacterium as the test subject (Pennisi, 2012 a). The bacterium was screened for a gene that coded for a single protein that had dual functions. A gene was found that coded for the synthesis of both tryptophan and histidine and this dual function gene was inserted into test bacteria. Under specific experimental conditions, and over the course of about 3000 bacterial generations, the investigators observed that the single copy of the dual-function gene had become amplified into multiple copies. Finally some of these dual copy genes mutated to actually form two separate genes each with a single function; tryptophan or histidine synthesis.

In summary, the genome project revealed layers of complexity not previously appreciated. Although the great majority of DNA bases are involved in transcription only a very small fraction of these transcripts express the function of (traditional) protein-coding genes. Many DNA sequences transcribe non-structural, non-coding RNAs (ncRNAs) which are believed to have important regulatory functions. The genome also contains structural variants varying in size from single nucleotide polymorphisms to larger structural DNA variants such as copy-number variants. The epigenome also regulates gene expression in response to environmental or developmental cues. Although the early steps in the sequence are not well understood the mechanisms by which gene expression is altered are chiefly through changes in the methylation state of DNA or post translational changes to histone proteins in the nucleosomes. These epigenetic mechanisms are a link between environmental variations and alterations in biological processes (Richards, 2006). Hence, phenotypic differences between individuals are based upon genomic/epigenetic variations between individuals such as single nucleotide polymorphisms, copy number variants and different genomic methylation states. That is why there is no such entity as a "wild type" human (Olson, 2011).

The biological significance of individual variation has been the subject of a number of publications, so I have arbitrarily chosen one study to illustrate the importance of this issue. Crawford and Oleksiak (2007) studied cardiac metabolism in sixteen male killifish, Fundulus heteroclitus. Metabolic rate (oxygen consumption) was measured in the isolated hearts from these fish as a function of three different substrates; glucose, fatty acid (FA) and lactate/ketones LKA). There was considerable variation across individual fish with respect to both cardiac metabolic rate (oxygen consumption) and the use of these three primary substrates to drive cardiac metabolism. In some individuals metabolism was primarily fueled by FAs whereas in others glucose was the primary fuel. Gene expression patterns (gene specific mRNA levels) also varied among the sixteen male fish but the subjects could be clustered into three main groupings on the basis of shared gene expression patterns. The gene expression patterns allowed the investigators to examine which pathways were important for substrate-specific cardiac metabolism across individuals. For example, for individuals in grouping one, 81% of the variance among individuals in cardiac metabolic rate measured with glucose as a substrate was explained by changes in the expression of genes involved in glycolytic pathways. By contrast, for individuals in groupings two and three, changes in the expression of glycolytic genes had little power to account for variation in glucose –specific cardiac metabolic rate among these individuals; for both of these groupings, changes in the expression of genes involved in the oxidative phosphorylation pathway better explained variation among these individuals in glucose-specific cardiac metabolic rate. These observations underscore that gene expression patterns responsible for variation in cardiac metabolism between individuals differ between these individuals. The investigators summarized their findings as follows; there exists significant individual variation in cardiac metabolism, which metabolic substrate was preferentially used and the pattern of cardiac metabolic gene expression. One implication of this data is that it is highly unlikely that one gene or a set of genes is responsible for the phenotypic variation (in this case cardiac metabolism represents the phenotype) among all individuals. This observation is consistent with data in humans that the genetic underpinnings of insulin resistance in individuals with impaired glucose regulation are not the same across these individuals; the mechanisms responsible for insulin resistance will be different in different individuals (discussed in the section; Diabetes Mellitus (Type 2); Insulin resistance). In essence, DNA polymorphisms or changes in expression result in changes in molecular phenotypes which in turn affect molecular and cellular processes that then lead to changes in physiological states. The important point is that a given physiological state (organismal phenotype) can be the result of more than one underlying molecular phenotype.

Since the genetic underpinnings of complex common diseases are believed to be identical to those of quantitative traits (Flint and Mackay, 2009), newer genotyping technologies have been used to search the genome for underlying “disease causing” genes. Genome-wide association (GWA) studies examine for statistical associations between DNA sequence variants at different chromosomal locations and disease phenotypes. Hundreds of thousands of single nucleotide polymorphisms (SNPs, single base pair substitutions) can be measured in individuals with and without the disease phenotype. SNPs have only two alleles and SNPs for which one variant is statistically more common in individuals having the disease phenotype are said to be associated with that disease (phenotype) (Donnelly, 2008). Association studies essentially identify a genomic location statistically related to a disease phenotype but provide little information on actual gene function and in fact some of the associated SNPs have been in genomic regions containing no known protein coding genes (Pearson and Manolio, 2008). As pointed out by Donnelly (2008), disease associated SNPs are often not the actual causal variants, but rather proxies for the true disease variants due to the phenomenon of linkage disequilibrium i.e. the causal variant and the associated variant on the same chromosome are inherited together more frequently than expected by chance. Genome wide studies can also be used to examine for particular regions of the genome that contain or are linked to genes that underlie a disease phenotype. This region is called a quantitative trait locus (QTL) and is generally a large stretch of DNA containing hundreds of genes. QLT mapping is done using a defined set of genetic markers. Rockman and Kruglyak (2006) and Flint and Mackay (2009) discuss effect sizes i.e. how much of the heritable variation in a quantitative trait or disease phenotype does each QTL explain. For both quantitative traits and disease phenotypes, the genetic architecture is characterized by small effect sizes (Flint and Mackay, 2009). In addition sample sizes (number of individuals in the study) need to be extremely large to detect QTLs with very small effect sizes. For the quantitative trait of height all known loci explain less than 5% of the variance and for the quantitative trait of obesity known loci account for less than 1%of the variance (Maher, 2008; Flint and Mackay, 2009). As noted by Donnelly (2008) and Flint and Mackay (2009) many quantitative trait nucleotides lie in regulatory regions of the genome although the nature of the regulatory role is unknown.

The limitations of genome wide association studies, including effect sizes, have been discussed by Goldstein in a recent publication (2009). In addition, two recent reports highlight other difficulties in interpreting the results of genome wide association studies.

Kong et al., (2009) have examined the parental origin of DNA sequence variants associated with several complex diseases. These investigators pointed out that the impact of parental origin of DNA sequence variants on the associations detected in genome wide association studies have largely been ignored. Kong et al., (2009) identified forty-eight genes in humans known to be imprinted. Imprinting is an epigenetic mechanism involving DNA methylation and histone modifications by which one of the alleles (maternal or paternal) of a given gene is silenced. Imprinted genes are essentially monoallelic, expressed only from the non-imprinted allele inherited from the mother or in other instances from the non-imprinted allele inherited from the father. In addition, most imprinted genes are found in clusters. The investigators examined for disease-SNP associations in DNA regions close to or encompassing known imprinted genes. Unoki et al., (2008) had documented that SNPs in the region of the gene KCNQ1 (chromosome 11) are associated with an increased risk for diabetes type 2. However, the strength of this association is influenced by whether the SNP is in the maternally or paternally expressed KCNQ1 allele (Kong et al., 2009).For example, in the case of the SNP rs2237892, the odds ratios for the association between this SNP and diabetes type 2 are 1.03 for the paternally transmitted allele and 1.30 for the maternally transmitted allele. Kong et al., (2009) also described another SNP with very striking parent-of -origin effects. This SNP (rs2334499) was located at the same chromosomal locus and close to two known clusters of imprinted genes. SNP (rs2334499) lies within the first intron of the gene HCCA2, a gene of unknown imprint status but close to clusters of known imprinted genes. The odds ratios for association between diabetes type 2 and this SNP were 1.35 for the paternally transmitted allele but 0.86 for the maternally transmitted allele. Hence when this SNP is in the paternally transmitted allele, the risk of diabetes type 2 is increased but when this SNP is transmitted in the maternal allele the risk was reduced; the SNP was protective.

In another recent report, MacArthur et al., (2012) examined for loss- of- function (LoF) variants in human protein coding genes. DNA sequence variants were chosen which had a high probability of completely disrupting gene function i.e. protein coding transcription. LoF variants are of considerable interest since they have been considered rare due to the severe deleterious effects that they can have as demonstrated by Mendelian disorders such as cystic fibrosis and forms of muscular dystrophy. The investigators examined for these LoF variants in 185 genomes from apparently healthy individuals. The data indicated that on average an individual carried 97 such LoF variants with 18 being present in a homozygous state. These results indicate that the majority of these LoF variants are probably found in "non-essential' genes and therefore there is a need for caution in assuming that even LoF variants in protein coding genes are diseases causing.

Part of the answer to this Mendelian puzzle has been discussed by Chakravarti and Kapoor (2012). Generally, not all family members with a Mendelian type mutation in a protein coding gene are equally affected. It appears that alterations in accompanying regulatory elements (which are much commoner variants) can alter the dosage of the mutated gene depending on whether the regulatory element is an enhancer, silencer or insulator. Hence the expression of a Mendelian mutation (rare on its own) requires an appropriate variant (quite common) in an associated regulatory element. The evidence suggests that deleterious protein coding gene mutations are rare because of a strong purifying (negative) selection mechanism whereas selection against variants in regulatory elements is much weaker allowing these types of mutations to be more common.

Two recent GWA studies have examined the frequencies of SNPs (Wellcome Trust Case Control Consortium, 2007) and CNV s (Wellcome Trust Case Control Consortium, 2010) in populations with common disease states compared to reference populations. In the SNP study, seven common diseases; bipolar disorder, coronary artery disease, Crohn's disease, hypertension, rheumatoid arthritis, and types 1 and 2 diabetes were chosen. The highest heterozygote odds ratio (2.08) was for bipolar disorder and an SNP on chromosome 16. In general, however, the variants uncovered had only modest predictive values (odds ratios in range of 1.2 -1.5). For any given disease phenotype, there appears to be few if any variants with a large effect, a handful with a modest effect and a large number of genes generating small or even very small increases in disease risk. In the CNV study, seven diseases were examined; bipolar disorder, breast cancer, coronary artery disease, Crohn's disease, hypertension rheumatoid arthritis, and types 1 and 2 diabetes. The investigators concluded that common CNVs detectable with today's technology were unlikely to have a major role in the genetic basis of common diseases.

GWA studies have defined statistical associations between DNA sequence variants and "disease" states but have not revealed the functional links between these variants and altered biological processes. To date, about 93% of "disease" and trait associated DNA variants examined in GWA studies lie within non protein coding genomic regions (Maurano et al., 2012).The ENCODE data base and newer genomic technologies have given investigators the tools to use GWA studies to actually explore connections between DNA variants and gene functions. Maurano et al., (2012) performed genome wide mapping in 349 cell and tissue samples including 85 cell types studied under the ENCODE project. They examined the genomic location for 5134 unique SNPs for 207 "diseases" and 447 quantitative traits. The investigators identified regulatory genomic regions (catalogued in the ENCODE project) that function as enhancers of transcription levels. They defined approximately 200,000 such regions per cell type. About 77% of all these non-coding disease and trait associated SNPs were either located in a genomic enhancer region or close to one. The investigators were able to define the gene targets for 419 genomic enhancer regions harboring SNPs. For about 40% of the 419 genomic enhancer regions containing SNPs, the distance between the enhancer region and target genes was greater than 250kb. The observations of Maurano et al., (2012) suggest that a large number of functional DNA variants of small quantitative effect act through modulation of regulatory DNA. Numerous genomic enhancer regions containing SNPs with associations to disease states are connected with the promoters of distant genes and disease states can be at least partly explained as a problem of disordered gene regulation.

Another important consideration that could confound the interpretation of GWA studies is that of epistasis. The definition of epistasis has changed over the years but this term generally refers to the observation that the phenotypic effect of a particular genotype is not independent of the overall genomic background or context. In its simplest form, epistasis describes an interaction between a pair of genomic loci in which the phenotypic expression of one locus depends upon the genotype at the second locus (Carlborg and Haley, 2004).

Breen et al., (2012) in a recent report documented the importance of epistasis in the molecular evolution of proteins. These investigators examined proteins encoded by sixteen housekeeping genes across different species. Since the genes had housekeeping functions they were not subject to strong environmental selection pressures. Their data set consisted of over 1000 unique orthologous proteins (from different species) for each gene. For each of these genes, when the orthologous proteins were aligned, they observed that the average number of different amino acids per position was about nine. This observation indicated that over the course of evolution, each amino acid position in one of these orthologous proteins could accept a substitution by eight other amino acids. The investigators calculated the ratio of the per position rates of non-synonymous to synonymous substitutions as a measure of the rate of molecular protein evolution. In a situation without epistasis, an amino acid that is acceptable at a given position in one species should be equally acceptable at the same position in the orthologous protein of another species. The non-epistatic model predicted a certain rate of protein evolution. However, the observed rate of protein evolution was about seven times smaller than that predicted by the non-epistatic model. This large difference between the two rates indicated that amino acid substitutions were not equally acceptable across orthologous proteins. For an amino acid substitution to persist on an evolutionarily relevant time scale the other amino acids within that protein must be the "correct" mix (Wagner, 2012). As stated by Breen et al., (2012), the evolutionary fitness of most amino acid substitutions depends upon the genetic context or background in which that substitution occurs. An amino acid substitution that is beneficial in one background would be expected to be detrimental in another background. They believe that their data indicated that epistasis was wide spread in the process of protein evolution. A feature of epistasis is that a given polymorphism (amino acid substitution) within a population could be beneficial (or neutral) to one individual but deleterious to another individual with a different genomic background making the interpretation of an association between this polymorphism and a "disease" state difficult.

One important "driver" behind genome wide association studies has been the concept of personalized medicine. Personalized medicine is based upon the premise that the sequencing of an individual genome can provide that individual with a measure of his/her risk for future occurrence of various diseases. Such a risk assessment is strongest with so-called Mendelian disorders and weakest for disorders with an underlying large polygenic basis. Such a personalized medical approach has been applied to the field of oncology where therapies have been directed at the genetic abnormalities detected in a biopsy of an individual's tumor (Longo, 2012). However, it turns out that even within a given tumor and its metastases there is extensive spatial heterogeneity in DNA mutations and in chromosomal number (Gerlinger et al., 2012). In addition different regions of the tumor can have different mutations in the very same genes. These findings indicate that the growing metastasizing tumor (which originated from normal tissue in that individual) evolves and "survives" through the selection of different mutations in different regions of the tumor. This highly complex tumor biology makes individual decision making with respect to chemotherapeutic agents very difficult. In addition this complex tumor genetic pattern starting from normal tissue is quite consistent with this process being an extreme breakdown of normal DNA repair mechanisms rather than being a so-called "disease".

This demonstration of genomic heterogeneity within a single tumor raises an interesting observation not necessarily related to the field of cancer. Imperfect DNA replication creates random variation and in essence imperfect DNA replication is the source of genomic heterogeneity within a single tumor (Shibata, 2012). The accumulation of mutations over time can eventually transform a single cell. The progeny of this first transformed cell expand by the process of bifurcating branching cell division to form a visible tumor population (Shibata, 2012). The occurrence of imperfect DNA replication during this process of branching cell division is responsible for a heterogeneous collection of DNA structural variants within the tumor. It is not unreasonable to expect imperfect DNA replication to result in de novo DNA structural variants within a replicating non-cancerous tissue within the body. Hence this mechanism could lead to genomic heterogeneity within a single non-cancerous tissue type and could lead to biological "diversity" within a single tissue.

Finally, another layer of complexity exists, at least at the cellular level, which has yet to be fully explored. Although it is known that single cells in a population can display variability in properties, such variability can also be observed in populations of monoclonal cells that have been cultured under identical conditions (Pelkmans, 2012). Phenotypic cell to cell variability among genetically identical cells can be deterministic and regulated. The mechanisms underlying this cell to cell variability have not been clarified but these mechanisms may be related to heterogeneity of cell microenvironments. Pelkmans speculates that perhaps a class of molecular regulators exist that have yet to be described.

As pointed out in an article in the New York Times, December 18, 2011, the amount of data on DNA, RNA, and proteins being collected is voluminous. All of this data has to be analyzed and integrated and this aspect has become a problem. "Data handling is now the bottle-neck" said David Haussler, from the University of California, Santa Cruz. "It costs more to analyze a genome than to sequence a genome." As a corollary to this issue of data interpretation, the rapid advances in genomic sequencing technologies have resulted in an exponential increase in the number of published papers reporting genomic –based studies. Initial interpretation of this data and its biological significance is generally somewhat superficial. Integrating this rapidly expanding new data into a coherent picture of genomic and epigenomic functioning will be a long term project. As such some of the interpretations of genomic and epigenomic data used in this book will no doubt change in the future. A case in point is our changing understanding of so-called "junk" DNA, transposable genetic elements (TEs; transposons and retro transposons) and epigenetic mechanisms. As discussed by Federoff (2012), transposon and retro transposon sequences constitute two thirds of the human genome and TEs are no longer simply considered selfish, parasitic DNA sequences. Previously epigenetic mechanisms were thought to have evolved as a gene silencing mechanism to protect the cell against the effects of TEs. Now, it is proposed that the evolution of epigenetic mechanisms have actually allowed genomes to grow and accumulate

TEs (Federoff, 2012). This is just one example of genomic data acquisition outstripping interpretation.

Phenotypic Plasticity

Broadly defined, phenotypic plasticity is the capacity of a given genotype to produce different phenotypes in response to different environmental conditions (Aubin-Horth and Renn, 2009; Kelly et al., 2012). For mammals, such as humans, it is important to remember that the environment extends to the intrauterine environment. During the intrauterine time frame, environmental factors can alter fetal development and this result has been termed developmental plasticity although this is just a specific example of phenotypic plasticity. Defining the underpinnings of phenotypic plasticity is an important research field since phenotypic plasticity encompasses the mechanistic link between environmental cues and behavioral, morphologic and physiological traits. Ultimately the underlying link is genetic and as a result of newer genomic and epigenomic techniques more information about this link is now available (Kelly et al., 2012; Bossdorf et al., 2008). Environmental cues induce the differential expression of suites of genes and regulatory factors. A few examples will illustrate these principles.

Social behavior (nursing versus foraging) is a plastic trait in honey bees (Singer, 2011). Whitfield et al., (2003; 2006) used the honey bee to examine the relationship between brain gene expression profiles and behaviors. During the first three weeks of life, worker bees perform nursing –type (brood care) activities inside the hive. At about three weeks, worker bees shift to doing outside the hive activities such as foraging. The actual timing of this behavioral change (nursing to foraging) is variable and dependent on the needs of the colony. To minimize the effect of genetic variation, Whitfield et al., (2003) used full sister nurses and foragers which are 75% related due to haplodiploidy. To avoid age as a confounder, individual brain gene expression profiles were obtained in age-matched nurses and foragers. The data showed a strong association between brain gene expression profiles and behavior (nursing versus foraging). In fact about 39% of the genome was differentially expressed between the nurse and forager stage. Whitfield et al., (2003) were able to identify a set of predictor genes expressed in the brain that could successfully classify 57 out of 60 individual bees with respect to their behavior (foraging or nursing). In a later study, Whitfield et al., (2006) showed that juvenile hormone was a key regulator of the behavioral transition of nursing to foraging and bees deprived of foraging experience but treated with a juvenile hormone analog showed forager-like brain gene expression profiles. In summary, these experiments demonstrate that in the honey bee an extensive rearrangement of genome activity underlies the plasticity of task-related behavior. However, what have not been clarified in this example are the environmental cues that trigger the behavioral change.

Whitehead et al., (2011) have examined the plasticity of the physiological response of killifish to habitats of differing osmotic states. Killifish occupy habitats varying from freshwater to seawater extremes of the saline continuum. The fish used in these experiments were from coastal New Hamphshire and were acclimated to artificial seawater for at least 3 months prior to the study. The experimental protocol consisted of exposing the acclimated fish to a hypo-osmotic shock by transferring them to fresh water. The immediate effects of the transfer were; a large decrease in plasma osmolality and plasma sodium concentration and a much lesser decline in plasma chloride concentration. By 72 hours, osmolar and electrolyte balance had been restored. The physiological processes responsible for the restoration of salt and water balance within this new fresh water habitat included; production of a hypo-osmotic urine by the kidney, reduction of water intake at the intestine and transformation of the gills from a salt secreting to a salt absorbing epithelium. The investigators found that 498 genes showed a significant change in expression following the osmotic shock and during the reparative period. The result of this differential gene expression profile was the restoration of salt and water balance. This restoration process included a dramatic change in gill morphology such that this structure became capable of actively absorbing sodium from the environment. As in the behavioral plasticity of the honey bee, the plasticity of the killifish's physiological acclimatization to varying habitat salinity is based upon a large genetic transcriptional response.

The two previous animal models illustrate examples of behavioral and physiological trait plasticity. The honey bee also demonstrates morphological plasticity. Nurse worker bees differentially feed genetically identical female larvae to create mainly workers and when needed, a few queens. Royal jelly is fed to larvae destined to become queens and a less sophisticated food is fed to the other larvae. Kucharski et al., (2008) investigated the genetic basis of this morphologic plasticity in response to the nature of the food ingested. They used RNA interference technology to silence the gene transcribing one of the DNA methylation enzymes in newly hatched larvae. This silencing resulted in profound morphological changes in the developing larvae. In the methylation silenced larvae, the majority developed into queens whereas in the control group the majority of larvae developed into workers. The investigators measured the methylation status of a specific gene, dynactin p62, known to be differentially methylated during development. In hive reared larvae, the heads of queens show less methylation at specific CpG exon coding sites in dynactin p62 than the heads of workers. Similarly, the heads of queens derived from methylation silenced larvae showed less methylation at these same CpG sites compared to the heads from control larvae. Hence, in the honey bee, caste (queen versus worker) morphology is plastic and the underlying genetic mechanism appears to be one of differential DNA methylation in response to a dietary cue.

A study performed by Borghol et al., (2012) raises interesting questions with regard to phenotypic plasticity in humans. These investigators used 3362 subjects of 42 years of age who had originally been enrolled in the perinatal mortality study in the UK. A childhood SEP (socio-economic position) score was calculated as well as a current SEP score at age 42 years. DNA was extracted from blood samples from these adult subjects and the methylation state of the promoters of about 2000 genes was measured. The investigators identified 1252 gene promoters whose methylation status was associated with childhood SEP; 666 more methylated in high childhood SEP and 586 promoters more methylated in low childhood SEP. They identified 545 gene promoters whose methylation status was associated with adulthood SEP; 336 more methylated in high adult SEP and 209 more methylated in low adult SEP. The interesting observation is that there was a statistically significant correlation between childhood SEP and a DNA methylation pattern obtained from these same individuals at age 42 years. However, since this is a cross-sectional study and blood was obtained for DNA analysis only in adulthood, it is not known at what life stage the association between childhood SEP and the DNA methylation pattern was established. Generally, SEP is viewed as a proxy for a certain set of environmental circumstances. Individuals with a low SEP are considered to have a higher probability of having poorer future health. It is difficult to frame the observations of Borghol et al., (2012) within the construct of phenotypic plasticity. The observations are interesting in that they support a link between an individual's childhood environmental circumstances and that individual's DNA methylation pattern as an adult. However, at this juncture, the nature or significance of this link is unknown.

Phenotypic plasticity, when defined broadly, is a very widespread phenomenon in nature since most biological processes are influenced to some extent by environmental cues. With the use of newer genomic techniques, the mechanistic basis of phenotypic plasticity is becoming better understood. The understanding of this phenomenon is at the heart of the field of integrative biology, since acquiring such understanding will require inputs from a number of separate fields such as genomics, physiology, ecology and evolutionary biology to name a few. Understanding the mechanisms underlying phenotypic plasticity is the key to understanding not only how environmental cues shape biological processes in general but also how the interaction between environmental cues and biological processes can have features which differ across individual members of a species.

Ageing

Although the literature on ageing (senescence) is extensive, the number of studies on ageing in natural animal models, particularly non- primates, is much more limited. In this section, some general features of ageing based on observations in natural animal models will be reviewed.

Central to the evolutionary theory of ageing is an animal's fitness, defined in terms of survival probability and reproductive success within that animal's environmental setting. The force of natural selection declines with age so that deleterious gene mutations, if they act later in life after the reproductive period, will most likely not be eliminated. Within the evolutionary model, the accumulation of late acting deleterious mutations underlies the ageing process (Singer, 2011). Rose (2009) has defined the evolutionary basis of ageing on a somewhat different basis. Again a key feature in his synthesis is the declining strength of natural selection with age. According to Rose (2009) ageing is not simply an accumulation of damage or disrupted high order signaling processes (although it does secondarily involve both of these mechanisms), but rather the absence of adaptive genomic information required for survival and functioning to later adult ages. Ageing is a period of progressively impaired adaptation that follows a period of adequate adaptation. However, in essence this absence of "adaptive genomic information" really implies a deficiency in repair processes.

Mechanistically, ageing can be thought of as consisting of two components; one at the species level and one at the individual animal level. This construct is an important conceptual framework for understanding the ageing process. Given that different species have ageing patterns that differ from that of other species, there must be a link between the developmental program (determined by evolution) that establishes the morphological and behavioral traits of a species and the rate of ageing observed in that species (de Magalhaes and Sandberg, 2005). In general, species which show a slow developmental phase until reproductive maturity is reached tend to have slower rates of age related declines in physiological/metabolic functions (i.e. ageing). The mechanistic links between morphological/behavioral developmental programs and ageing will set the boundaries of the ageing process for a given species. For example, among rodents, naked mole rats as a species are developmentally programmed to be exceptionally long lived and to display negligible senescence. Among primates, humans are developmentally programmed to live longer than other primates. At the level of the individual animal, the ageing phenotype will have both the general features characteristic of that species and individual variation in the rate of ageing. Individual variation is due to the integrated consequences of accumulated genomic mutations (structural DNA variants), experience - induced changes in epigenetic marks (DNA methylation, histone methylation, acetlylation and deacetylation), cellular damage (from intrinsic and extrinsic causes) as well as the results of imperfect repair of this damage. An illustrative example of this mix of species and individual components of the ageing process is the dog. This species has a developmentally set ageing and life span pattern, but through artificial breeding and selection there is also a wide range of individual variation in both life span and the ageing phenotype.

Can developmentally set ageing at the species level be modified? Can the maximum lifespan developmentally programmed for humans be increased? I would suggest that the answer is no.

However, developmentally set ageing at the species level and individual level ageing are clearly mechanistically intertwined and in essence inseparable. Natural selection acts on individual phenotypes (including the "ageing phenotype") which are determined by the genetic variation across individuals. Eventually as a result, the species to which those individuals belong will evolve further or a new species will develop. Regardless, as the existing species evolves further or a new species appears, the modified developmental programs for that further evolved species or for the new species will set new ageing patterns and boundaries at the species level.

Within the evolutionary framework, the strength of repair processes will diminish with age, particularly in the post-reproductive period. A number or repair processes have been studied in some detail and one of these is that of DNA repair. Nuclear DNA exists in large scale aggregates known as chromosomes. A chromosome is made up of chromatin which consists of arrays of nucleosomes; DNA wound up around bead-like proteins called histones. Whenever a cell needs to access genetic information, it will unravel the required section of DNA, read it and then wind the DNA back into its protective chromosomal configuration. DNA structural variants (mutations) can occur as a result of endogenous metabolic by-products such as reactive oxygen species or as the result of mistakes made during DNA replication. DNA mutations can also be induced by exogenous agents such as radiation (ionizing, ultraviolet), plant toxins and mutagenic chemicals and drugs. De novo DNA mutations such as single nucleotide polymorphisms (discussed in a subsequent paragraph) are predominantly transmitted by the father by virtue of the many replicative steps involved in spermatogenesis. The structural changes to the DNA can be single or double stranded and in the case of double stranded DNA breaks, one repair process involves non-homologous end joining (NHEJ). In this repair process, the two ends of the break are rejoined. However, there are often DNA sequences lost during this process and so this repair process is itself mutagenic. The DNA damage response pathways coordinate cellular DNA repair activities following DNA damage detection and transiently arrest cell cycle progression in proliferating cells until DNA damage has been removed (Fumagalli et al., 2012).

Herbig et al., (2006) and Jeyapalan et al., (2007) have reported the occurrence of an increased prevalence of unrepaired double stranded DNA breaks in dermal fibroblasts of ageing non-human primates (baboons). Interestingly, these breaks occurred preferentially at the telomere region of the chromosome. The mechanism underlying this observation has been explored in more detail by Fumagalli et al., (2012). In one series of experiments, these investigators exposed non-proliferating human fibroblasts to ionizing radiation. The ionizing radiation induced DNA damage and the investigators monitored the occurrence of double stranded DNA breaks (DSB). Despite an initial efficient repair response, a small but significant number of DSB persisted in about 70% of the irradiated cells even four months following the radiation exposure. The overall number of DSB per cell fell progressively with time after radiation, but the persistent DSB co-localized to telomere regions of the chromosome. Telomeres are genomic loci composed of repetitive DNA sequences coated by specific proteins that inhibit DNA repair at chromosomal ends to prevent chromosomal fusions and genome instability particularly during cell replication. The preferential localization of persistent DSB at telomeres was due to a physical association. To confirm these observations in vivo, the investigators exposed mice to whole body irradiation and then examined hippocampal neurons for DSB. Three months after irradiation, most of the DSB had been repaired but about one to two DSB persisted in most of the cells and these breaks in 40% of the cells localized to telomeres. In addition, there was no preferential localization of DSB at short telomeres; i.e. persistent DSB caused by exogenous radiation is not triggered by critically short telomeres. In summary, agents that damage DNA, generate DSB throughout the genome. The repair process "removes" the great majority of these DSB. However, a few of these DSB will occur at telomeres and will not be repaired. These persistent unrepaired DSB will put these cells into a senescent state (Fumagalli et al., 2012). Complementing the observations of Herbig et al., (2006) and Jeyapalan et al., (2007), Fumagalli et al., (2012) also reported persistent DSB in hippocampal neurons and hepatocytes of aged baboons. Both of these tissues are non- proliferating.

The observations of Fumagalli et al., (2012) provide an example of an interesting trade-off. Trade-offs are a key feature of the evolutionary process. In this case, irreparability of DNA damage at telomere sites may be the direct and unavoidable consequence of the function of telomeres to prevent chromosomal fusions. Telomere DNA repeats resist non homologous joining of the two ends of the DNA break. As a consequence DNA double stranded breaks that occur at telomeres will not be repaired. Persistence of these unrepaired DSB in the cell will result in arrest of cell cycle progression and put the cell in a senescent state.

Another interesting "trade off" involves the structure of telomeres themselves. Telomeres consist of long tracts of G-rich repeats terminating in a 3' single strand extension known as the G overhang (Nelson and Shippen, 2012; Kazda et al., 2012). This extension serves as a primer for telomerase, as a binding site for specific DNA binding proteins and as a site for forming secondary DNA structures such as t-loops. The G overhang is a by- product of the mechanism of DNA replication and exon nucleolytic processing (Nelson and Shippen , 2012). Kazda et al., (2012) have shown that angiosperm plants, unlike vertebrates, contain two distinct populations of telomeres terminating with either a long 3' G overhang or a blunt end. The point is that blunt ended telomeres represent an evolutionary solution to the DNA replication and end protection problem in this plant but not a satisfactory solution in vertebrates. Nelson and Shippen (2012) speculate that the extended proliferative capacity of blunt ended telomeres might be less attractive to mammals subject to malignant transformation of cells.

In essence, mutations due to extrinsic or intrinsic factors are the cornerstone of genetic variation and genetic variation is the substrate on which natural selection acts. Since mutations will vary in their adaptive advantage, ageing becomes an inseparable component of the living state. The rate and spectrum of mutations arising in the human genome, particularly those occurring spontaneously, has become an important issue since the advent of newer genomic technologies. This topic is central to both evolution and the ageing process. Mutations cover a wide range of DNA changes; base substitutions, insertions, deletions and copy number variants to name a few. The mutation rate varies considerably between germ line and somatic cells with somatic cells having a mutation rate between 4 to 24 times that of germ line cells (Lynch, 2010). Even non proliferating somatic cells accumulate mutations although the rate in proliferating somatic cells is approximately 1.6 times greater (Lynch, 2010).

Recently, Kong et al., (2012) used newer genomic techniques to measure the rate of de novo germ line cell mutations by sequencing the entire genomes of 78 Icelandic parent-offspring trios. The focus was SNP mutations. A de novo mutation was defined as a mutation observed in the offspring but not in the parents. A newborn's genome sequence contained about 60 de novo SNPs, but this number was strongly dependent on the age of the father at the time of conception. The number of de novo mutations increased with father's age at the time of conception with an estimated effect of 2.01 mutations per year of father's age. The number of de novo SNPs transmitted by the mother was not age related and was always about 14. For example, a child born to parents of age 20 years would have about 54 de novo SNPs with about 40 being paternal in origin and about 14 maternal in origin. A child born to a father of 40 years of age would have about 94 de novo SNPs; 80 from the father and again about 14 from the mother. The dominant effect of the male in terms of transmitting de novo base substitution mutations (SNPs) is the result of the many more divisions that germ line cells undergo in the male than in the female. In the female, all germ line cell mitotic divisions and chromosome replications are completed before birth; there is no increase with post natal age. In the male, sperm cells are produced continuously throughout reproductive life so the number of cell divisions and chromosome replications that have occurred increases with age (Crow, 2000). Germ line cell base substitution mutations (SNPs) occur primarily in males and the mutational rate increases with age probably due to mistakes occurring during the many DNA replications and the weakening of repair mechanisms with age (Crow, 2000).

Kong et al., (2012) also noted that about two thirds of the mutations were transitions and one third was trans versions. Rates of mutation were much higher at CpG sites compared to non CpG sites; for transitions the CpG sites had a rate 18 times that of non CpG sites and for trans versions the ratio was 2.55 times. These observations can be combined with the data of Li et al., (2012) discussed in the section; Genetics. Li et al., (2012) showed that in male germ line cells, hotspots of structural mutability were regions of the genome with the lowest levels of DNA methylation i.e. so-called methylation deserts. Hence, it would appear that the de novo SNPs that are passed from father to offspring at the time of conception (Kong et al., (2012) probably arise in the father's germ line cells at CpG islands in unmethylated genomic regions.

In summary, about fifty de novo mutations (SNPs) occur on average in each individual genome between generations with about 80% transmitted by the male germ line (Kong et al., 2012). This de novo mutation rate is in agreement with the revised published human mutation rates summarized by Scally and Durbin (2012).The rates measured in these summarized studies were based upon changes in individual nucleotide bases. About 10% of the human genome is structurally polymorphic at the submicroscopic level (Li et al., 2012) so that a comparison of two individual genomes will reveal considerable divergence. This divergence represents the mutations (variants) that have accumulated in the lineages of the two individuals. For example, on average one SNP is present every 300 nucleotides (Feuk et al., 2006). Sequencing of 185 human genomes detected 28,025 copy number variants; 22,025 deletions, 501 duplications, 5371 mobile element insertions and 128 novel sequence insertions (Mills et al., 2011). Korbel et al., (2007) sequenced the genomes of two different females, one of European and one of African ancestry. They detected 1297 structural variants between the two genomes; 853 deletions, 322 insertions and 122 inversions. About 45% of the structural variants were shared between the two individuals. The human genome also contains on average about 97 loss of function variants (Mac Arthur et al., 2012). Not all regions of the human genome are equally mutable; methylation deserts (1% fraction of human genome with lowest methylation status) in the male germ line are particular hot spots of mutability (Li et al., 2012). The rate of de novo mutations between generations plus the structural DNA variations that exist within the human genome (transmitted from previous ancestors in the lineage)are important considerations not only for understanding the ageing process but also for charting the course of human evolution (Gibbons, 2012).

As noted by Lynch (2010), these observations underscore the enormous mutational burden faced by somatic and germ line cells of a long lived animal such as the human. Since deleterious mutations are much more common than beneficial ones (Kondrashov, 2012), this cumulative mutational burden will set an upper limit to human life span as well as shaping the ageing process. Another important observation is that advances in human culture and societal organization (agriculture, industrialization and sophisticated medical care) have mitigated the ecological pressures faced by humans resulting in a relaxation in the strength of natural selection against mildly deleterious mutations (Crow, 2000). In addition, advanced medical interventions by prolonging productive life spans in individuals carrying mutations with more major morphological and physiological defects have protected these mutations from elimination by natural selection (Lynch, 2010). The effects of relaxed selection pressures on organismal fitness have been documented in fruit flies (Shabalina et al., 1997). In these experiments, measures of fitness (survival and reproductive success) showed about a 2% decline per generation in flies subjected to relaxed natural selection pressures.

The relatively high mutation rate in humans, the corresponding relaxation of the strength of natural selection due to our societal organization coupled with the age-related decline in the force on natural selection observed in all animals will all conjoin to determine our species maximum life span, re- shape the course and boundaries of our ageing process as well as lead to a progressive decline in human (Darwinian) fitness per generation (Lynch, 2010). To compensate for this reduction in the strength of purifying selection (selection that eliminates deleterious mutations) will require further modifications in our environment plus an enormous and probably unrealizable investment into medical interventions and pharmaceutical agents in order to ameliorate or buffer the effects of these mutations.

Senescence is clearly a polygenic complex process which represents the trade-off or cost for investing somatic resources into the early part of life during which there is a high probability of survival and reproduction (Singer, 2011). However, a more pragmatic definition of senescence is an age-dependent variable decline in the physiological function of organs and systems with death the ultimate end point. Within this latter definition of senescence, a survey of different natural animal models illustrates some general features of the ageing process.

The life history of the ageing process is quite variable. Some animals have a very long life span characterized by slow almost negligible senescence. One such animal is the mammal Heterocephalus glaber, commonly known as the naked mole-rat (Buffenstein, 2008; Csiszar et al., 2007). The insect queens in social insect colonies (ants, bees) have much longer life spans and a slower rate of senescence than worker insects of the same colony (Keller and Genoud, 1997; Page Jr and Peng, 2001). Many marine invertebrates are extremely long lived and grow and reproduce throughout their lifespans; features characteristic of negligible senescence (Bodnar, 2009). Birds generally live longer than mammals of similar body mass, but also display a wide range of life spans and rates of ageing among different species (Singer, 2011; Holmes and Austad, 1995). On the other hand, the Pacific salmon (Oncorhynchus nerka) has a life history in which breeding is followed by a rapid, catastrophic senescence and death (Singer, 2011).

The remarkable diversity of life spans and rates of ageing across different species can be used as a natural experiment to test various mechanistic explanations with regard to the developmentally- set ageing process at the species level (Austad, 2010). In particular, species that are exceptionally long-lived can give important insights into the categories of mechanisms thought to underlie age-dependent declines in physiological and metabolic functions. Some of the proposed general mechanisms include; oxidative stress, shortened telomeres and cellular senescence, imperfect repair of genomic damage and changes in protein stability. As Austad (2010) points out, no one of these different categories alone can account for the wide range of life spans observed in nature across different species. Most likely variable combinations of these mechanisms or other as yet undefined mechanistic categories are operative across different species.

Before leaving this topic of diverse animal life spans, one animal group in particular is noteworthy. The polyp hydra, a solitary fresh water member of the phylum Cnidaria, displays a radically different ageing pattern (Baudisch and Vaupel, 2012). Martinez (1998) measured the age-specific mortality rate in groups of Hydra vulgaris and observed that it was essentially zero indicating that this very simple multicellular animal was immortal and by inference experienced not simply negligible senescence but no senescence. Tissue function and body maintenance in hydra is based upon three tissue-specific types of stem cells; ectodermal epithelial, endodermal epithelial and interstitial (Watanbe et al., 2009; Bosch, 2009). All three stem cell types are capable of unlimited self- renewal and subsequent differentiation into one or more specific cell types. Interestingly, stem cells of these three co-existing lineages have never been observed to transform from one lineage into another (Bosch, 2009).

The study by Martinez (1998) used hydra maintained in an asexual reproductive state. Hydra usually reproduces asexually by budding, but various environmental factors such as a change in temperature can induce sexual differentiation in several species. Yoshida et al., (2006) examined the effects of sexual differentiation on ageing of hydra. They used male and female cohorts of Hydra oligactis and induced sexual differentiation by lowering the ambient temperature from 18 oC to 10 oC. Following the temperature change, males and females ceased budding and formed testes and eggs respectively. This sexually differentiated hydra showed definite features of ageing. Most animals survived the first 60 days after the temperature change but thereafter there was a rapid increase in mortality such that by 150 days there were very few survivors. There was also an associated decline in physiological functions such as food capturing, body movements and digestion. Cellular events associated with the process of sexual differentiation showed an interesting pattern. By day 30 after the temperature change, the number of interstitial stem cells and somatic cells showed a significant reduction whereas germ cells had increased in number by day 30. After day 30 the number of germ cells also decreased. Yoshida et al., (2006) proposed that sexual differentiation was associated with a directional change in the fate of interstitial stem cells; stem cells selectively differentiated into germ cells at the expense of forming somatic cells and self-renewal. The decrease in somatic cell numbers and the stem cell pool leads to a decline in physiological functions and ultimately death of the animal. In summary, hydra in an asexual reproductive state, appear to be immortal with little or no manifestations of ageing whereas hydra in a differentiated sexual state senesce and die.

These observations raise a number of interesting questions. What are the genomic and metabolic mechanisms by which an environmental cue such as a change in temperature can alter the differentiation pattern of stem cells in hydra? What are the links between this change in the differentiation trajectory of stem cells and the decline in multiple physiological functions?

The indefinite renewal capacities of the three stem cell lineages are clearly the basis for the apparent immortality of asexual hydra (Watanabe et al., 2009). An important question is whether asexual hydra reflects a very unique and specific ageing process or does the biology of this animal give insights into general relationships between stem cell numbers and function and the pattern of senescence in more complex animals (Bosch, 2009). As reviewed by Wehrwein (2012), the involvement of stem cells in the ageing process is both complex and multifaceted. Stem cells also senesce as a result of intrinsic cellular events as well as alterations in their microenvironment (ecological niche). Niche effects appear to be mediated by epigenetic mechanisms. Stem cell senescence and its relationship to the ageing process in general represent an important research area.

The sequencing of the human genome has spurred the sequencing of other genomes including those of non-human primates. Comparing human and non- human primate genomes has the potential to give important insights into the process of human evolution as well as provide a better understanding of the genetic underpinnings responsible for the phenotypic differences, such as lifespan and senescence, between us and our closest "cousins". Chimpanzee maximum life expectancy is less than 50 years even for those in captivity with available modern veterinary care and chimpanzees display an obvious ageing process that is evident by the age of 20-25 years (Finch, 2010). For example, a decline in cognitive functioning has been well documented in ageing Rhesus monkeys (Herdon et al., (1997). The temporal course of decline varied for different cognitive skills but all monkeys that survived to age 29 years showed a significant impairment in all of the cognitive skills tested. The causes of mortality in wild chimpanzees include; infections 67%, violence and accidents 32% and senescence 1% (Finch, 2010).There appears to be a number of biomedical differences between humans and great apes (Orangutan, gorilla, chimpanzee and bonobo) such as a lower incidence of "Alzheimer disease" pathology, myocardial infarctions and cancer in the great apes (Finch, 2010; Olson and Varki, 2003).

What has been learned by a comparison of human and non-human primate genomes (Olson and Varki, 2003; Marques-Bonet et al., 2009)? Differences in protein coding genes across primates have not turned out to be as significant as originally expected. Gene expression differences between human and chimpanzee genomes appear to play a much more important role in the phenotypic differences. A comparison of the expression profile of 1000 orthologous genes in the human, chimpanzee, orangutan and macaque genomes showed a greater enrichment of transcription factors among genes up regulated in humans. This finding is consistent with the notion that regulation of gene expression patterns is a key process in the differences between human and non-human primate phenotypes. In addition there are substantial structural variations in both human and chimpanzee genomes; insertions, deletions, duplications and inversions as well as single base pair changes (Marques-Bonet et al., 2009). Compared to other mammalian genomes, primate genomes are enriched with larger more complex segmental duplications which tend to be hotspots of genomic structural variations including sites for the emergence of new genes. However, as pointed out by Marques-Bonet et al., (2009) much more data are needed before significant progress can be made in defining the genomic basis underlying the phenotypic differences (including the ageing phenotype) between humans and non-human primates.

The ageing process is both plastic and partially reversible. In the honeybee (Apis mellifera), senescence is determined chiefly by the social task of the bee (Singer, 2011). Queen bees, as already noted, have a long life span and negligible senescence. Worker bees have much shorter lifespans than queens and among worker bees, foragers display much more evidence of ageing than nurse bees. Foragers show cognitive senescence and immunoscenescence, but these features of ageing in foraging worker bees can be partially reversed by inducing the foragers to revert back to nursing activities. In birds, the processes of neurogenesis and recruitment of new neurons into the forebrain show evidence of ageing as well as plasticity. Short term survival of new neurons recruited into the forebrain and hippocampal complex of sexually mature male zebra finches is strongly influenced by the social complexity of the bird's environment (Singer, 2011).

As already alluded to, an age-dependent decline of physiological functions has been well described in natural animal models. For example, cognitive decline has been well described in the honeybee (Singer, 2011) and zebra fish (Yu et al., 2006), immunosenescence in the honeybee (Singer, 2011) and neuroendocrine ageing in birds (Singer, 2011). Many of the features of ageing in these natural animal models are due to epigenetic modifications of gene expression patterns. An epigenetic mechanism would underlie features such as the link between ageing in the honeybee and social task, the influence of social environment on the survival of new neurons recruited into the forebrain of birds and the partial reversibility of ageing in forager worker bees if they revert to performing nursing tasks. Since epigenetic mechanisms do not change DNA sequences, they are potentially reversible.

One other important consideration is that the specific features of the ageing process are not necessarily "transferrable" between species. Observations in rodents have indicated that reducing food consumption increased longevity and modified aspects of the ageing process in these mammals. However, a recently reported study in rhesus monkeys did not replicate these observations in this primate (Mattison et al., 2012). Male and female monkeys were enrolled in the study at young, middle and older ages. Experimental monkeys were subjected to a 30% calorie reduction (CR) in an otherwise nutritious diet. CR did not improve life span outcomes but did modify the ageing process. Starting CR in young aged monkeys reduced the incidence of malignancy and glucose regulatory dysfunction but interestingly did not alter the incidence of cardiovascular disease. As discussed by Austad (2012), the contrasting results between CR in rodents and primates with respect to life span extension and modification of the ageing process raise some very important questions. What might be the differences in physiology underlying these contrasting results? Are there subtle differences in the insulin/IGF 1 signaling networks between rodents and primates that could be responsible for these observations? At the moment these questions are unanswerable.

In summary, the features of ageing in natural animal models are very similar to those observed in the human. As in natural animal models, human ageing is also characterized by plasticity (modification by environmental cues) and partial reversibility. In addition, epigenetic mechanisms will be very important in shaping these particular features of the ageing process.

Chapter II

Atherosclerotic Vascular Disease

Atherosclerotic vascular disease has become a worldwide human health problem, responsible for damage and dysfunction in many organs; e.g. ischemic heart disease, renal failure, strokes and loss of limbs. However, this is not a new problem. Computed tomographic assessment of the vasculature of ancient Egyptian mummies (1981 BCE to 334 AD) showed calcifications in the aorta and medium sized peripheral arteries (Allam et al., 2009). In addition, vascular calcifications have been documented in a Tyrolean Copper age Iceman who lived 5300 years ago in the Italian Alps (Keller et al., 2012).

Atherosclerosis occurs in large and medium sized arteries and characteristically begins focally in sites having non laminar complex blood flow patterns such as bifurcations, branch points and areas of high curvature (Glagov et al., 1988; Weninger et al., 1999).Some vascular beds including the coronary and internal carotid arteries show the greatest predilection for development of atherosclerotic lesions (Weninger et al., 1999; Glagov et al., 1988). For example, blood flow in the coronary arteries differs from that of other organs in that it is intermittent; during systole the contracting heart compresses intramyocardial vessels (Velican and Velican, 1979 a). In addition coronary arteries are subject to unusual biomechanical forces such as torsion, bending and spiral twisting with every myocardial contraction (Velican and Velican, 1979 a). The nonrandom distribution of atherosclerotic lesions (i.e. specific vascular beds and localized arterial areas within these vascular beds) has led to the concept that biomechanical processes are crucial initiating factors since known systemic risk factors such as hyperlipidemia and hypertension have a uniform distribution throughout the circulation. As reviewed by Hahn and Schwartz (2009), complex blood flow patterns (low flow, oscillatory flow or other flow patterns that involve changes in flow direction and magnitude) as occurs for example at arterial bifurcations and areas of high curvature, change fluid shear stress and endothelial cells in these regions develop an activated "pro-inflammatory" phenotype. This endothelial cell phenotype makes the arterial wall susceptible to the development of atherosclerosis. Hence characterizing the mechanoreceptors responsible for sensing disturbances in shear stress and defining the mechanisms and events by which these mechanical signals are "converted" into biochemical processes which alter endothelial cell morphology and function, have become an important area of vascular research (White and Frangos, 2007; Hahn and Schwartz, 2009). However, arterial bifurcations, branch points and other regions of complex blood flow patterns are present in all animal vascular systems and yet atherosclerosis appears to be limited to mammals, largely humans and domesticated animals. Why is atherosclerosis not a widespread feature of animals in general? Experimental studies using traditional laboratory animals (chiefly rodents) that have been genetically altered cannot give a clear answer to this question since these animals are not in their natural state. However, examining the morphology and physiology of the arterial tree in natural animal models can give clues as to the answer to this question.

Natural Animal Models

The collection of data on the occurrence of vascular lesions in natural animals presents many technical barriers. In addition, studies that have been done are difficult to compare because experimental details are not necessarily consistent across these different studies. Most studies have been carried out on domestic animals or captive wild animals (zoo animals) as opposed to animals in their natural habitat because of the obvious difficulty studying free living animals in their own environment. Unfortunately, both the domestication process and the zoo environment modify the biology of animals (Schmidt et al., 2009; Vastesaeger and Delcourt, 1962). Perhaps the best studied natural animal, certainly with respect to coronary artery lesions, is the fish although data for other vertebrates are also available.

Focal myointimal arterial lesions have been described in teleosts; the trout and salmon family (Genus Oncorhynchus) and in several elasmobranch species; Chimaera monstrosa L. (rabbitfish) and Scyliorhinus canicula (dogfish). Focal intimal thickenings have been most thoroughly described in the coronary arteries of these fish, although Robertson et al (1961) did observe lesions in the arteries of the pancreas of spawning male Steelhead trout. Histologically, the intimal changes are generally comprised of; thinning, breaking or replication of the inner elastic lamina; focal intimal cellular proliferation, probably of smooth muscle cells; increase in collagen and elastic fibers. The endothelial layer generally remains intact.

In teleosts, the incidence and severity of intimal thickenings increase with body size (age), but are independent of whether the fish are hatchery- raised or wild-caught and independent of the lipid composition of the fish diet (Farrell, 2002; Seierstad et al., 2008). In addition, mechanical perturbations and changes in shear stress secondary to altered blood flow patterns are considered to be the initiating factors in the development of these coronary artery thickenings (Farrell, 2002; Seierstad et al., 2008).

With respect to elasmobranchs, the coronary vessels of the dogfish show numerous intimal thickenings, with lesion severity significantly correlated with fish body length, a proxy for age (Garcia-Garrido et al., 1993). Lesions occurred at branch points and in intramyocardial vessels subject to significant mechanical stresses. In the rabbitfish, the formation of coronary artery intimal thickenings is age related and the distribution of lesions is consistent with the notion that mechanical stress is a key etiological factor in their genesis (Duran et al., 2010).

Koppang et al., (2007) reported the occurrence of a small number of immunoreactive cells and possibly foam cells in the coronary artery thickenings of Atlantic salmon, but in general the focal intimal lesions in fish never develop the complex histological changes characteristic of atherosclerotic lesions observed in mammals.

The presence of arteriosclerosis has also been reported in the arterial vessels of wild African elephants residing in East Africa (McCullagh, 1972). This mammal has a long life span (about 70 years) and is a herbivore consuming a very low fat diet. This study was undertaken during 1966 and 1967 as part of a research program associated with the planned reduction cropping of the elephant populations in Kenya and Uganda. McCullagh performed post mortem examinations of the arterial trees of 467 elephants; males and females ranging in age from about 10 to 60 years of age. Blood samples were collected from elephants immediately prior to death and serum lipids were measured.

Arteriosclerotic “lesions” were found in the aorta, carotid, brachial, renal, iliac and coronary arteries. Histologically, small lesions were simple focal intimal thickenings composed of fibroblast-like cells with increased connective tissue and ground substance. Larger plaque-like lesions were also seen. These plaques contained cellular necrosis and connective tissue hyalinization. The sub-endothelial layers contained plasma cells and lymphocytes and extracellular lipid deposits were observed in the middle layers of the plaque. The majority of cells in these plaques were fibroblasts. As the investigator noted the main common histological characteristic of all of these “lesions” small and large was their highly fibrous nature. Interestingly, in the elephant, the occurrence of thickenings and plaques in the coronary arteries was much less frequent than in the aorta and other peripheral arteries. Not unexpectedly, the severity of aortic “lesions” (measured as percentage surface area involvement) increased significantly with age; increasing by greater than four times over the age range 10 to 60 years.

Serum lipid measurements (cholesterol, triglycerides, and free fatty acids) were made in these elephants but there was no correlation between serum lipid concentrations and the severity of arteriosclerotic “lesions”.

McCullagh concluded that these “lesions” were of “mechanical” origin. Lesions were focal in distribution and in the aorta, the site with generally the most extensive occurrence and severity of thickenings and plaques, the “lesions” were situated immediately posterior to the orifices of branch arteries (e.g. intercostal, mesenteric, renal) or at the bifurcation of the abdominal aorta. The sites of lesions corresponded to regions of altered laminar blood flow i.e. areas in the arterial tree where mean fluid shear stress would be reduced. McCullagh viewed these “lesions” as being part of the repair process in response to (hemodynamic) mechanical vascular injury.

Vastesaeger (1965) described coronary artery lesions in 1404 wild vertebrates; 100 fish (94 bony, 6 cartilaginous), 52 reptiles, 530 birds and 722 mammals. The source of the animals is not specified. Vastesaeger (1965) noted that the primary process involved the intima and consisted of an alteration of the internal elastic lamina. Other secondary processes included fibrosis and elastosis. Vastesaeger also observed that atherosclerosis (identified by its lipid component) always developed in vessels previously damaged by sclerosis of the intima. The coronary arteries of eighteen of the one hundred fish examined showed focal cushions of intimal sclerosis as already described in previous sections. Atherosclerotic lesions, defined as the presence of extracellular lipid deposits, were seen in only two immature Bluefin tunas (Thunnus thynnus). Coronary lesions were rare in the reptiles examined and occurred in only three of fifty-two specimens. Coronary intimal sclerotic lesions were observed in nearly twenty percent of the 530 bird specimens, while atherosclerotic lesions had a frequency of only 1.3%. In the group of mammals, atherosclerotic coronary artery lesions were rare with an occurrence of about 3%, whereas the frequency of coronary intimal sclerosis was not given. Vastesaeger described the effects of the domestication process by comparing the coronary lesions between domestic swine (50 animals) and the wild boar (50 animals). In the case of the wild boar, there was an 80% frequency of intimal sclerosis but only a 6% occurrence of atherosclerotic lesions. Domestic swine showed a 60% incidence of intimal sclerosis but a 33% incidence of atherosclerotic coronary artery lesions.

In an earlier publication, Vastesaeger and Delcourt (1962) presented similar findings based upon a sample of 403 captive wild vertebrates that died in the zoo of Antwerp and a second group of 144 vertebrates living in freedom and killed in their natural habitat. Fatty streaks were relatively common in the aorta of wild mammals and birds, both captive and free living specimens. Coronary intimal sclerosis was much more common than atherosclerotic lesions in captive mammals and birds. Animals "shot in freedom" also showed evidence of coronary intimal sclerosis but no evidence of coronary atherosclerosis.

In addition, there are observations from specific mammals that indirectly reflect on the genesis of atherosclerotic lesions. Goetz and Keen (1957) comment that the arteries (including coronaries) of giraffes (Giraffa camelopardalis) they had examined showed no signs of any degenerative lesions even though one of the giraffes was an old bull. In addition, Maluf (2002) in a published study of the histology of the giraffe kidney noted that the aorta and visceral distributing arteries of the bull giraffes in the sample showed no evidence of atherosclerosis. These are interesting observations given that the giraffe is a physiologically hypertensive mammal (Singer, 2011) and hypertension is considered a significant risk factor for the development of atherosclerosis. In the long-lived naked mole rat (Heterocephalus glaber) which displays negligible senescence (Buffenstein, 2008), arterial endothelial function (measured as the relaxation response to acetylcholine) was well maintained even in old animals whereas control laboratory rats showed a drastic decline in arterial endothelial function with increasing age (Csiszar et al., 2007). In addition, autopsies on two old female naked mole rats which died at ages 29 and 30 years showed minor histological changes in the heart. There were an increased number of cardiomyocytes as well as cardiac cells with enlarged nuclei. Lipofuscin was observed in the cytoplasm. There were also increased amounts of fibrous tissue in the heart (Edrey et al., 2011 a)). However, a detailed histological analysis of specific vascular beds such as the coronary arteries has not been done in the naked mole rat.

In humans, intimal coronary artery thickenings have been observed in fetuses and generally in regions of bifurcations and emergence zones (Velican and Velican, 1979 b; Neufeld et al., 1962; Velican and Velican, 1976). Similar but less extensive thickenings have been found in the basilar and renal arteries of a full term fetus (Velican and Velican, 1976). Weninger et al., (1999) described intimal thickenings in the (parasellar) internal carotid artery of human infants. They observed a correlation between the developmental shape of the parasellar internal carotid artery and the degree of intimal hyperplasia. These shape changes would be associated with changes in blood flow pattern and hence would alter mean vessel wall shear stress.

In summary, the available data from a wide variety of non- human vertebrates, both captive and free, and humans indicate that arteriosclerosis (focal arterial intimal thickenings and fibrous plaques) particularly of the coronary arteries is quite common, but that the occurrence of atherosclerotic lesions (presence of intra and extracellular lipids and associated thrombus formation, hemorrhage, rupture) is quite uncommon except in humans and domesticated animals. A current model is that these focal intimal sclerotic lesions develop at sites of altered biomechanical forces and Stehbens (1996) has proposed that arterial intimal thickenings actually represent a reparative process.

Influence of Social Environment

Zoo animals represent a rather unique population and observations collected by Ratcliffe and co-workers raise the issue of non-dietary environmental influences as important factors in the genesis of vascular lesions in mammals and birds. Over a forty year period (1916 to 1956), Herbert Fox and after his death H. L. Ratcliffe and co-workers collected data on the health, nutrition and causes of death of mammals and birds in the Philadelphia zoo (Ratcliffe and Cronin, 1958; Ratcliffe et al., 1960; Ratcliffe, 1965). Between 1916 and 1935, nutritional diseases were a common cause of mortality in the zoo and arteriosclerosis (intimal thickenings) relatively uncommon. In 1935, the traditional and inadequate zoo diet was replaced by a more adequate controlled diet with the result that the occurrence of nutritional diseases fell but interestingly arteriosclerosis developed much more frequently (Ratcliffe and Cronin, 1958). The vascular beds examined at autopsy by these investigators were chiefly heart, kidney and spleen. For example, for the mammal population, between 1916 and 1920 the occurrence of arteriosclerosis was 3.5% while the frequency, between the years 1951 to 1955, was 25.5%. For the bird population, the corresponding figures were 0.45% and 21.7%. In a later publication, Ratcliffe (1965) presented data for the period 1944 to 1964. He discussed the increasing occurrence of coronary arteriosclerosis and myocardial fibrosis and infarction observed in the zoo population of mammals and birds over this time period. The coronary lesions were most frequent in the intramural branches and consisted of intimal thickening, fragmentation of elastic fibers and proliferation of fibrous tissue and smooth muscle cells. The myocardial infarcts were not associated with occlusive coronary artery lesions. Thrombi were observed only in the arteries included within the infarcts. Ratcliffe (1965) explored factors that he thought might be responsible for this increased occurrence of coronary and myocardial lesions. Since the zoo diet had been improved in 1935, nutritional factors were probably not a primary cause. Ratcliffe (and co-workers) speculated that the changing social environment within the zoo over this time frame, associated with efforts to assemble and maintain breeding stock, had resulted in a greater intensity of social interactions and that this change in the social environment was an important factor in the recent increases, within the animal population, of coronary artery and myocardial lesions.

Ratcliffe and Synder (1964) explored the influence of social environment on the occurrence of coronary arteriosclerosis and myocardial infarction in a series of experiments using caged chickens. Single-comb White Leghorns (Hy-line strain) male and female, were caged either alone or in various groups (2 to 24 chickens); uni-sexual and heterosexual. All-cause mortality in males was significantly higher in heterosexual groups and pairs than for males caged singly or for males grouped without females. For females, all-cause mortality increased step-wise with group size. Myocardial infarcts were limited to males of heterosexual pairs and groups and to females of groups that contained 24 chickens. Myocardial infarcts were invariably associated with advanced grades of coronary arteriosclerosis although these lesions did not result in complete coronary occlusion. These experimental observations support the notion that the details or complexities of the social environment can somehow promote the occurrence of coronary arteriosclerosis and myocardial infarctions in a group of animals, in this case chickens.

A study exploring the effects of the social environment of chickens on adrenal function was reported in 1961 by Flickinger. He observed a correlation between the intensity of social interactions and histological evidence of adrenal gland hyper functioning. The data of Ratcliffe and Flickinger would be consistent with a mechanistic link between adrenal cortical stress hormones, stimulated by the pressures of complex social interactions, and coronary arteriosclerosis. The influence of stress hormones is explored in a subsequent separate section.

Finally a short report by Sikes (1968), also implicated the nature of the social environment as an important determinant of arteriosclerosis in wild animals. Sikes compared the occurrence of aortic arteriosclerosis in two populations (number of elephants in each population not given) of wild East African elephants. One population resided in their natural habitat while the second population had been "forced" to reside in a contracted habitat (due to continually encroaching human settlements) which had resulted in overcrowding with all of its consequences; changing patterns of mating, breeding and migration and reduced nutritional resources. Uncomplicated focal arterial intimal lipid deposits were observed in the aorta and muscular arteries of all elephants. However, elephants living in the contracted habitat showed more severe lesions characterized by intimal hyperplasia, hyaline degeneration, and disruption of the internal elastic lamella, hyaline degeneration and intimal calcification.

There are other examples in which social environment can significantly influence animal biology although not specifically vascular biology. For honeybees (Apis mellifera), social task is a primary determinant of senescence and the worker honeybee has emerged as a versatile model animal for studying the underlying links between social context, behaviors and senescence and the mechanisms underlying the plasticity of senescence (Singer, 2011). In adult sexually mature male zebra finches, the complexity of the social environment sets the survival outcome of newly formed neurons (Singer, 2011). In addition, it is now appears that the evolutionary pressure driving the evolution of large brains in some groups of animals, notably primates, is the demands of the complex social interactions which occur within groups of these animals (Dunbar and Shultz, 2007).

The observations of Seierstad et al., (2008) in fish, Ratcliffe and co-workers in the mammal and bird populations of the Philadelphia Zoo and McCullagh in elephants, indicate that dietary factors are probably not a primary causative agent in the development of arteriosclerosis. The observation that the coronary arteries of the giraffe are free of atherosclerotic lesions implies at least, that a markedly elevated mean arterial pressure in natural animals is not a primary determinant for progression of coronary artery arteriosclerosis (focal intimal thickenings) to atherosclerosis. Finally, the data collected by Ratcliffe and co-workers on the changing frequency of coronary arteriosclerosis in the mammal and bird populations of the Philadelphia Zoo and the observations of Sikes on arteriosclerosis in wild elephants, suggest that the nature of the social environment of an animal group can have a significant influence on the incidence of arterial intimal lesions within that group.

Mechanisms by which environmental changes (e.g. the nature of the social environment) can influence biological processes have been partially defined. For example, differential feeding of royal jelly to honeybee female larvae can alter the pattern of gene expression creating workers or queens by the selective methylation of DNA (Kucharski et al., 2008; see section, Background; Phenotypic plasticity). Interestingly, the component in royal jelly (a 57-kDa protein called royalactin) responsible for caste (queen/worker) differentiation has been isolated (Kamakura, 2011). In a study by Borghol et al., (2012), early childhood socioeconomic position was associated with a differential methylation signature for DNA regulatory regions measured in later life, consistent with the notion that epigenetic mechanisms contribute to the link between early life socioeconomic circumstances and adult health (see section, Background; Phenotypic plasticity). These observation are consistent with the notion that epigenetic mechanisms such as differential DNA methylation and post-translational modifications of core histone proteins (Richards, 2006), are an important mechanistic link between environmental variation and alterations in biological processes.

The observation that focal intimal arterial lesions are quite common in vertebrates whereas atherosclerotic lesions are almost exclusively found in humans and domesticated animals appears to be a paradox. Why do humans and domestic animals develop atherosclerotic lesions in contrast to most other vertebrates? The answer to this question is rooted in the interaction between the biological constraints of the arterial tree and the nature of the environmental setting of the modern human; how do these environmental factors modify gene expression (epigenetic effects). The environment of the modern human comprises in general, a large urban social setting with its attendant “social pressures” and complex interactions among groups of people. Ageing is also an important factor since atherosclerosis is more common in humans of advanced chronological age. In essence atherosclerosis rather than being a “disease” can be considered a component of the ageing process with the epigenetic effects of environmental factors responsible for the difference in lesion severity across individuals. In the next sections the interplay between vascular biology, genetics and environmental influences are discussed in more detail.

Biology of the Arterial Vasculature

There is an array of interconnected factors and processes which regulate the structure and function of the arterial tree. Probably the best described of these processes is the mechanosensory-transduction mechanism; mechanosensors within the vessel wall, detect sustained changes in hemodynamic forces and activate signaling pathways which lead to modifications in vascular morphology (remodeling) in response to these changes. However, this is but one defined process involved in arterial remodeling. The actual morphology of the vessel wall is determined by the dynamic summation of the individual effects of all component processes in this array. Other defined component processes and factors include the effects of molecular clocks and stress hormones. Ultimately, the connections within this interwoven array of processes and factors are specific gene expression patterns. The next sections review; what is known about the genetic underpinnings of atherosclerosis and the effects on vessel wall morphology of the mechanosensory-transduction mechanism, molecular clocks and stress hormones.

The overall sequence of steps leading to atherosclerosis can be summarized as follows; sustained changes in hemodynamic forces, subsequent development of focal arterial intimal thickenings and progression of these focal thickenings into atherosclerotic lesions in the human. This sequence of events can be reframed as a repair process initiated by altered hemodynamic forces which in the human has been significantly altered by the epigenetic effects of environmental factors (defined in the broadest sense).

Mechanosensor-transduction Mechanism

Considerable information has accumulated regarding both the molecular sensors which monitor mechanical forces on the vessel wall (circumferential stretching secondary to intraluminal pressure and fluid shear stress resulting from the friction of blood flow against the vessel wall) and the cellular signaling processes initiated by these sensors (Lehoux et al., 2006; Hahn and Schwartz, 2009; White and Frangos, 2007). As reviewed by Lehoux et al., (2006), endothelial and vascular smooth muscle cells have receptors in the plasma membrane (integrins, ion channels , receptor tyrosine kinases, G-protein coupled receptors, adhesion molecules) that allow them to detect and respond to the mechanical forces generated by intraluminal pressure and blood flow. Most likely, specific receptors respond to only one of the mechanical forces (pressure induced stretching or fluid shear stress), although such a characterization is still in its early stages. However, a mechanosensory complex has been identified, located at cell-cell junctions, which responds to alterations in shear stress (due to low fluid flow or changes in flow direction) by activating a number of shear-dependent signaling pathways (Tzima et al., 2005; Woodfin et al., 2007). This complex consists of PECAM1 (platelet endothelial cell adhesion molecule 1), VE-cadherin (vascular endothelial cell cadherin) and VEGFR2 (vascular endothelial growth factor receptor 2). All three components are trans membrane proteins with cytoplasmic and extracellular domains. The nature of the association between these three molecules is unknown, but it has been proposed that PECAM1 directly transmits mechanical force, VE-cadherin acts as an adapter bringing PECAM 1 and VEGFR 2 together and VEGFR2 promotes activation of a phosphatidylinositol-3-OH kinase (PI3K) following application of force to PECAM 1 (Tzima et al., 2005). PI3K probably leads to activation of integrins and is also linked to a diverse group of cellular functions (Tzima et al., 2005).

Another pathway that has been shown to be involved in the process of arterial vascular repair is the Notch signaling pathway. This pathway and its role in vascular repair is discussed in the section Hypertension; Natural experiments; a) Postnatal pulmonary and systemic arterial pressure changes.

The response to increased intraluminal pressure includes smooth muscle cell hyperplasia and hypertrophy plus increased extracellular matrix resulting in thickening of the media of the vessel wall (Lehoux and Tedgui, 2003). This response helps to normalize tensile (pressure) stress (Lehoux and Tedgui, 2003). On the other hand, arterial endothelial cells chronically exposed to alterations in fluid shear stress due to low flow, oscillatory flow or other flow patterns that involve changes in flow direction and magnitude (e.g. at vessel bifurcations or regions of high curvature) demonstrate an increased cell turnover, loss of alignment, a more rounded shape and an increased rate of proliferation (White and Frangos, 2007). This response to low mean wall shear stress leads to the development of focal arterial intimal thickenings in areas of bifurcations and regions of high curvature (White and Frangos, 2007).

Most of the data on vascular mechanosensory-transduction mechanisms have been collected from experiments using traditional laboratory animals. Very little experimental data are available for other vertebrates. However, several reports imply that similar mechanosensory- transduction mechanisms exist in other vertebrates. A recent study by Huhtala et al., (2005) has reported that integrins are widely distributed across vertebrate species. In addition, tissue –type VEGF's share more than 90% nucleotide and amino acid identities between snakes and humans (Yamazaki et al., 2009). Even though the comparative biological data on arterial mechanosensors are limited, it would seem reasonable to assume that vertebrates in general have an arterial mechanosensory-transduction mechanism similar to that described for the experimental laboratory rodent.

It has been proposed that the phenotype (high cell turnover, increased rate of proliferation, loss of alignment and altered shape) expressed by arterial endothelial cells in vascular regions chronically exposed to reduced mean fluid shear stress (due to low fluid flow or changes in flow direction) is associated with a high susceptibility to the development of atherosclerotic lesions in these regions (Hahn and Schwartz, 2009). The focal intimal thickenings formed in these regions of altered fluid shear stress have been considered pre-atherosclerotic. However, the comparative physiology data reviewed in the section "Natural animal models" are not consistent with this proposal. Focal arterial intimal thickenings (particularly in the coronary tree which is the vascular bed that has been most extensively studied) have been observed in fish (teleosts and elasmobranchs), birds, reptiles and wild mammals. Yet the incidence of atherosclerotic lesions in these groups is quite low. Two notable examples among mammals are the giraffe and naked mole-rat. Even old giraffes show no evidence of coronary artery atherosclerosis despite having physiological hypertension. The long lived naked mole-rat which shows negligible senescence, maintains near normal arterial endothelial function even at an advanced age. Although focal arterial intimal thickenings have been considered the soil in which atherosclerotic lesions develop, this progression is observed almost exclusively in humans and domesticated animals.

The mechanosensor-transduction complexes that detect reductions in mean positive shear stress (due to low fluid flow or a change in direction of flow) should be regarded as part of a repair process. Most of the studies defining the molecular details of these complexes and the resulting changes in endothelial cell phenotype have been done in vitro and have examined very short time periods (Tzima et al., 2005; Davies, 1995). The comparative physiology data are most consistent with the proposal that focal arterial intimal thickenings found in sites of bifurcations and regions of high curvature actually represent a reparative process (physiological adaptation) in response to the chronically low mean shear stress found in these sections of the arterial tree. A comparison with an analogous condition, the vascular remodeling observed in a physiological hypertensive state will help illuminate this point. The giraffe has a very high mean arterial pressure and this high pressure acting on pressure sensitive mechanosensory-transduction complexes in the arterial wall results in a remodeling of arterioles (thickening of media) in kidney, lung, heart and liver (Mitchell and Skinner, 2009). The morphological features of this arteriolar remodeling resemble the morphological changes observed in humans and animal models with hypertension and which have been linked to the organ failure observed in humans with an elevated mean arterial pressure. Yet in the giraffe this arteriolar remodeling is clearly a physiological adaptation not a pathological structural change. By analogy, focal arterial intimal thickenings represent a physiological and not a pathological adaptation to the chronic exposure of the arterial vessel wall to a low mean shear stress.

Genetics

The genetic underpinnings of atherosclerosis are believed to be the same as that of quantitative traits and genome wide studies have been done to look for associated DNA polymorphisms and QTLs. O'Donnell et al., (2007) in a genome-wide association study, used participants of the Offspring Cohort of the Framingham Heart Study to examine for statistical associations between measures of atherosclerotic disease, the "phenotypes" (carotid artery intimal thickening, coronary artery and abdominal aortic calcification and ankle-brachial systolic arterial pressure index) and SNPs. There were a limited number of associations detected. However, they did observe a number of SNPs that were near to 28 candidate genes previously reported to be associated with atherosclerotic vascular disease. The Wellcome Trust Case Control Consortium (2007) reported a genome wide association study covering seven common diseases in which approximately 2000 individuals suffered from coronary artery disease. A strong statistical association was detected for SNPs on chromosome 9, particularly SNP rs1333049. The risk odds ratios for this SNP were heterozygote 1.47 and homozygote 1.9.

Wang et al., (2005) reviewed the use of mouse to human comparative genetics in identifying genes associated with atherosclerosis. Studies with gene-knockout or transgenic mouse models have identified more than 80 genes associated with atherosclerotic vascular lesions. Nine genome wide scans in humans with atherosclerotic diseases have detected 27 unique QTLs distributed on 27 chromosome locations. Six candidate genes with confirmed association with atherosclerotic vascular disease lie in 6 of the 27 QTLs. Half of the human "atherosclerotic" QTLs have no obvious candidate genes. A total of 15 studies using mouse models of atherosclerosis have detected 21 unique QTLs. The causal genes underlying two of the 21 mouse atherosclerotic QTLs have been identified. Finally, 17 (63%) of the 27 human QTLs are located in regions homologous to mouse QTLs. Wang et al., (2005) proposed that genes associated with atherosclerosis in humans will be found most efficiently by first finding their orthologs in homologous mouse QTLs. Effect sizes are not given in these reports, but since atherosclerosis can be considered analogous to a quantitative trait, most likely many SNPs and QTLs with small effect sizes have not been detected. Given the complexity of the genome and epigenome (Background; Genetics), it is apparent that genome wide association studies have given very limited information as to the genetic mechanisms underlying vascular remodeling. Certainly, there is no justification for ascribing a causal relationship to these associations. What these genome wide association studies have done is direct investigators to specific regions of the genome where causative genes are most likely to be found.

Molecular (Circadian) Clocks

Circadian rhythms are regulated by molecular clocks and in the mammal the master clock is located in the suprachiasmatic nucleus (SCN) of the hypothalamus. Core clock genes have been identified and the basic "structure" of the clock consists of three negative and one positive loop of transcription, translation and posttranslational events (Reilly et al., 2007). Briefly, the three period genes (Per 1,2,3) display robust circadian rhythms in both the SCN and peripheral tissues (Yamamoto et al., 2005). Per 1 transcription is activated by the binding of CLOCK-BMAL 1 protein dimers to the Per 1 promoter region. The protein product of Per 1 is post translationally modified and together with other clock proteins is transported into the nucleus to suppress its own transcriptional activation by inhibiting the activity of the CLOCK-BMALI 1 dimers. Gradual loss of Period proteins leads to de-repression and then the daily cycle starts anew. A similar model applies to the auto regulatory loops involving other clock genes. Among mammalian Per genes, the expression of Per 1 and Per 2 are induced by light but Per 3 is not.

Recent experimental studies have begun to unravel the links between clock genes and target genes (Doherty and Kay, 2012; Koike et al., 2012). The core clock machinery consists of the transcriptional activators CLOCK, BMAL 1 and NAPS 2 which activate target genes and PER 1, PER 2, PER 3, CRY 1 and CRY 2 which act as repressors of the same target genes. These seven factors bind to a DNA regulator sequence known as an enhancer box (E box) as well as to nuclear receptors. Koike et al., (2012) measured circadian gene expression rhythms in the mouse liver; the target genes examined were enriched for metabolic pathways and the insulin signaling network. These investigators noted that transcriptional activity of target genes occurred in three phases. First there was a transcriptionally poised state when both activators and repressors occupied regulatory elements. As the extent of binding of repressors decreased, a second activation state occurred characterized by target gene transcription. The third stage was one of repression of target gene transcription as CLOCK and BMAL 1 occupancy decreased and repressor factors accumulated at regulatory element sites. The transcriptional activity of 3408 cycling genes was examined. In 458 of these genes pre mRNA expression (nascent transcription) and mRNA (mature mRNA) expression were phase correlated suggesting that transcriptional cycles primarily drive these mRNA rhythms. These 458 genes were enriched for circadian clock genes and high amplitude cycling target genes. In 1579 genes, nascent transcription did not show cycling but mRNA expression did, suggesting that the phase rhythms for these genes were due to mRNA post transcriptional regulatory processes (e.g. circadian changes in mRNA splicing). In 913 genes nascent transcription (pre RNA expression) showed cycling but mRNA expression showed much dampened oscillations. A surprise finding was the presence of rhythms for RNA polymerase II occupancy and promoter region histone acetylation and methylation marks in thousands of expressed genes irrespective of whether or not these genes displayed mRNA cycling. The significance of these genome wide circadian rhythms in RNA polymerase II occupancy and histone modifications which occurred in the presence and absence of mRNA transcript cycling is currently unknown.

Although the master clock is in the hypothalamus, molecular clocks are also distributed widely throughout peripheral tissues including the cardiovascular system (Davidson et al., 2005; Reilly et al., 2007). The biological importance of molecular clocks is underscored by the observation that subterranean mammals, which are not exposed to light and dark variation, still have functional molecular clocks. For example, the naked mole-rat (Heterocephalus glaber) displays active circadian rhythms for biological functions such as body temperature, metabolic rate and loco motor activity (Riccio and Goldman, 2000 a, b). Blind subterranean mammals of the Spalax ehrenbergi super species , which live their entire life underground and in darkness, have circadian clock genes (period 1, 2 and 3) in the suprachiasmatic nucleus, retina and in peripheral tissues such as the liver (Avivi et al., 2002). The three Period genes showed robust circadian expression patterns. In this same mammalian Spalax family, the (circadian) genes for transcription factors CLOCK and MOP3 have been identified not only in the suprachiasmatic nucleus but also in peripheral tissues such as kidney, liver and heart. Arteries and veins were not examined (Avivi et al., 2001).As in other mammals, Spalax Clock gene does not oscillate but Spalax Mop3 gene does oscillate.

The wide spread tissue distribution of molecular clocks suggests that this mechanism is fundamentally encoded within every cell (Barnard and Nolan, 2008). The rhythms of individual cellular clocks are not externally driven but rather coordinated by the output of the "master" SCN clock and the rhythms of individual clocks can be region specific (Bell-Pedersen et al., 2005; Dibner et al., 2010). The circadian system must also be sensitive to environmental cues such as prevailing day and night cycle, food resources and social interactions. The process of synchronization of circadian rhythms with external environmental cues is known as entrainment. In summary, the generation of metabolic and physiological circadian rhythms and the synchronization of these rhythms with environmental cues require a complex system of molecular clocks.

Cardiovascular functions such as arterial blood pressure and heart rate show well defined circadian rhythms and molecular clocks are present in the heart and vasculature (Davidson et al., 2005; Reilly et al., 2007). Davidson et al., (2005) demonstrated the presence of the molecular clock gene Period 1 and its rhythmic expression in rat heart and a variety of arteries and veins. Arteries generally showed more robust rhythms than veins. Rudic et al., (2005) examined global expression profiles in mouse aorta and identified 330 genes with a circadian expression pattern. The products of many of these "oscillating" genes are endothelial and smooth muscle cell proteins involved in vascular function and structure such as smooth muscle cell contractile proteins, extracellular matrix components, and endothelial cell specific junctional adhesion molecules. Cheng et al.,(2011) have documented the role of vascular molecular clocks in the biology of vascular remodeling. These investigators used a mouse model in which a section of aorta from a donor mouse was grafted into the course of the common carotid artery of a recipient mouse of the same strain and sex. The size difference between the aortic and common carotid sections causes an alteration in blood flow pattern which leads to remodeling of the aortic graft; narrowing of the lumen diameter and an increase in wall thickness. In one set of experiments, knockout mice with deletions of either the molecular clock gene Bmal 1 or the gene Period were used as recipients. In this experimental model in which an aortic section from a wild-type mouse was grafted into the common carotid artery of a molecular clock gene knockout recipient mouse, the features of aortic vascular remodeling were similar to that observed in wild-type donor-recipient pairs. In a second set of experiments an aortic section from a knockout mouse was grafted into the common carotid artery of a recipient wild-type mouse. In this experimental model, aortic vascular remodeling was much more extensive and included intimal hyperplasia, perivasculitis and histologically macrophage infiltration. These changes were not mediated by B or T lymphocytes. This hyperplastic vascular remodeling was not dependent on changes in blood flow pattern since these same features also occurred when a common carotid artery from a knockout donor mouse was grafted into the common carotid artery of a wild-type recipient mouse. These observations of Cheng et al., (2011) implicate tissue-specific vascular molecular clocks in regulating the morphological features and extent of vascular remodeling.

In addition, since tissue specific molecular clocks form a network with each other and with the master clock in the hypothalamus, the effects of molecular clocks on vascular structure are probably much more diverse than indicated by the experimental observations of Cheng et al., (2011).

Stress Hormones

Cortisol is a major stress hormone in salmonid fish and in the human and the production of cortisol is under the control of the hypothalamus-pituitary- adrenal/interrenal (fish) axis (Aluru and Vijayan, 2009). In the mammal, an increased amount of aldosterone is also secreted in response to stress (Thomson and Geraci, 1986) whereas there is conflicting evidence as to whether fish actually synthesize aldosterone (Greenwood et al., 2003). Corticosteroids, such as cortisol and also aldosterone, bind to specific nuclear receptors which represent the largest family of transcription factors found in metazoans (Bookout et al., 2006). Although the corticosteroid- receptor interaction is the focus of this discussion, there is evidence that many nuclear receptors cross-react with each other's DNA binding sites and can activate similar signaling cascades. Hence the family of nuclear receptors should be viewed as a hierarchical transcriptional regulatory network (Bookout et al., 2006). This broader context should be remembered, even when the discussion is limited to a specific nuclear receptor group, the corticosteroid receptors and its ligands, cortisol and aldosterone.

Recent experimental observations in salmonid fish have defined an association between post-stress cortisol levels and the degree of associated cardiac remodeling (Johansen et al., 2011).This is an interesting study since the surge in cortisol in these fish follows a stressful experience and hence the experimental situation in this study can be considered quite physiologic. Although the arterial vasculature is the focus of this discussion, there are no comparable experimental data that I am aware of, in which repetitive stressful experiences have been correlated with arterial vascular morphological changes. Hence, I will make the extrapolation that the stress- cortisol- nuclear receptor mechanism responsible for cardiac remodeling can activate a comparable sequence of events in the arterial vessel wall which results in morphological alterations.

Johansen et al., (2011) examined cardiac morphology and cardiac gene expression patterns in two strains of rainbow trout (Oncorhynchus mykiss) which significantly differ in their cortisol levels following a standardized confinement stress. These two strains have been denoted as high (high post stress cortisol levels, HR) and low (lower post stress cortisol levels, LR) responders. Average heart size was greater in HR fish than LR fish and this difference was due to a greater amount of compact myocardium in the HR fish. Gene expression patterns indicated that myocyte hypertrophy rather than hyperplasia was the chief mechanism for the structural change. The hearts of HR fish showed a moderate amount of collagen deposition in the ventricles, but no collagen was found in the hearts of LR fish. HR ventricles also showed a higher degree of vascularization than LR ventricles.

In terms of gene expression profiles, the expression of cortisol receptors (mineralocorticoid receptor, glucocorticoid receptors 1 and 2), activity of the NFAT – calcineurin pathway and expression of the VEGF (vascular endothelial growth factor) gene were all higher in HR hearts compared to LR hearts (Johansen, et al., 2011). NFAT (nuclear factor of activated T cells) signaling is initiated by a rise in the intracellular calcium concentration sufficient to activate calcineurin (Wu et al., 2007). Once activated, calcineurin interacts with NFAT proteins to expose a nuclear import sequence. The NFAT proteins translocate into the cell nucleus where they combine with partner proteins to form transcriptional complexes. NFAT signaling is involved in the development of many organs as revealed by studies in mice with mutations in different calcineurin and NFAT genes (Wu et al., 2007). For example, calcineurin-NFAT signaling is involved in cardiac valve morphogenesis as well as in the development of the myocardium. On the other hand, in mice subjected to cardiac pressure overload by aortic constriction, the ensuing pathological cardiac hypertrophy was accompanied by up regulation of cardiac calcineurin-NFAT signaling suggesting that this pathway may be involved in the pathological cardiac remodeling associated with pressure overload (Wilkins et al., 2004).

However, experimental observations of Cerra et al., (2004) on the changes in cardiac remodeling and function in the growing eel (Anguilla Anguilla L.) heart are not completely consistent with the conclusion of Wilkins et al., (2004). Eel ventricular growth was achieved by an increase in both the thickness of the compact layer and in the trabecular diameters of the spongiosa layer. In addition, collagen was deposited in the ventricles of the larger hearts of the more fully grown eels, but not in the smaller hearts of less fully grown eels. However, unlike the situation in the human in which cardiac collagen deposition impairs function, collagen deposition in the larger eel hearts was actually associated with enhanced cardiac performance. Larger eel hearts which contain increased amounts of collagen (improves structural resilience) were able to maintain a constant stroke volume when subjected to a high applied afterload which in small eel hearts caused a fall in stroke volume.

In summary, rainbow trout which show a large surge of cortisol production in response to a confinement stress have larger hearts than rainbow trout with a much lower post confinement stress cortisol production response. The increase in heart size is due to hypertrophy and collagen deposition, but there is no evidence that these structural changes lead to functional cardiac impairment.

Corticosteroid receptors have been identified in the endothelial and smooth muscle cells of mammalian arteries (Yang and Zhang, 2004) and specific in vitro studies have been reported using bovine coronary artery endothelial cells (Rogers et al., 2002), sheep uterine artery rings (Xiao et al., 2002) and rabbit aorta, femoral and carotid arteries (Kornel, 1993). As reviewed by Yang and Zhang (2004), the binding of cortisol to its receptor in endothelial and vascular smooth muscle cells leads to a reduction in the expression of endothelial nitric oxide synthase, reduced endothelial formation of nitric oxide and an increase in agonist-induced (e.g. norepinephrine) contraction of smooth muscle cells. There are limited data, linking cortisol to vascular remodeling (Sugiyama et al., 2005) but there are a number of experimental observations that the mineralocorticoid, aldosterone, is involved in remodeling arterial blood vessel structure.

There are two classes of corticosteroid receptors; the glucocorticoid receptor (GR) and the mineralocorticoid receptor (MR). Unlike the human, the fish contains multiple GRs and four have been identified in a cichlid fish (Haplochromis burtoni) (Greenwood et al., 2003). Although fish do have a distinct MR, it is still controversial whether fish actually synthesize aldosterone (Greenwood et al., 2003). Both MR and GR have a widespread tissue distribution (Greenwood et al., 2003; Bookout et al., 2006) .This widespread distribution indicates that even this set of nuclear receptors affects a number of physiological processes involving metabolism, circadian clocks and cardiovascular function (Bookout et al., 2006).In the human, both the MR and GR genes transcribe multiple mRNA isoforms and hence multiple protein (receptor) variants (Viengchareun et al., 2007; Tallec and Lombes, 2005). Both the mammalian GR gene and MR gene contain a number of promoter regions through which other factors regulate expression of these genes (Viengchareun et al., 2007; Weaver et al., 2004). In their non- ligand bound state; the MR and GR are located in the cytoplasm attached to a large variety of proteins including chaperone proteins. Ligand free receptors are phosphorylated with additional phosphorylation occurring in conjunction with ligand binding. Upon hormone binding, the receptor undergoes conformational changes, dissociates from these attached proteins and the ligand-receptor complex trans locates into the cell nucleus. Within the nucleus, the ligand-receptor complex forms a homodimer as well as interacting with various co-regulators (activators and repressors) to ensure appropriate transcriptional regulation. The complex of homodimer and coregulators binds to specific hormone responsive elements located upstream or downstream from transcriptional start sites in the target genes (Viengchareun et al., 2007; Aluru and Vijayan, 2009).

Since both aldosterone and cortisol bind to (human) MR with equal affinities how is receptor specificity determined? In aldosterone responsive epithelial tissues, the cortisol inactivating enzyme 11B-hydroxysteroid dehydrogenase is expressed. This enzyme converts cortisol to an inactive form (cortisone) that has a much lower affinity for MR. However, other tissues such as the central nervous system and vascular tissue express very low levels of this enzyme, so other mechanisms must exist to confer receptor specificity (Tallec and Lombes, 2005). At the receptor level, aldosterone and cortisol do induce ligand specific conformational changes even though their binding affinities are similar and hence this is one mechanism responsible for receptor specificity. In addition, it appears that MR recruits distinct co-activators and co-repressors which results in transcription selectivity.

Some of the target genes for MR have been elucidated. Nakamura et al., (2006) demonstrated that the aldosterone MR complex increased the expression of the gene NDM2 in human cultured vascular smooth muscle cells (VSMC) and in VSMC in human small resistance arteries. The protein product of this gene is involved in regulating the cell cycle and proliferation of VSMC and hence the up regulation of this gene by aldosterone could explain the arterial vascular remodeling observed in states with hyperaldosteronism. Grossmann et al., (2007) using human aorta smooth muscle cells, showed that aldosterone up regulated the gene coding for epidermal growth factor receptor (EGFR) and resulted in an EGFR dependent increase in fibronectin. This mechanism could be another link underlying aldosterone induced arterial remodeling in conditions of hyperaldosteronism. Another target gene of both MR and GR is the one coding for angiotensin converting enzyme (ACE). Sugiyama et al., (2005) using cultured rat aortic endothelial cells which express both MR and GR, showed that the expression of ACE was up regulated by both aldosterone and dexamethasone through binding to their respective receptors. The effect of aldosterone was both dose and time dependent. Activation of the renin- angiotensin system has been implicated in the development of atherosclerotic lesions and in the genesis of pathological cardiac hypertrophy. In keeping with this notion, clinical studies have shown that the aldosterone receptor inhibitor spironolactone can improve the prognosis of patients with congestive heart failure (Funder, 2001).

Although the nuclear receptors (NR) of particular interest with respect to vascular remodeling are GR and MR, the function of MR and GR need to be viewed within a broader context as noted previously. Bookout et al., (2006) examined the anatomic al expression and function of 49 members of the nuclear receptor family in 39 tissues from two different strains of the most widely used mouse models. These investigators were able to group the various nuclear receptors into hierarchical clusters. Group 1 contained NRs that had an abundant central nervous system expression as well as being expressed in most other tissues as well. Some of the members of this group are crucial in maintaining global basal metabolism. MR is a member of this group and as already discussed MR is also an important regulator of cardiovascular function. GR is a member of group 2, which contains NRs involved in specialized aspects of fuel utilization such as fat storage, cholesterol and glucose metabolism. According to the analysis of Bookout et al., (2006), group 1 NRs are predominantly involved in central nervous system function and reproduction while group 2 NRs are chiefly involved in nutrient metabolism and immunity. Bookout et al., (2006) concluded that NRs function together in specific groupings as part of higher order regulatory networks. The ligands (dietary factors, endocrine factors) which bind to members of the NR family traverse the body through the blood stream conveying information from the central nervous system to peripheral tissues. In these tissues, ligands bind to specific NRs, forming complexes which function as transcription regulators of various target genes. Ligands acting through this family of NRs permit the integration and communication of information between the central nervous system and peripheral organs and tissues.

Within this broader context, the experimental observations of Yamamoto et al., (2005) define a possible mechanism by which the glucocorticoid receptor in particular, could link molecular clocks and vascular remodeling. These investigators examined behavioral rhythms (free- running periods) as well as the expression of peripheral tissue molecular clock genes in mice subjected to a physical restraint stress protocol. The acute restraint stress did not alter the circadian activity rhythm or the temporal expression of clock genes in peripheral tissues (liver, heart, and kidney). However the acute physical stress did increase the amount of mRNA transcribed by the clock gene Per 1 but not by the other clock genes examined. Yamamoto et al., (2005) found that the promoter region of Per 1 but not the other clock genes contained a glucocorticoid response element (GRE). Hence in response to stress or other equivalent environmental situations that result in elevated glucocorticoid levels (cortisol in humans and fish, corticosterone in birds, rodents and reptiles), the glucocorticoid-GR complex will bind to the GRE in the Per 1 promoter region and increase transcriptional activity of the Per 1 gene. This enhanced transcriptional activity of Per 1 does not appear to influence overall clock regulation and as such, is probably involved in non-clock physiological functions.

How might these observations of Yamamoto et al., (2005) relate to vascular remodeling? As discussed in the section; Molecular (circadian) clocks, vascular tissues (arteries, veins and the heart) contain molecular clocks and clock genes including Per 1 (Reilly et al., 2007; Davidson et al., 2005; Rudic et al., 2005). As noted by Davidson et al., (2005), the rhythmic expression of Per 1 was more robust in arteries than veins or the heart. Cheng et al., (2011) documented that vascular molecular clocks can regulate the morphology and extent of vascular remodeling. These observations can be summarized as follows; transcripts of many genes involved in maintenance of vascular structure and function, oscillate in a circadian rhythm (Rudic et al., 2005); the clock gene Per 1 is present in vascular tissue and Per 1 contains a functional glucocorticoid response element (GRE) in its promoter region; binding of the glucocorticoid-GR complex to this GRE activates transcription of the Per 1 gene. Given these observations, a reasonable hypothesis is that the glucocorticoid-GR complex acts as a functional link connecting environmental stressors, vascular molecular clocks and vascular remodeling.

It is also important to remember that stress (as measured by glucocorticoid hormone levels) can also be associated with an increase in animal fitness. The stress response is not always maladaptive in nature. Bonier et al., (2011) measured baseline corticosterone (the primary glucocorticoid in birds) levels in female tree swallows (Tachycineta bicolor) before and after experimentally enlarging or reducing brood sizes. These investigators found that females with experimentally enlarged broods had a greater increase in baseline (before brood was enlarged) corticosterone levels and fledged more offspring than females who had their brood size reduced. Also, females who demonstrated a greater increase in baseline corticosterone levels after brood size manipulation demonstrated higher offspring provisioning rates than females with smaller increases in baseline corticosterone levels after brood size manipulation. The investigators concluded that a greater increase in maternal stress as measured by the magnitude of increase in corticosterone levels was associated with a more successful reproductive outcome and hence an enhancement of animal fitness.

Finally, what are the factors which set the stress response of a given animal? Since no two individual animals are genetically identical, there will be natural variation in the magnitude of the stress response among individuals. In fact, selective breeding of rainbow trout demonstrating a high and low cortisol response to confinement stress within the range of natural variation, is how the two strains of rainbow trout used in the study of Johansen et al., (2011) were developed.

In the rat, maternal care of offspring during their first week of postnatal life can significantly modify the stress response of these offspring as adults. Hence the stress phenotype is plastic. Mother-pup contact in the rat occurs within the context of a nest bout, which begins when the mother licks and grooms the pups while also nursing. The two forms of behavior generally considered are licking and grooming (LG) and arched back nursing (ABN) and there are natural variations in the frequency of these two forms of maternal behavior over the first ten days of postnatal life. Liu et al., (1997) studied the effects of maternal behavior on the stress response of offspring in Norway rats. Mothers were classified as demonstrating either high LG-ABN or low LG-ABN behavior based upon the number of LG-ABN episodes over the 10 days of the study. As adults (male and female), the offspring of high LG-ABN mothers showed significantly lower blood levels of ACTH and corticosterone in response to a standardized restraint stress than the offspring of low LG-ABN mothers. Adult offspring of high LG-ABN mothers also showed lower levels of hypothalamic corticotropin releasing hormone (CRH) mRNA than the adult offspring of low LG-ABN mothers. CRH is a hypothalamic factor which regulates the secretion of ACTH and via this mechanism, the secretion of glucocorticoids. Finally, the hippocampus of offspring of high LG-ABN mothers showed increased amounts of GR (glucocorticoid receptor) mRNA compared to offspring of low LG-ABN mothers.

In a subsequent publication, Francis et al., (1999) using cross-fostering studies, demonstrated non genomic transmission across generations of maternal and offspring behaviors. The adult female offspring (F2) of high LG-ABN mothers showed significantly more licking/grooming and arched-back nursing than did the adult female (F2) offspring of low LG-ABN mothers. Also the level of fearfulness in response to a novel situation demonstrated by the adult (male and female) F3 offspring of these F2 mothers differed; the level of fearfulness was higher in the F3 offspring of low LG-ABN F2 mothers compared to the F3 offspring of high LG-ABN F2 mothers.

The epigenetic mechanisms underlying these maternal and offspring behaviors were investigated by Weaver et al., (2004). The increased hippocampal GR gene expression observed in the offspring of high LG-ABN mothers (compared to the offspring of low LG-ABN mothers) is regulated by a serotonin /serotonin receptor interaction with subsequent activation of cAMP dependent protein kinase activity. There is also an accompanying increase in the hippocampal expression of the gene for the transcription factor, nerve growth factor-inducible protein A (NGFI-A). Hippocampal GR has a promoter region (exon 1/7) which contains a binding sequence for NGFI-A. The expression of GR mRNAs containing this promoter region (exon 1/7) is increased in the offspring of high LG-ABN mothers. Maternal care alters cytosine methylation at specific sites in the hippocampal GR promoter region in offspring. The exon 1/7 promoter region includes 17 CpG dinucleotides and sites 16 and 17 lie within the NGFI-A binding sequence. The CpG dinucleotide at site 17 is always methylated regardless of the nature of maternal care whereas the CpG dinucleotide at site 16 is fully methylated in offspring of low LG-ABN mothers but rarely methylated in offspring of high LG-ABN mothers. Hence the type of maternal care has a pronounced effect on the methylation status of the CpG nucleotide at site 16 within the NGFI-A binding region. This effect of maternal care on differential methylation of CpG dinucleotides in the hippocampal GR gene promoter region is established in the offspring within the first six days of postnatal life and the effect on methylation persists for the life of the animal. Site specific changes in methylation of CpG dinucleotides within the promoter region of the GR gene result in the recruitment of proteins which modify histone acetylation. Chromatin structure is altered thereby modifying gene transcription activity. In summary, the maternal care provided by the high LG-ABN mother (compared to the low LG-ABN mother) results in demethylation of site specific CpG dinucleotides (site 16) within the NGFI-A binding sequence of the offspring hippocampal GR gene. Chromatin structure is changed, binding of the transcription factor NGFI-A to the GR promoter region is enhanced and transcriptional activity of the GR gene is increased. The increased transcriptional activity of the GR gene results in glucocorticoid negative feedback which inhibits CRF synthesis and release, thus dampening of the hypothalamic-pituitary-adrenal response to stress (Weaver et al., 2004).

In a more recent report, Weaver et al., (2007) further characterized the epigenetic mechanism linked to maternal care. These investigators proposed the following sequence of events. The maternal handling of offspring by high LG-ABN mothers (compared to low LG-ABN mothers) is associated with increased expression of hippocampal NGFI-A and increased expression of GR mRNA containing the exon 1/7 promoter region. This promoter region contains the binding site for NGFI-A. Increased serotonin and cAMP dependent protein kinase activity mediate the increased expression of hippocampal GR transcripts and the expression of NGFI-A transcription factor. On the day of birth, in the pups of both high and low LG-ABN mothers, the CpG nucleotides in the GR exon 1/7 promoter region are hypermethylated. Over the first week of postnatal life, the site 16 CpG nucleotide in the promoter region of offspring of high LG-ABN mothers, becomes progressively demethylated. This demethylation is mediated by binding of NGFI-A to the GR promoter binding sequence. The progressive demethylation of the site 16 CpG nucleotide enhances NGFI-A protein binding to the GR promoter region. Furthermore, NGFI-A binding, recruits histone acetyltransferases which alter chromatin activity. The sum total is that maternal care provided by high LG-ABN mothers (in the first week of postnatal life) sets in place a cascade of intracellular events; an increase in hippocampal GR and NGFI-A expression, site specific demethylation of the promoter sequence of GR, an increase in NGFI-A binding with an alteration in chromatin activity and an increase in transcriptional activity of GR. This increase in transcriptional activity results in an enhanced glucococorticoid negative feedback with reduced CRF secretion and a reduction in the magnitude of the stress response.

The experimental observations of Liu et al., (1997), Francis et al., (1999) and Weaver et al., (2004; 2007) demonstrate that maternal nursing behavior can epigenetically modify specific gene expression patterns in her offspring resulting in a change in the stress response phenotype of the offspring. The epigenetic mechanism underlying these observations represents a specific example of a more general model as to how the nature of an animal's social environment can modify the expression of specific genes in that animal and hence alter that animal's phenotype. In fact, some investigators argue that epigenetic mechanisms are the core processes underlying phenotypic plasticity.

The plasticity of the stress response in offspring as a function of variations in maternal-infant interactions has also been documented in primates. Bardi et al., (2005) studied 73 mother-infant baboon pairs all born in captivity. The offspring remained with their mothers until they were weaned at the age of 12- 15 months at which time they were placed in social groups with other juveniles and several unrelated adult female "nannies". At 18 months of age the offspring were subjected to a "stress" test which consisted of separating the juvenile from its social group and placing it in a small cage. The juvenile was kept isolated for 15 minutes after which the juvenile was sedated and a blood sample was obtained for a cortisol level determination. Maternal- infant interactions as well as the responses of the juvenile to the isolation stress test were classified using a series of standardized behaviors as references. The juvenile stress responses fell into four reasonably distinct patterns; vigilant/vocalizing (alert), passive/nervous (anxious), attempt to find a way out of cage (fight) and running away response (flight). The first two responses were associated with low blood cortisol levels while the latter two responses (fight/flight) were associated with high blood cortisol levels. An even more interesting finding was that the four behavioral responses of the juvenile baboons were tied to their interactions with their mothers and to maternal rank. Juveniles whose mothers displayed high levels of maintaining contact with their infants and directed grooming, watching and lip-smacking behaviors towards their offspring, responded to the isolation stress with higher levels of vigilance and resting type of behaviors. These juveniles had the lower blood levels of cortisol. Juveniles whose mothers expressed more stress related behaviors toward their offspring and were of lower rank, showed a flight type of response to the isolation stress and also displayed higher levels of blood cortisol. The investigators concluded that when juvenile baboons are confronted with a source of psychological stress, they display a multidimensional behavioral response and that different components of this behavioral response are determined by the natural variations in quality and quantity of interactions they experienced with their mothers during early life. Infants that received higher levels of watching, grooming, lip-smacking behaviors and contact from their mothers are better able to cope with stress in a more measured manner than infants whose mothers are of low dominance rank and showed higher levels of stress related behaviors towards their offspring. These results are quite similar to the observations made in rats. The genetic mechanisms underlying the plasticity of the stress response in primates has not been clarified but it is reasonable to assume that an epigenetic mechanism similar to that described in the rat is probably operative.

Tobacco Smoke Exposure

Chronic exposure to tobacco smoke has been described as a risk factor for the development of atherosclerosis on the basis of a number of clinical studies. The mechanistic link between tobacco smoke and vascular disease has not been defined, but one possibility is that tobacco use alters the methylation status of DNA i.e. changes an individual's epigenome. Although this mechanism has not been examined with respect to smoking exposure and vascular remodeling, it has been examined in other contexts. Suter et al., (2011) looked at the methylation pattern of placental DNA and the correlation of this pattern with maternal smoking history (smokers versus nonsmokers). They found a significant correlation between placental transcription regulation and differential CpG methylation in the promoter regions of 25 genes among nonsmokers but in 438 genes among smokers. The 438 differentially methylated genes in smokers were associated with disruption of metabolic pathways resulting in alterations in cell development, cell morphology, cell survival and cell to cell signaling. The investigators concluded that maternal smoking exposure deregulated placental DNA methylation in a CpG site specific manner, thus modifying placental gene expression, and that this change in methylation pattern resulted in meaningful alterations in gene expression along important pathways involved in cell signaling and function. In addition, as the investigators noted, there are data going back many years linking maternal tobacco use and delivery of small for gestational age infants. Similarly, in this study, gestational age at birth was comparable for mothers who were smokers or nonsmokers, but the average infant birth weight was significantly lower in the smoking group. The effect of tobacco exposure on the fetus is consistent with the construct of developmental plasticity; a developmental phenotype (birth weight) has been changed in response to an environmental cue (intrauterine tobacco smoke exposure).

These observations suggest at least two pathways by which tobacco smoke exposure could adversely affect biological processes. First, maternal smoke exposure by changing (epigenetically) the expression pattern of placental genes would modify the fetal intrauterine environment, most likely in a deleterious way. This mechanism would account for the low birth weight of infants born to mothers who smoke and in addition, a "sub optimal" intrauterine environment has been considered a significant risk factor for future health issues across the life span of the offspring. Secondly, tobacco smoke exposure could epigenetically modify the expression of genes directly involved in arterial remodeling.

Summary and Perspectives

When we weave all these informational threads together, what does the composite tell us about whether atherosclerosis is a "disease" or a component of the ageing process? In this summary atherosclerosis will be considered to be a morphological variant of arterial vessel wall remodeling within the context that the specific injury inducing the remodeling is a focal change in shear stress. The terms remodeling and atherosclerosis will be used interchangeably.

Observations made in natural animal models and zoo populations indicate that focal arterial intimal thickenings are present in most if not all vertebrates and that these thickenings occur at arterial sites where there is an alteration in laminar blood flow. The coronary arterial bed is particularly prone to the development of these thickenings since these arteries are subject to unusual biomechanical forces due to their intramyocardial location. Similar focal arterial thickenings have also been found in the coronary arteries of human fetuses. These observations are consistent with the proposal that these thickenings represent a repair process initiated by the vascular mechanosensor-transduction mechanism in response to a reduction in mean positive shear stress. In essence, the underlying basis of the "injury" rests with the actual anatomy of the arterial tree. Sites where bifurcations occur, branch points intersecting at rather acute angles and regions of high curvature create non laminar blood flow and a reduction in mean positive shear stress. One would expect these thickenings to change with age. In fish the incidence and severity of coronary artery intimal thickenings increase with age. In wild elephants, the severity of arteriosclerotic thickenings and plaques in the aorta increases with chronological age. In addition, observations in mammals such as the giraffe and naked mole-rat illustrate that a "hypertensive" state (giraffe) or extreme old age (naked mole- rat) do not in themselves lead to occlusive lesions in large and medium sized arteries.

A second observation arising from the study of zoo populations, wild elephants residing in a "contracted" habitat and domesticated animals, is that the complexity of an animal's social environment is a key determinant of progression of arterial focal thickenings to atherosclerotic type lesions. In addition, studies in chickens and fish strongly suggest that stress hormones (glucocorticoids and mineralocorticoids) are the link between social environment and the extent of vascular remodeling.

Glucocorticoids and mineralocorticoids play a central role in vascular remodeling. First, the complexes formed by binding of these hormones to specific nuclear receptors, function to regulate the transcriptional activity of "vascular" genes directly involved in arterial remodeling. Secondly, these hormones indirectly modulate vascular remodeling through their interactions with other nuclear receptor-ligand complexes and with clock genes. Finally, the social environment of the animal can influence vascular remodeling through an epigenetic mechanism which directly modifies the magnitude of the stress response. In rats, the nature of maternal care given to offspring at a critical time window can modify the magnitude of the stress response in those offspring for the duration of their life.

The epigenetic effects of social environment could also modify vascular remodeling through pathways not necessarily directly involving the stress response. As noted in the section; Influence of social environment, Borghol et al., (2012) observed a correlation between early childhood socioeconomic position and the differential methylation pattern for 1252 gene promoter regions measured in those individuals as adults. A low socioeconomic position in childhood is associated with more extensive physiological dysfunction (earlier ageing) in those individuals as adults. Maternal smoking during pregnancy alters the methylation status of the promoter regions of a number of placental genes. Such an epigenetic change in gene expression probably explains the low birth weight (for gestational age) of such fetuses and as well the "sub optimal" intra uterine environment of these fetuses would increase the occurrence of greater physiological dysfunction in adult life. The poorer "health status" of adults who had a low early childhood socioeconomic position or whose mothers smoked during pregnancy, often includes significant vascular atherosclerosis. The pathways that might link the epigenetic effects of maternal smoking or one's early childhood socioeconomic position to vascular remodeling are presently unknown.

From this discussion, it is clear that numerous genes underlie the process of vascular remodeling. There will be the genes associated with the mechanosensor-transduction mechanism, the nuclear receptor family, and molecular clocks. Since nuclear receptors are also transcription factors, there will also be a number of downstream target genes involved in the process of vascular remodeling. In addition, the social environment through epigenetic mechanisms will change the expression pattern of suites of other genes. Given this complex polygenic basis, why do we call vascular remodeling/atherosclerosis a disease? Vascular remodeling starts as a focal repair process, which in the human is overlaid by the epigenetic effects of the social environment. These environmental cues modify the repair process such as to make the structural changes more extensive over the life time of the individual. In essence, vascular remodeling rests upon the cumulative results of numerous gene- environment interactions although for the modern human the environment has become dominated by the complexities of social interactions among large numbers of individuals living within a relatively small space.

Finally, no two individuals have the same genome and epigenome. Individuals differ in terms of structural variations in DNA sequences (SNPs, copy number variants) and in terms of DNA methylation patterns and histone epigenetic marks. These genomic and epigenomic differences account for phenotypic variation among individuals and also variation among individuals in the extent of vascular remodeling despite exposure to the same social environmental cues.

Chapter III

Hypertension

In humans, a chronic elevation in arterial blood pressure in the absence of obvious kidney or endocrine dysfunction has been defined as primary or essential hypertension. There are several problems with this definition. First, what is the reference arterial blood pressure value that is considered normal? Secondly, how does arterial blood pressure vary with age in humans? These questions are not that easy to answer although clearly without defining a "normal" arterial blood pressure range one cannot diagnose a state of hypertension. A few examples will illustrate the difficulty in obtaining answers to these questions.

Kean and Hammill (1949) summarized blood pressure data from a number of sources available at that time. In the United States on the basis of over 150,000 measurements by Insurance companies, systolic pressure increased from a mean of 123 mmHg in the young (15-20 years of age) to a mean value of 135 mmHg in those between 60-65 years of age. Over the same age range, mean diastolic pressure increased from 79 mmHg to 86 mmHg. Blood pressure measurements taken in native Kenyans showed no increase with age. Chinese in rural areas had low arterial pressures with no increase with age while Chinese from wealthier areas showed a moderate increase with age. Poulter et al., (1984) measured blood pressure in members of the Luo tribe in Kenya. They compared a sample living in their traditional rural environment with a sample that had migrated from that rural area to Nairobi. The urban sample demonstrated a higher mean systolic and diastolic blood pressure at all ages than the rural sample and the increase in systolic and diastolic blood pressures with age was greater in the urban group compared to the rural group. Page et al., (1974) examined cardiovascular parameters in six Solomon Islands societies which differed in their degree of acculturation. Acculturation status of these societies was based upon cultural, demographic and population physical data. The investigators noted that an increase in acculturation was associated with an increase in total serum cholesterol, a reduction in serum uric acid and an age related rise in blood pressure which expressed itself earliest and most noticeably in the females. The investigators also pointed out that the society with the highest systolic and diastolic pressures (in both sexes) had the highest salt intake. The importance of salt intake is exemplified by the Yanomamo Indians of South America (Oliver et al., 1975). This population subsisted on a sodium intake of approximately 2 mmoles per day. Mean arterial pressure (systolic mmHg/diastolic mmHg) was about 100/65 for both males and females and actually appeared to decrease with age. In addition, urinary aldosterone excretion rates and plasma renin activity measured in a sample of the Yanomamo population were exceedingly high compared to a control sample of Caucasians on a general "North American" diet. Finally, the INTERSALT STUDY (Stamler, 1997), examined the relationship between salt intake and blood pressure in more than 10,000 males and females aged 20-59 years from 52 diverse sites in 32 countries worldwide. In brief the study findings indicated that much of the total overall increase of systolic and diastolic pressure with age (20-59 years) could be attributed to a high salt intake.

This brief survey points out the difficulty in defining an upper limit for "normal" arterial pressure in humans since mean values in a given population will be affected by; diet (particularly salt intake), age/sex of the group and social environment. However, since the current construct is that a causal relationship exists between the magnitude by which blood pressure is increased above normal and the extent of tissue and organ damage, it becomes necessary to set an upper limit for "normal" arterial pressure. This construct forms the justification for the use of antihypertensive medications (Alderman, 2004).

Another approach to establishing "normal" blood pressure values in the human is to define physiological blood pressure ranges using comparative biology since the physiology of the human cardiovascular system is an adaptive modification of the basic vertebrate cardiovascular system.

Comparative Biology of the Cardiovascular System

Complex multicellular organisms require a highly integrated cardiovascular system to deliver nutrients to all the cells in the body. Pressure is one attribute of this system and its value is shaped by a number of determinants. In this discussion, steady state resting arterial pressure is the parameter being considered. Obviously in a given animal, arterial pressure can vary considerably if that animal is in a very stressful situation such as under attack by a predator. This type of variation under states of "emergency" is controlled by short term regulatory mechanisms. Acute fluctuations in arterial pressure are not the consideration in this review. The focus in this discussion is defining the factors that determine steady state blood pressure values in various animals but in particular mammals.

During the course of evolution, the transitions from an aquatic to a terrestrial mode of life and from a land (walking) to an air (flying) habitat were associated with significant changes in the impact of gravity. These transitions required adaptations in both structure and function and one of these adaptations was a change in mean arterial pressure. Land animals must do more antigravity muscular work than aquatic animals and flying animals must do more antigravity muscular work than land animals (Poupa and Lindstrom, 1983). These habitat transitions from water to land and land to air resulted in increases in mean arterial pressure and the relative size of the heart. The link between these two parameters is cardiac output (Harris, 1983). The greater antigravity muscular work associated with these habitat transitions necessitated greater blood flows, larger cardiac outputs and hence higher mean arterial pressures. Analogous physiological circumstances occur in the trained athlete and in "athletic" animals e.g. hare versus tame rabbit, falcon versus hen (Ford, 1976; Poupa and Ostadal, 1969). Birds compared to mammals of similar size, have a higher mean arterial pressure and a greater heart mass (Grubb, 1983; Seymour and Blaylock, 2000). Mean arterial pressures in snakes also illustrate the important influence of gravity. Mean arterial pressure is significantly lower (22-38 mmHg) in aquatic snakes than in terrestrial snakes (49-74 mmHg) (Seymour and Lillywhite, 1976; Lillywhite, 1996). Arboreal snakes by virtue of their tree climbing activities, have the highest mean arterial pressure (80-95 mmHg) as a consequence of the additional hydrostatic pressure generated by the vertical column of blood between head and heart (Lillywhite, 1996). This effect of gravity due to an extended vertical distance between head and heart is most pronounced in the giraffe whose cardiovascular physiology is reviewed in a subsequent section.

The evolution of thermoregulation in animals and thus the ability to maintain a "constant" core body temperature also required increased blood flows and hence a higher cardiac output. As in the transitions between water and land and air habitats, a larger cardiac output necessitated an increase in relative cardiac size and resulted in an increase in mean arterial pressure. Mean arterial pressure is higher in homoiotherms than in poikilotherms (Poupa and Lindstrom, 1983) and relative heart weight is significantly greater in birds and mammals than in fish, amphibians and reptiles (Poupa and Lindstrom, 1983).

Another broad determinant of mean arterial pressure is animal mass. Seymour and Blaylock (2000) examined the allometric scaling of cardiovascular variables in mammals and birds based on a data set of 24 mammalian species and 12 species of birds. For example, systolic blood pressure has a scaling coefficient of 0.05 for mammals and 0.02 for birds against body mass. Using the allometric equation calculated by Seymour and Blaylock (2000) for systolic blood pressure, an elephant weighing 4000kg will have a predicted systolic blood pressure of 174 mmHg whereas a 30 gram mouse will have a predicted systolic blood pressure of 97 mmHg. For comparison, this allometric equation predicts a systolic blood pressure of 142 mmHg for a 70 kg human.

Hence, from an evolutionary perspective, determinants such as animal habitat (water/land/air), metabolic rate (or more specifically the presence or absence of the capacity to thermoregulate) and animal mass set broad boundaries as to permissible ranges of physiological arterial pressure. Thus in general, a relative large bird capable of flying would require a higher mean arterial pressure than a similar sized land mammal and would require a much higher mean arterial pressure than a similar sized aquatic reptile. The bird would be expected to have the largest relative heart weight and also the highest cardiac output on a unit weight basis compared to the similar sized land mammal and aquatic reptile. However, this generalization has many exceptions and one particular outlier that is discussed in a subsequent section is the giraffe. This mammal by virtue of the post natal growth of its neck requires as an adult, a mean arterial pressure much higher than other land mammals of equal or greater mass.

Another consideration is whether the mechanical and structural properties of the conduits in the vascular system, the elastic arteries, give information about permissible physiological pressure ranges? Are the structural and mechanical properties of the proximal elastic arteries "programmed" for specific arterial pressures across different species?

The closed circulatory system of vertebrates can be regarded as a pump and a set of conduits to circulate the blood. Since the pump contracts cyclically, the flow of blood will be pulsatile. In order to ensure a reasonably steady flow of blood through the peripheral capillary beds, the larger proximal arteries have elastic properties which allow them to store a portion of the stroke volume with each systole and discharge that volume with diastole (windkessel effect) (Wagenseil and Mecham, 2009). The mechanical properties of the proximal arteries are determined by a composite of elastin and collagen deposited by smooth muscle cells in the medial layer. Stress is the force applied to an object divided by the surface area over which that force is applied while strain relates the deformed dimensions of an object to the undeformed dimensions. For materials like the arterial wall, the relationship between stress and strain is nonlinear. When volume change in an isolated artery like the carotid is plotted against inflation pressure, the greatest change in compliance occurs at an inflation pressure coinciding with the normal physiological range of arterial pressure (Shadwick, 1999). Isolated aortas show an approximately linear increase in incremental elastic modulus with an increase in inflation pressure, although the characteristics of the relationship vary considerably across different vertebrates (Shadwick, 1999; Wagenseil and Mecham, 2009). However, the differences essentially disappear if the inflation pressures are normalized to the mean arterial pressures characteristic of the different species (Shadwick, 1999; Wagenseil and Mecham, 2009). In a plot of normalized pressure versus incremental elastic modulus, the value of the incremental elastic modulus at a normalized pressure of "one" converges towards a common value. To achieve this result each organism must adjust its mix of extracellular components to achieve the appropriate mechanical properties. The data indicate that elastic arteries from a variety of animal groups have similar mechanical properties at their mean physiological arterial blood pressures. This comparative biological data confirm that different ranges of mean arterial pressure are developmentally set in different species and that the structure and composition of the elastic arteries have evolved to provide similar mechanical properties across these different ranges of mean arterial pressure.

A similar conclusion is supported by the observations of Wolinsky and Glagov (1969) with respect to the structure of the aorta in different mammals (mouse to horse series). These investigators considered the media of the aorta to be comprised of lamellar units consisting of muscle, collagen and elastin. Using isolated aortas (thoracic and abdominal); they calculated total medial tension as well as the number of lamellar units. Estimated mean medial tension per lamellar unit varied by less than a factor of two across these different mammals despite a weight spread of approximately 15,000 fold (30 gram mouse to 450 kilogram horse).

An interesting experiment described by Wagenseil and Mecham (2009), underscores the significant consequences between setting arterial pressure during development as opposed to during adult life. Mice with one functional elastin allele (Eln+/-) have half as much elastin in their vessels but live a normal life span. Eln+/- mice have a mean arterial pressure about 30-40 mmHg higher than wild type (WT) mice, but despite the elevated arterial pressure they show minimal cardiac hypertrophy. Arterial walls are thinner and circumferential wall stress is higher in Eln+/- mice compared to WT mice. Yet the Eln+/- mice do not show vascular remodeling in response to this elevated arterial pressure. However, if the arterial pressure in an adult Eln+/- mouse is further increased (by clipping a renal artery), the expected cardiac hypertrophy and vascular remodeling do occur. The Eln+/- mouse is born with an increased number of arterial lamellar units so even though circumferential stress is higher than in WT mice the tension per lamellar unit is the same in Eln+/- and WT mice and in fact similar to the tension to lamellar unit ratio in other mammalian species (Wolinsky and Glagov, 1969). Despite the high mean arterial pressure of the Eln+/- mice, there is no significant increase in collagen or elastin concentration in the arterial wall. Vessel walls are thinner not thicker and the vessel thickness –to- lumen ratio is about the same as in WT mice; cardiac hypertrophy is minimal. The authors point out that the structural and compositional characteristics of the cardiovascular system in the Eln+/- mouse are established during the fetal (developmental) stage and these characteristics are programmed to accommodate the increased arterial pressure in the Eln+/- (compared to WT) mouse. If the incremental elastic modulus of the isolated Eln+/- mouse aorta is plotted against inflation pressure normalized to the mean arterial pressure of the Eln+/- mouse, the incremental elastic modulus converges towards the same common value as observed across the other vertebrate species at their respective mean arterial pressures (i.e. at a normalized pressure of "one"). Hence, the mechanical properties of elastic arteries in the Eln+/- mouse are similar to those of other vertebrates although the structural and compositional features of its elastic arteries differ. The differential consequences of setting arterial pressure during fetal as opposed to adult life are dramatically illustrated in the Eln+/- mouse strain. When exposed to high arterial pressure during embryonic development, the cardiovascular system of the Eln+/- mouse undergoes a physiological adaptation to function at a higher pressure. When the arterial pressure is raised even higher during adult life (through renal artery clipping), the cardiovascular system shows a different type of adaptation characterized by thicker, stiffer, collagen-rich vessels and significant cardiac hypertrophy. This different type of adaptation can be considered as an injury/ repair response.

Changes in the mechanical properties of elastic arteries also occur with age as documented by Learoyd and Taylor (1966). These investigators examined postmortem arteries (aorta, iliac, femoral, carotid) in two groups of males and females; a "young" group ages 11-20 years and an "old" group ages 36-52 years. Grossly atheromatous vessels were discarded. The differences between old and young arteries can be summarized as follows. The ratio of wall thickness to mean diameter was greater in the "old" vessels. The "young" group showed an increasing wall stiffness (based upon measurements of circumferential incremental elastic modulus) as one proceeded from aorta towards peripherally situated arteries whereas in" old" arteries the opposite trend was found. These results indicate that changes in arterial viscoelastic properties occur with age, at least in humans. However, as calculated by Wagenseil and Mecham (2009) using the data of Learoyd and Taylor (1966), the incremental elastic modulus of the aortas of young and old humans plotted against normalized inflation pressure converges towards the same common value as calculated for the aortas of other vertebrates at a normalized pressure of "one". (I should add that Wagenseil and Mecham do not detail as to whether they used different mean physiological pressures for the young and old subjects). Hence, the differences noted by Learoyd and Taylor (1966) in the viscoelastic properties between young and old human aortas may not have a significant physiological effect on the overall mechanical properties of aged human elastic arteries.

The structural and functional changes in the cardiovascular system observed with ageing have been reviewed by Wilson et al., (2010). Maximal heart rate, peak exercise stroke volume and maximal aerobic capacity (VO2 max) all decline with age. Although resting left ventricular systolic function does not change with age there is a reduction in left ventricular diastolic function in normal ageing. This change in left ventricular diastolic function is thought to be due to a general increase in ventricular stiffness with age. Structural changes have also been noted in the myocardium with ageing. These changes include fibrosis and fat within the conduction system and an age-related increase in right atrial fibrosis. With respect to the observed myocardial fibrosis noted in "older" hearts, one possible mechanistic link is the effects of cortisol since as discussed in the section; Atherosclerotic Vascular Disease: Stress hormones; fish that respond to stress with large surges in cortisol develop cardiac fibrosis. As noted in the preceding paragraph, the compliance of large elastic arteries decreases with age and the peripheral arteries show an age dependent increase in wall thickness and a wall thickness to lumen ratio that increases with ageing. Finally global cerebral blood flow declines with age. As reviewed by Wilson et al.,(2010), cerebral blood flow velocity falls by almost 50% over the ages 20 to 80 years.

The transition of animals from water to land to air habitats, the increase in size of animals and the capacity of animals to maintain a near constant body temperature were all evolutionary milestones that required adaptations in the evolving cardiovascular system. These directional changes in animal habitat and animal size as well as the capacity of animals to thermoregulate mandated increases in blood flow to tissues and this increased blood flow required correspondingly greater cardiac outputs and relative heart weights. Increases in cardiac output resulted in increases in mean arterial pressure. Since the vertebrate cardiovascular system is closed and characterized by pulsatile blood flow, as part of the adaptation of this system the elastic arteries evolved similar mechanical properties when referenced to each species mean appropriate physiological arterial pressure. Across species, mean physiological arterial pressure is "set" developmentally. For example, fish because of their habitat, size and biological characteristics have a mean arterial pressure range physiologically appropriate for this vertebrate. Mammals because of their specific habitat, size, and biological features require a much higher arterial pressure range than fish. These phylogenetic differences in mean arterial pressure ranges are developmentally programmed and "set" by the mix of cardiac output, relative heart size and peripheral resistance to flow necessary in each species to supply nutrients to tissues and organs. Arterial pressure ranges can therefore be defined across species based upon evolutionary principles. However, these species- specific arterial pressure ranges can be considered as "background" reference ranges since they do not take into account the effects of specific environmental influences on mean arterial pressure in animals. Integrating environmental cues into the regulation of arterial pressure requires both sensing and regulating mechanisms. What is known about such mechanisms?

Pressure Mechanosensors

Intraluminal pressure causes circumferential vessel wall stretching. According to the principle of Laplace, circumferential tension on the walls of blood vessels is proportional to the product of intraluminal blood pressure and vessel radius. In more exact equations, tension is replaced by stress which is defined as the force per unit cross-sectional area (distance between inner and outer vessel radius) (Seymour and Blaylock, 2000). If pressure rises, circumferential stress can be normalized by decreasing vessel inner radius and/or increasing vessel wall thickness.

There are probably a variety of molecular complexes that react to intraluminal pressure and these molecular complexes would be located in smooth muscle cells. However, several specific complexes have garnered attention as likely pressure mechanosensors; TRP channels and the angiotensin II receptor, AT1 (Sharif-Naeini et al., 2010).

TRP (transient receptor potential) channels constitute a family of channels composed of six trans membrane segments and a single pore. There are 33 TRP channel genes in mammals. Studies by Welsh et al., (2002) and Spassova et al., (2006) support the hypothesis that the TRPC6 channel, a nonselective cation channel which is highly expressed in the arterial vascular smooth muscle cell membrane responds directly to pressure induced stretch. Spassova et al., (2006) proposed that pressure induced stretching thins the membrane lipid bilayer. This effect directly opens the TRPC6 channel leading to membrane depolarization, the opening of voltage gated calcium channels and an increased vascular smooth muscle contraction. This sequence underlies the well described vascular myogenic response (Davis and Hill, 1999).The data of Spassova et al., (2006) indicate that the TRPC6 channel is opened at a threshold pressure of about 85 mmHg. As further suggested by Spassova et al., (2006), this same mechanism is also involved in the vascular remodeling that occurs with chronic elevations of intraluminal pressure. However, as reviewed by Sharif-Naeini et al., (2010), recent experiments in a variety of mammalian cells transfected with the TRPC6 channel have not supported a direct mechanosensor action by this channel.

Another potential pressure mechanosensor is the angiotensin II type 1 (AT1) receptor. Cell stretch, as would occur with pressure, induces a conformational change in this trans membrane receptor in the absence of ligand (angiotensin II) binding (Sharif-Naeini et al., 2010). This conformational change activates the receptor and leads to activation of downstream signaling cascades that result in cardiovascular remodeling.

Ozaki et al., (1999) measured the effect of pressure on DNA synthesis by human aortic smooth muscle cells (HASMC). DNA synthesis was measured over a three hour period. Cells exposed to a pressure of up to 120 mmHg showed no increase in DNA synthesis compared to control cells subjected to a pressure of zero mmHg. Between pressures of 140-180 mmHg, there was a roughly linear increase in DNA synthesis by HASMC. Higher pressures actually caused a falloff in the synthesis of DNA.

Lehoux et al., (2005) have presented evidence using rabbit aorta that the mechano-transduction mechanism for steady versus pulsatile pressure changes are probably different. Although these investigators did not address the question whether different mechanosensors were involved in detecting changes in steady or cyclic stretch, they did demonstrate that the resulting downstream events were different between steady and pulsatile pressure.

Finally, Ingber (2006) has discussed the role of mechanical forces as developmental regulators. On the basis of his discussion, one could postulate that in the developing animal, mechanosensors in arterial smooth muscle cells regulate the mix of elastin and collagen in the matrix of elastic arteries such as to achieve the appropriate mechanical properties of these arteries at the developmentally “set’ physiological mean pressure for that animal species.

Hence, (vascular) smooth muscle cell pressure sensitive- mechanosensors appear to have a number of biological functions. These sensors initiate the myogenic response (pressure dependent contraction) which is important in regulating regional blood flows and overall peripheral resistance to flow. They are also involved in the structural remodeling of arteries in response to sustained changes in mean arterial pressure and they are probably instrumental in establishing the mechanical properties of the elastic arteries in the developing animal.

How is this complex cardiovascular system regulated in the whole animal? What mechanism(s) put all the pieces together?

Regulating Mechanisms

a) Kidney

The kidney has long been recognized as an important regulator of mean arterial pressure (Guyton, 1987). The kidney is characterized by a pressure-natriuresis mechanism such that a function curve can be described relating increases in mean arterial pressure with increases in urinary sodium output. At a fixed sodium intake, this curve will define a specific mean arterial pressure such that sodium intake and sodium output are in balance. If mean arterial pressure rises but sodium intake remains unchanged, sodium (and water) output will become greater than input. The negative balance of sodium and water will restore mean arterial pressure back to its previous level. Conversely, a fall in mean arterial pressure will lead to reduced urinary sodium excretion, sodium retention and volume expansion with an increase in cardiac output. This sequence of events will restore arterial pressure back to the previous set value. With time peripheral resistance to flow increases and cardiac output returns to its previous level. According to Guyton (1987), the pressure-natriuresis function of the kidney is a key factor in all types of long term arterial pressure regulation. On the basis of this mechanism, hypertension is then explained as a right resetting of the pressure-natriuresis curve. Such a resetting means that for a given sodium intake, a higher than "normal" mean arterial pressure is required to increase sodium excretion so that sodium balance is restored.

Coffman and Crowley (2008) have explored the roles of the AT1 receptor and the kidney in blood pressure regulation using genetically altered mice. AT1 receptors are widely distributed in many tissues; heart, kidney, blood vessels, adrenal glands, and central nervous system. Mice with a targeted disruption of the gene for the AT1 receptor (total KO)(Ito et al., 1995)were transplanted with a wild-type kidney to create a population of mice with kidney AT 1 receptors but no extra renal AT1 receptors (systemic KO). Wild-type mice were transplanted with an AT1 deficient kidney to create a population of mice lacking AT 1 receptors in the kidney only (kidney KO). Hence, there were four populations of mice; wild-type (WT), those completely lacking AT1 receptors (total KO), those lacking extra renal AT1 receptors (systemic KO), those lacking renal AT1 receptors only (kidney KO). Overall blood pressure regulation required both renal and extra renal AT1 receptors. Systemic and kidney KO mice had lower arterial pressures than WT mice, but total KO mice had even lower blood pressures. Infusion of angiotensin II into wild mice causes a chronic elevation of arterial pressure. No elevation in arterial pressure occurs with angiotensin II infusion in total KO mice and the extent of the blood pressure increase was much less in kidney KO mice. Only the group systemic KO had a blood pressure rise with angiotensin II infusion comparable to the wild-type. Hence, kidney AT 1 receptors must be present for an angiotensin II infusion to cause a significant elevation of mean arterial pressure. The infused angiotensin II binds to AT1 receptors in the kidney leading to reduced sodium and water excretion, weight gain and an elevated arterial pressure. This alteration in renal sodium handling is in the "direction" predicted by the hypothesis of Guyton but overall regulation of arterial pressure requires both renal and systemic AT1 receptors.

However, the results of this elegant experiment may not be transferrable to the human. AT1 receptor gene number and structure differ between rodents and humans. The rodent genome contains two distinct AT1 receptor genes; AT1aR and AT1bR whereas the human genome has only a single AT1R gene (Elton and Martin, 2007). The two rodent genes are composed of three exons while the human gene contains four exons and the human gene transcribes four alternatively spliced mRNAs whereas each of the rodent genes transcribes three alternatively spliced mRNAs (Elton and Martin, 2007). The functional implications of these differences between rodent and human AT1R genes are unclear. However, as noted by Elton and Martin (2007), the relative abundance of AT1R mRNA splice variants in humans appears to control AT1R protein levels and the strength of the angiotensin II response since the different splice variants have differing affinities for angiotensin II.

b) Brain

Are there sufficient data to suggest that the brain is the regulator of mean arterial pressure? One strong piece of evidence is based upon the sequence of events associated with the postnatal elongation of the giraffe neck (Paton et al., 2009). As the neck of the giraffe elongates, mean arterial pressure will have to rise in order to maintain cerebral blood flow. In order to maintain adequate cerebral blood flow as the neck lengthens, the giraffe's heart hypertrophies and peripheral resistance to flow increases. The most parsimonious hypothesis is that this sequence of events in the giraffe is orchestrated by the brain. Hence there would have to be a brain "sensor" to monitor cerebral blood flow and effector mechanisms to continuously reset cardiac output, peripheral resistance to flow and the renal pressure-natriuresis function curve to allow the giraffe's mean arterial pressure to increase during the time period that its neck is growing. The cardiovascular physiology of the giraffe will be reviewed in a subsequent section.

"Hypertensive" states in humans are usually accompanied by elevated sympathetic nerve activity (Guyenet, 2006) and the brain centers that regulate sympathetic nerve activity are located chiefly in the rostral ventrolateral medulla (RVLM), spinal cord, hypothalamus and the nucleus of the solitary tract (NTS) in the brain stem. This system is highly complex but some of the salient features are as follows (Guyenet, 2006). The NTS receives sensory inputs from pressure receptors and other mechanoreceptors (e.g. volume receptors) in the cardiopulmonary region. Multiple regions of the brain including the NTS and hypothalamus are also "influenced" by the effects of circulating factors such as angiotensin II, interleukin- 1 and aldosterone. The RVLM pressure sensitive neurons receive inputs from the NTS and other brain areas (e.g. hypothalamus) and a large subset of the neurons feeding into the RVLM can also synthesize epinephrine. The RVLM pressure sensitive neurons are the chief source of sympathetic efferents which innervate numerous Ponto medullary regions as well as sympathetic preganglionic neurons. Parasympathetic neurons that control the heart are located in the same brain region. Postganglionic sympathetic neurons innervate the heart, kidney, adrenal gland and blood vessels. Although the RVLM is probably the most important nodal point in this network, the NTS is also a very important integrative center. An important component of this complex network is the regulation of sodium reabsorption by the kidney (Guyenet, 2006). A feedback loop involving atrial volume receptors, the NTS, the paraventricular nucleus of the hypothalamus and the renal sympathetic nerves is an important regulator of sodium handling by the kidney. Through such a feedback loop, brain and kidney regulation of blood pressure can be integrated.

Additional experimental data supporting the hypothesis that the central nervous system regulates mean arterial pressure and that there is a neural set point for arterial pressure have been reviewed by Schreihofer et al., (2005) and Osborn et al., (2005).

Another possible mechanism, although speculative, is involvement of glucose sensing neurons in the regulation of arterial pressure. (The topic of glucose sensing neurons is discussed in the section; Diabetes Mellitus; Biology of glucose regulating mechanisms.) The circulatory system evolved to distribute nutrients to the various tissues and organs in multicellular organisms and therefore changes in the nutrient "status" within an animal could require an adjustment in cardiovascular function. The glucose sensing or perhaps more accurately, the nutrient sensing neurons in the hypothalamus could play a key role in this regulatory function. These neurons are spatially and functionally organized to integrate various signals reflecting nutrient state and their connections to the autonomic nervous system would give these neurons a mechanism by which to co-ordinate a physiological response (e.g. a change in cardiac function or peripheral resistance to flow) to a change in the animal's nutrient state. Experimental observations reported by Levin and Sullivan (1987) support this possibility. These investigators infused glucose into rats and noted an increase in plasma levels of norepinephrine associated with the glucose infusion. As a control, an iso-osmolar infusion of mannitol did not cause any change in plasma norepinephrine levels.

Another system involved in arterial pressure regulation is that of molecular clocks; this system consists of a master clock in the suprachiasmatic nucleus of the brain plus molecular clocks in most peripheral tissues. (This topic of molecular clocks was discussed in a previous part of the section on Atherosclerotic Vascular Disease.) Curtis et al., (2007) observed that deletion of both copies of the clock gene Bmal 1 in mice (Bmal 1 -/-) completely abolished the circadian rhythm for arterial pressure and heart rate, but in addition Bmal 1 -/- mice also had a lower mean arterial pressure than wild-type mice. Hence this gene, at least in mice, appears to be involved not only in establishing the circadian rhythm for arterial pressure but also in maintaining a normal level of mean arterial pressure. Bmal 1 -/- mice also displayed reduced expression of catecholamine biosynthetic enzymes in the heart and adrenal gland. Hence, the molecular clock exerts its effects on the vasculature and arterial pressure by modulating the synthesis and disposition of catecholamines. There is also evidence of an anatomical connection between the suprachiasmatic nucleus (site of the master clock) and the adrenal gland via sympathetic nerves (Curtis et al., 2007).

Hence, molecular clocks and the brain centers controlling the sympathetic nervous system comprise an interconnected system that is probably the dominant regulator of mean arterial pressure.

c) Renin Angiotensin System (RAS)

The RAS does not comprise an actual anatomical system for arterial pressure regulation such as the brain, but rather this system functions as a messenger "service" to coordinate the cardiovascular and renal determinants of mean arterial pressure. The RAS is a very old system from an evolutionary perspective and elements are found in vertebrates and invertebrates (Breno et al., 2007). This system has been best characterized in mammals, particularly the angiotensin receptors (ATR). In non-mammalian vertebrates distinct ATR have been identified and the consensus is that a prototype ATR evolved in early vertebrates which then diverged into more than one type of ATR during speciation (Breno et al., 2007). However, there are limited data concerning the structure of ATR in non-mammals and for example, the ATR has not been cloned in reptiles. Much more is known about the comparative structure of angiotensin across different species. Angiotensins I and II are well conserved throughout the phylogenetic tree. In the mammal, angiotensin II not only has vasopressor effects but can modulate other cellular processes such as cell growth, apoptosis, cell migration and matrix deposition (vascular remodeling) (Elton and Martin, 2007). In the snake, angiotensin II has a vasopressor action which is due to a combination of direct effects of angiotensin II on the vasculature plus the effects of angiotensin II- induced release of catecholamines (epinephrine and norepinephrine) (Breno et al., 2007).

Carroll and Opdyke (1982) examined the pressor response and catecholamine releasing activity of angiotensin II in a variety of non-mammalian vertebrates. Plasma catecholamine levels significantly increased following administration of angiotensin II in the lumpfish, bullfrog, turtle and chicken. In all animals tested (hagfish, dogfish, lumpfish, bullfrog, turtle, chicken and rat) angiotensin II elicited a significant rise in arterial pressure. By using an alpha adrenergic blocking agent, phentolamine, the investigators were able to partition the pressor response into how much was due to a direct action of angiotensin II and how much was due to the action of released catecholamines. The partition was quite variable. In the dogfish, hagfish and chicken the pressor response appeared to be completely due to the action of released catecholamines. In the lumpfish and rat 90% of the pressor effects of angiotensin II were a direct action of this agent on the vasculature. In the turtle and frog the partition was about 50/50 between a direct action of angiotensin II and the action of released catecholamines. The data of Carroll and Opdyke (1982) clearly demonstrate a very close interplay between the renin angiotensin system and the sympathetic system in the control of arterial pressure and this inter-relationship between the RAS and the sympathetic nervous system is a highly conserved feature across vertebrate species.

In recent years our understanding of the components and functions of the renin angiotensin system particularly in mammals has been greatly extended with the identification of new angiotensins and receptors (Phillips and de Oliveira, 2008; Chappell, 2007). The RAS is not only involved in the regulation of cardiovascular function but also in brain functions such as learning and memory. However, only those parts of the RAS relevant to arterial pressure control will be considered.

The rodent genome codes for two distinct AT1 receptors, AT1aR and AT1bR whereas the human genome codes for a single AT1R. AT1R are found in the brain, adrenal glands, heart, vasculature and the kidney. Davisson et al., (2000) studied the effects of mouse brain AT1aR and AT1bR on mean arterial pressure and volume balance. Mice with targeted deletions of the AT1aR gene or AT1bR gene were given intracerebroventricular (IVC) injections of angiotensin II. Basal mean arterial pressure was similar in wild-type mice and AT1bR-/- mice but significantly lower in AT1aR -/- mice. IVC administration of angiotensin II caused a significant increase in mean arterial pressure in wild-type and AT1bR -/- mice but only a minor increase in AT1aR -/- mice. IVC injection of angiotensin II elicited a robust drinking response in wild-type mice, a somewhat diminished drinking response in AT1aR -/- mice and a very limited drinking response in AT1bR -/- mice. Hence, at least in the rodent, AT1a and AT1b brain receptors sub serve different functions with AT1aR involved in blood pressure regulation and AT1bR primarily involved in the regulation of drinking and water balance.

A homolog of the enzyme angiotensin converting enzyme (ACE), named ACE2 has been identified which mediates the conversion of angiotensin II to angiotensin- (1-7) (Hocht et al., 2009). Angiotensin- (1-7) binds to a receptor termed Mas receptor which is a member of the G protein coupled receptor superfamily and is expressed in heart, blood vessels, brain and reproductive organs. The physiological effects of the angiotensin- (1-7)-Mas receptor interaction include vascular endothelium dependent vasodilatation (NO mediated), an ant proliferative effect on vascular smooth muscle cells and a lowering of arterial pressure through an effect on the brain. These physiological actions of the angiotensin- (1-7)-Mas receptor complex appear to counterbalance many of the actions of the angiotensin II-AT1 receptor complex. However, there is not yet a clear picture as to the suite of physiological effects resulting from the binding of angiotensin (1-7) to the Mas receptor and a number of conflicting observations have been noted (Pinheiro and e Silva, 2012; Hocht et al., 2009; Chappell, 2007).

Finally, the RAS can also be modulated by glucocorticoids. Corticosterone (rat major glucocorticoid) and aldosterone both potentiate the angiotensin II stimulated constriction of rat aortic rings (Ullian et al., 1996). In addition these investigators found that corticosterone and aldosterone up regulated angiotensin II binding by cultured rat aortic vascular smooth muscle cells. Consistent with these observations, Gou et al., (1995) found that the transcription of the rodent AT1a R gene was increased by glucocorticoids. Guo et al., (1995) identified a glucocorticoid response element (GRE) in the promoter region of the rat AT1a receptor gene upstream from the transcription start site. The glucocorticoid-GR complex binds to this GRE in the promoter region thus enhancing the transcription of the AT1a receptor gene. No GRE was found in the promoter region of the AT1b receptor gene. Unlike the rat receptor gene, the human AT1 receptor gene contains a number (three) of GRE half sites in the promoter region (Nawata et al., 1995). Hence, glucocorticoid up regulation of the human AT1 receptor gene may be mediated by multiple ½ GREs or a ½ GRE plus an additional accessory element (Elton and Martin, 2007).

d) Dopaminergic System

Dopamine and dopamine receptors comprise a system that is also involved in arterial pressure regulation. Like the RAS, the dopaminergic system should be viewed as acting in a supporting role to the dominant regulator of arterial pressure, the brain. Dopamine is synthesized in neural and epithelial tissues with the immediate precursor being L-DOPA (Zeng and Jose, 2011). Dopamine receptors are part of the superfamily of G-protein coupled receptors. Mammals possess five dopamine receptor subtypes which are generally grouped into D1-like receptors (D1 and D5) and D2-like receptors (D2, D3 and D4). D1-like receptors activate adenylyl cyclases while D2-like receptors inhibit adenylyl cyclases (Zeng et al., 2008). Dopamine receptors are expressed in the central nervous system, kidney, heart and vascular tissue and the observation that receptor null mutant mice (D1,2,3,4 or 5) are hypertensive compared to wild-type litter mates substantiates the role of the dopaminergic system in arterial pressure control. The actions of dopamine are a function of the tissue site and the receptor subtype involved. In general, dopamine- receptor interactions in the kidney lead to an increase in sodium excretion as a result of inhibition of epithelial ion transport processes (Zeng et al., 2008). In the central nervous system, dopamine-receptor interactions decrease the activity of the sympathetic system.

The complexity of the dopaminergic system is compounded by the observation that dopamine receptor subtypes can physically interact to form heteromeric protein complexes. There is also extensive "cross talk" between the dopaminergic and renin angiotensin systems (Zeng et al., 2008). Finally, there are a number of experimental observations pointing to a significant interplay between glucocorticoids and the dopaminergic system (Van Craenenbroeck et al., 2005). Zhou et al., (1992) have described a potential glucocorticoid response element in the rat dopamine D1 receptor gene.

The data strongly support the role of the central nervous system as the dominant regulator of mean arterial pressure. The most likely regulatory centers in the brain are those that control the sympathetic and parasympathetic nervous system. Efferents from these centers can alter the pressure-natriuresis mechanism in the kidney thereby integrating brain and renal regulation of mean arterial pressure. Interacting with these brain centers are at least three other systems which help to regulate mean arterial pressure; molecular clocks and the renin angiotensin and dopaminergic systems. In addition glucocorticoids can input into the renin angiotensin and dopaminergic systems by acting as transcription regulators of the angiotensin II AT1 receptor gene and probably also of dopamine receptor gene(s).

Although the mean arterial pressure (or perhaps more accurately the mean arterial pressure range) for a given species is developmentally set, programmed events can occur post-natal which necessitate "resetting" of the mean arterial pressure and as a result adaptations in cardiovascular structure. Two such "natural experiments" are; the changes in pressures in the pulmonary and systemic vascular circulations that occur after birth and the changes in systemic arterial pressure that occur in the giraffe after birth with growth and elongation of its neck.

Natural Experiments

a) Postnatal Pulmonary and Systemic Arterial Pressure Changes

A critical adaptation in the evolution of vertebrates with high oxygen demands was the complete separation of the pulmonary and systemic circulations (West, 2011). In fish, gill capillaries are exposed to the full intraluminal pressure of the dorsal aorta while, in amphibians and non-crocodilian reptiles partial separation of the pulmonary and systemic circulations occurs. However, only in the fully endothermic mammal and bird is there complete separation of these two circulations (West, 2011). This separation permits the development of a blood-gas barrier of high diffusion features (large surface area and thin walled capillaries) while protecting this delicate blood-gas diffusion barrier from the mechanical stresses of a high vascular intraluminal pressure. A similar sequence of events occurs when the mammalian fetus transitions from the intra- to extra-uterine environment after birth (Gao and Raj, 2010). During embryonic development, the pulmonary and systemic circulations are only partially separated. The fetal pulmonary circulation is characterized by a high vascular resistance and low blood flow to the lung. A major fraction of the (right sided) cardiac output is diverted away from the lung to the systemic circulation via the foramen ovale and the ductus arteriosus. At birth with the establishment of respiration, there is a dramatic decline in pulmonary vascular resistance. The entire cardiac output of the right ventricle goes to the lung and the foramen ovale and ductus arteriosus close.

Pulmonary and systemic arterial hemodynamic parameters have been measured across the transition from fetus to newborn (Gao and Raj, 2010; Emmanouilides et al., 1964). Mean fetal pulmonary arterial pressure is about 55 mmHg while that of the newborn is about 20-25 mmHg. Pulmonary blood flow almost doubles from 138 to 245 ml/min/kg from fetus to newborn and pulmonary vascular resistance falls from 0.4 to 0.08 mmHg/ml/min/kg across the transition from fetus to newborn. Aortic pressure increases from about 45-50 mmHg in the newborn to about 60-65 mmHg by 60 hours after birth. In summary, at birth with the onset of breathing, the lung replaces the placenta as the organ of gas exchange. Pulmonary blood flow increases to now encompass the total cardiac output; pulmonary artery pressure gradually decreases while systemic pressure increases. As soon as systemic pressure and resistance become greater than that in the pulmonary circulation, the foramen ovale and ductus arteriosus close. In essence, at the transition from the intra- to extra-uterine environment, there occurs a significant "resetting" of the pulmonary mean arterial pressure with a quantitatively smaller "resetting" of the systemic mean arterial pressure.

The dramatic hemodynamic changes occurring when the fetus assumes its extra-uterine existence are accompanied by structural changes (remodeling) in the aorta and pulmonary vasculature. Leung et al., (1977) examined postnatal structural changes in the rabbit ascending aorta and pulmonary trunk. At birth the medial lamellar structure of the two vessels as well as the elastin and collagen content (relative to tissue dry weight) were similar. Within two weeks of birth, elastin content had increased significantly in the ascending aorta but only marginally in the pulmonary trunk. After two weeks, elastin content remained constant in the ascending aorta but gradually fell in the pulmonary trunk. By contrast over the first two weeks, collagen content increased more in than pulmonary trunk than in the ascending aorta and after two weeks the content of collagen remained relatively constant in both vessels. Leung et al., (1977) calculated total medial tangential tension (using the Laplace relationship) in both vessels; total tangential tension increased progressively by a factor of ten in the ascending aorta over the first two months of postnatal life but remained essential stable in the pulmonary trunk over the same time frame.

The smaller pulmonary arteries also show significant remodeling after birth (Gao and Raj, 2010; Haworth et al., 1987; Michel et al., 1991). Haworth et al., (1987) examined the structure of peripheral pulmonary arteries in pigs varying in age from newborn to six months. Wall thickness abruptly decreased during the first 30 minutes of life and thereafter arterial vessel wall gradually thinned over the next 21 days. Arterial lumen increased over a similar time frame of postnatal life. The major histological change responsible for the decrease in wall thickness was a remodeling of smooth muscle cell morphology; these cells became thinner and increasingly separated from each other as if these smooth muscle cells had "spread" within the vessel wall (Haworth et al., 1987; Gao and Raj, 2010). A morphological study in lambs from newborn to one month of age by Michel et al., (1991) gave essentially similar results. Arterial medial muscle thickness in all pulmonary vessels greater than 100 microns in diameter decreased over the first month of life and these arteries also showed an increase in lumen size over this same time frame. The percentage of muscular arteries (versus non muscular and partially muscular) in the more distal pulmonary vasculature decreased significantly between ages 2-4 days and two weeks.

Hence, in the post natal period significant remodeling occurs in the pulmonary trunk and intra pulmonary arteries. This remodeling consists of a decrease in elastin content and an increase in collagen content of the pulmonary trunk compared to the ascending aorta and an increase in lumen size and reduction in medial wall thickness of the intrapulmonary arteries. In the immediate post natal period a suite of hemodynamic changes take place; large reductions in pulmonary vascular resistance and pulmonary artery pressure and a significant increase in pulmonary blood flow. These hemodynamic changes result from a number of birth related events; ventilation, oxygenation, increased shear stress due to the greater pulmonary blood flow and changes in the activities of a number of vasoactive agents and their signaling pathways (Gao and Raj, 2010). The remodeling of the ascending aorta and pulmonary vasculature is a physiological adaptation to the changes in circumferential tension (the result of decreased pulmonary artery intraluminal pressure and increase aortic intraluminal pressure) and shear stress (the result of increased pulmonary artery flow).

Although, Gao and Raj (2010) discussed some of the signaling pathways and vasoactive agents involved in the hemodynamic changes associated with the intra- to extra-uterine transition, there are little data as to the genetic underpinnings of the programmed vascular remodeling that occurs as a result of these hemodynamic changes. A likely player in this remodeling process is the Notch signaling pathway. This highly conserved fundamental signaling pathway is critical for embryogenesis of the cardiovascular system (High and Epstein, 2008). In addition, there are data that the Notch pathway is also important for cardiovascular remodeling post-natal (Hoffman and Iruela-Arispe, 2007; Lindner et al., 2001). This pathway comprises five ligands (delta-like 1,3,4 and jagged 1, 2) as well as four Notch receptors (notch 1-4). Notch receptors and ligands are both single-pass trans membrane proteins that enable the Notch pathway to transduce signals between neighboring cells i.e. activation generally requires cell to cell contact (High and Epstein, 2008). Binding of the ligand to a Notch receptor triggers a proteolytic cleavage which releases the Notch intracellular domain (NICD) into the cytoplasm. The NICD trans locates to the nucleus where it forms an active transcriptional complex with the DNA binding protein RBPJ and other co-activators. In the absence of NICD, RBPJ acts as a transcriptional repressor of Notch target genes, but the binding of NICD acts as a transcriptional switch converting RBPJ from a repressor to an activator. The Notch pathway is extremely sensitive to spatial and temporal cues. The Notch pathway is required for proper development of the cardiac outflow tract which involves septation of the atria and ventricles and remodeling of the outflow tract to form a separate aorta and pulmonary artery. The ligand jagged 1 and the Notch receptor 2 appear to be particularly important in this developmental process (Jain et al., 2010). Deletion of the ligand jagged 1 or inhibition of Notch signaling in the second heart field (progenitor cells originating in the pharynx) result in outflow tract abnormalities such as persistent truncus arteriosus (failure of separation of aorta and pulmonary artery) and double outlet right ventricle (Jain et al., 2010).

In addition to cardiac embryogenesis, Notch signaling is also critical for the reorganization of vessels that derive from the primitive vascular plexus (Hoffman and Iruela-Arispe, 2007). During this developmental reorganization, the primitive vascular plexus is remodeled into a hierarchic network. Notch receptors are expressed in both endothelium (Notch 1 and 4) and arterial smooth muscle cells (Notch 1and 3). Expression of Notch receptors and ligands are found predominantly in the arterial vascular tree although smaller amounts have been detected in veins and capillaries. Activated Notch 1 receptor has also been detected in the endothelial and smooth muscle cells of adult arteries in adipose tissue, kidney, brain and lung (Hoffman and Iruela-Arispe, 2007). Given the critical role that the Notch signaling pathway plays in cardiovascular development and the observation that activated Notch receptor is expressed in adult arteries suggest that this signaling pathway may also be important in regulating the response of "adult" cardiovascular tissue to injury.

Lindner et al., (2001) have experimentally tested this hypothesis. These investigators used a balloon catheter technique to denude the endothelial lining of rat carotid arteries. The ligands jagged 1 and jagged 2 were expressed to a limited degree in normal endothelium but the expression of both genes was dramatically enhanced in regenerating endothelial cells. This expression was seen predominantly in the endothelial cells at the migrating front of the wound. This enhanced expression lasted for the time period (about four weeks) over which the repair process (active migration and proliferation of endothelial cells) lasted and then diminished. A similar expression pattern and time course for jagged 1 and 2 was observed for smooth muscle cells. There was also an increase in the expression of Notch 1-4 receptors in regenerating endothelial and smooth muscle cells after the vascular injury. The spatial pattern of expression in endothelial and smooth muscle cells suggested that cell contact between endothelial cells, at the regenerating margin of the wound and smooth muscle cells regulated the levels of receptor expression in the smooth muscle cells.

The establishment of a normal cardiac outflow tract with a separate aorta and pulmonary trunk is due to a developmental program critically dependent upon the Notch signaling pathway. At birth, abrupt and significant hemodynamic changes occur as already discussed. In response to these hemodynamic changes, remodeling of the aortic and pulmonary trunks as well as the intrapulmonary arterial vessels takes place. Hence this remodeling is a vascular adaptation to the altered circumferential tension and shear stress. A reasonable proposal is that the Notch signaling pathway which is of fundamental importance to cardiac embryogenesis plays a key role in the postnatal remodeling of the aortic trunk and pulmonary vasculature.

b) Postnatal Growth of the Giraffe

The postnatal growth of the giraffe represents a second example in which there occurs a "resetting" of mean arterial pressure. However, unlike the situation described in the previous section where the "resetting" in mean arterial pressure occurs within a very short time span, growth of the giraffe with elongation of its neck leads to a progressive gradual "resetting" of mean arterial pressure. The high mean arterial pressure in the adult giraffe is a consequence of gravitational effects on the vertical column of arterial blood in its long neck. In addition, the progressive "resetting" of systemic mean arterial pressure is accompanied by significant cardiac and vascular remodeling. Since the cardiovascular physiology of the giraffe has been discussed in a previous publication (Singer, 2011) only the salient features will be reviewed here.

Mitchell and Skinner (2009) collected cardiovascular variables from 56 giraffes; 10 fetuses and 46 postnatal animals varying in age from 0.4 to more than 20 years. Mean systemic arterial pressures were calculated based on body mass and neck length. Mean pulmonary artery pressures were calculated using Laplace's principle. In the postnatal giraffes, calculated mean arterial pressure varied from 147 mmHg in the youngest to 237 mmHg in the oldest while for fetuses calculated mean arterial pressure was about 100 mmHg. For a 775kg giraffe, calculated mean arterial pressure would be 208 mmHg which agrees with a mean arterial pressure of 203 mmHg derived from measurements previously published in the literature. The predicted mean arterial pressure for a 775 kg mammal based upon the allometric equations calculated by Seymour and Blaylock (2000) would be 127 mmHg; clearly the giraffe is an outlier. Mean pulmonary artery pressures calculated by Mitchell and Skinner (2009) were 35-49 mmHg in the postnatal giraffes and 54-68 mmHg in fetuses; higher than values for mammals of equivalent body mass. By contrast, using values published in the literature, Mitchell and Skinner (2009) calculated mean arterial pressure in the giraffe at the level of the brain in the head- up posture to be 100 mmHg which is similar to that of other mammalian species.

As a result of high mean arterial pressures in both the systemic and pulmonary circulations (based upon a mammal of equivalent body mass as a reference), the giraffe demonstrates considerable structural remodeling of its cardiovascular system. Although relative heart mass is comparable to that of mammals of equivalent body mass (Mitchell and Skinner, 2009; Perez et al., 2008; Brondum et al., 2009), the giraffe's heart shows considerable hypertrophy of the left ventricular, interventricular and right ventricular walls (Mitchell and Skinner, 2009; Goetz and Keen, 1957). In addition, the extreme elliptical shape (Gothic shapaae) of the giraffe's left ventricle (compared to that of the human) allows the left ventricle to generate the pressures necessary to maintain cerebral perfusion (Coghlan and Hoffman, 2006). The remarkable strength of the Gothic left ventricle is the result of its geometry and myocardial fiber orientation. Using the fetal vasculature as a reference, the arterial tree of the adult giraffe shows significant structural changes. Arterioles in the kidney, heart, lung, liver and mesentery of the adult giraffe display considerable thickening of the media and a reduction in luminal diameter compared to similar vessels in the fetus (Mitchell and Skinner, 2009). In the adult giraffe, the posterior tibial artery shows a pinpoint lumen and an extremely thickened media whereas in the same animal the carotid artery (in the head), which has a comparable external diameter, shows a much larger lumen and much thinner walls (Goetz and Keen, 1957). Similarly, arteries in the foot skin of the adult giraffe have thick walls and small lumens whereas comparable foot skin arteries in the newborn have larger lumens and thin walls (Hargens et al., 1988).

The cardiovascular remodeling observed in the giraffe is a physiological adaptation to the high mean arterial pressure. The parts of the arterial tree that display the greatest structural changes (thickening of the media and reduction in luminal diameter) are the vessels subjected to the highest mean arterial pressures; vessels at or below the level of the heart. The carotid artery shows very little remodeling since this artery is in a region of much lower intraluminal pressure. The structural changes are "driven" by the principle of Laplace; thickening of the vessel wall and reduction in the diameter of the vessel lumen help to reduce circumferential stress when intraluminal pressure rises. In fact despite a high mean arterial pressure, left ventricular wall stress in the giraffe is actually in the lowest quartile for all mammals (Seymour and Blaylock, 2000).

A fascinating and very informative "experiment" would be to reconstruct the physiological events that occur within the cardiovascular system of the giraffe as this mammal grows and its neck elongates. The start and end points of this experiment are known. The newborn giraffe weighs about 100 kg (Van Sittert et al., 2010), has a mean arterial pressure of about 100 mmHg and has an arterial tree containing vessels with thin walls and large lumens. The mature adult giraffe has a mean arterial pressure of about 200 mmHg, a heart with greatly thickened walls and an arterial tree containing extensively remodeled vessels in regions exposed to the high arterial pressure. Unfortunately longitudinal cardiovascular physiological measurements have not been made in the growing giraffe. However, since both systemic mean arterial pressure at the level of the heart and left ventricular and interventricular wall thicknesses directly correlate with neck length (Mitchell and Skinner, 2009); indirect information about these physiological events can be obtained by looking at the postnatal development of the giraffe neck itself.

Van Sittert et al., (2010) examined the development of the giraffe axial skeleton from fetus to mature adult. Giraffes have 7 cervical, 14 thoracic and 5 lumbar vertebrae. Compared to the trunk (thoracic plus lumbar regions), postnatal giraffes display a differential increase in the dimensions of the cervical vertebrae. The neonatal cervical spine increases markedly in the first six months of life from about 116% to 122% of the thoracic plus lumbar spine length. The mature adult giraffe has a cervical spine 139% of the thoracic plus lumbar spine length. The newborn giraffe has cervical vertebrae of about 100 mm in height whereas in the mature adult the height is about 300 mm. In the post natal period, vertebral body height shows continuous growth with the curve being steepest in the neonatal period and then slowing down as a mature adult stage is reached. It is not clear from the data when cervical vertebrae elongation plateaus. Axial skeletal development with selective elongation of the cervical spine is clearly a programmed process but the genetic underpinnings are presently unknown. Transcribing this data to the cardiovascular system means that mean arterial pressure and cardiac wall thickness increase continuously from birth to mature adulthood.

The following sequence of cardiovascular events would seem reasonable. In this discussion it is important to distinguish physiological events that are involved in the setting of the mean pressure level and physiological events that occur as an adaptive response to the rising mean arterial pressure. At birth, the giraffe's mean arterial pressure of about 100 mmHg is developmentally set as discussed in previous sections. The increasing mean arterial pressure as the giraffe grows and its neck elongates is a consequence of gravitational effects on a lengthening vertical column of blood in its neck. As the giraffe's neck elongates cerebral blood flow will be reduced to the brain "arterial pressure" sensor center(s). These center(s) integrate inputs from a number of sources such as molecular clocks and the renin angiotensin and dopaminergic systems and have efferents that regulate the autonomic nervous system. The reduction in blood flow is detected by a neural sensor and appropriate adjustments to the outflow from the brain center(s) controlling the autonomic nervous system will occur (Paton et al., 2009). As discussed in the section Regulating mechanisms; b) brain, the existence of a specific neural center that regulates long term arterial pressure is still controversial. In addition, the signal to such a neural center/sensor could be the reduced blood flow itself or a reduction in delivered nutrients (e.g. oxygen, glucose) as a result of the diminished blood flow. Mean arterial pressure is ultimately a function of both cardiac output and total peripheral resistance to flow. Currently the best data is that cardiac output in the postnatal giraffe is comparable to other mammals of equivalent mass (Mitchell and Skinner, 2009). However, calculated total resistance to flow is higher in the giraffe than in mammals of equivalent body mass. Hence the driving parameter for the increase in mean arterial pressure with neck elongation appears to be greater sympathetic outflow, enhanced vascular smooth muscle myogenic tone and hence increasing total peripheral resistance to flow. In addition, this increasing sympathetic outflow will alter renal function and in particular reset the renal pressure-natriuresis mechanism. In the mature giraffe, the forceful expulsion of blood by the extreme Gothic shaped heart into an arterial tree with an appropriate total resistance to flow is able to generate a mean arterial pressure of about 200 mmHg at the level of the heart. In the upright standing posture, gravitational effects account for the measured gradient in mean arterial pressures (Hargens et al., 1987); 100-110 mmHg at the base of the head (same as that in all other mammalian species; Mitchell and Skinner, 2009), 200 mmHg at the level of the heart and 260 mmHg at the level of the foot. The extent of arterial remodeling follows this pressure gradient with the greatest remodeling in the arteries in the foot and the least remodeling in the arteries of the neck such as the carotid. A similar gradient of arterial remodeling has been documented in humans since gravitational effects are also important in human cardiovascular physiology but clearly not to the same extent as in the giraffe. Based upon ultrasound measurements in healthy humans of various ages, average luminal diameter was smaller in the anterior tibial artery compared to the radial artery and the ratio of intimal thickness to lumen diameter was larger in the anterior tibial artery versus the radial artery (Osika et al., 2007).

The data of Wolinsky and Glagov (1969) cited in a previous section (Comparative biology of the cardiovascular system) indicate that medial tension per lamellar unit has a similar value in aortas from a wide variety of mammals. I am not aware of similar data for smaller arteries. However, extrapolating from this data, it would appear that a certain limited range for permissible values of circumferential wall stress has been evolutionarily selected. The remodeling that occurs in arteries in response to changes in intraluminal pressure is due to a local sequence of events initiated by vessel wall pressure mechanosensors which leads to a “normalization” of circumferential wall stress.

What about the giraffe heart? As the giraffe grows and its neck elongates, mean arterial pressure at heart level must increase from 100mmHg to 200 mmHg to ensure adequate cerebral perfusion. To accomplish this task, the heart must do more work and the data of Mitchell and Skinner (2009) show that left ventricular and interventricular wall thicknesses increase linearly with neck length. The hypertrophied heart can perform increased work as measured by the integral of pressure developed with respect to volume of blood ejected (Grossman, 1980). Gunther and Grossman (1979) studied left ventricular function in 14 patients with isolated aortic stenosis of varying severity. They observed that left ventricular midwall circumferential (wall) stress (a function of left ventricular pressure, wall thickness and ventricular cavity size) was an excellent predictor of left ventricular functional characteristics such as ejection fraction and the velocity of circumferential fibre shortening. Ventricles with thicker walls and a smaller cavity size i.e. lower wall stress had better overall cardiac performance with a greater velocity and extent of myocardial fiber shortening than ventricles with higher wall stress i.e. thinner walls and larger cavity size. Seymour and Blaylock (2000) calculated left ventricular wall stress using a data set that included 24 species of mammals and 12 species of birds. Left ventricular wall stress displayed a very small range across all of these species of varying body masses and the value for the adult giraffe was well within this range. Seymour and Blaylock's data plus the observations of Gunther and Grossman (1979) imply that there is an optimal range of myocardial fiber shortening characteristics that have been evolutionarily selected and that can be captured by measurement of wall stress. Hence as the giraffe grows and its neck elongates, the heart walls must continuously hypertrophy while cavity size remains relatively small (wall stress remains unchanged) so that the heart can perform more work and thus generate an ever greater mean arterial pressure.

The cardiovascular physiology of the giraffe teaches us several very important lessons. First, the center or centers that regulate arterial pressure long term must reside in the brain. If for some reason, mean arterial pressure becomes reset to a higher value, this resetting must occur in this center(s). Secondly, the remodeling of peripheral arteries is strictly a response to the change in intraluminal pressure and this arterial remodeling is not responsible for the increase in total peripheral resistance to flow characteristic of the giraffe's "hypertensive" state. Thirdly, the cardiac hypertrophy observed in the giraffe is a necessary physiological adaptation to allow its heart to generate and maintain the required mean arterial pressure. The degree of cardiac hypertrophy i.e. size in other animals will depend upon the level at which their mean arterial pressure has been set.

A similar phenomenon of postnatal growth resetting arterial pressure occurs in other species such as the human, but clearly not to the same extent as observed in the giraffe. deMan et al., (1991) pooled the arterial blood pressure readings from six European studies that in total contained measured arterial pressures in 28043 children over the age range 4-19 years. Separate plots of systolic and diastolic blood pressure versus age showed an increase in both variables with age in both males and females, although the slopes appeared steeper with systolic compared to diastolic pressure. The authors also plotted systolic and diastolic pressure versus height in the same data set of children. The plots of systolic or diastolic pressure versus age or height look identical. Using the giraffe as a construct, this human data set indicate that with postnatal growth in the human, the vertical distance between the heart and brain increases mandating a continuous resetting of arterial pressure until growth ceases. This human growth-blood pressure data set would be consistent with a brain location for the arterial pressure "resetting" center(s).

In summary, for each species, mean arterial pressure (or more accurately pressure range) is developmentally set. This set range represents the byproduct of a number of integrated developmental programs; a heart of the appropriate size, structure and function to supply the requisite forceful expulsion of blood, a system of blood vessels with congruent mechanical properties and kidney structure and function with the capacity for appropriate regulation of salt and water balance. After birth, events can occur which lead to further changes in arterial pressure and cardiovascular structure. Two such events were discussed; changes in pulmonary and systemic arterial pressures and flows that occur at the time of birth and postnatal growth of the giraffe with differential elongation of its neck. These natural experiments reveal that the center(s) for long term regulation of mean arterial pressure reside in the brain and that cardiovascular remodeling involves local mechanisms and is strictly a response to the changes in intraluminal pressures and flows. Clearly, the human species is also bound by these developmental considerations. However, an equally critical variable is the influence of environmental cues on the function and structure of the cardiovascular system.

Environmental Cues

Before discussing environmental cues, the importance of genetic diversity across individual humans needs to be emphasized. As reviewed in the section Background; Genetics, the phenotypic diversity across humans reflects underlying diversity across genomes and epigenomes. As a result, every individual will respond differently to the same environmental cue. The situation is radically different in inbred strains of laboratory animals where the genetic and epigenetic diversity across individual animals has been greatly diminished. This distinction has to be kept in mind when extrapolating from experimental situations involving genetically simplified laboratory animals.

Social Environment

In this section, environmental influences limited to the postnatal period will be discussed. However, it is important to remember that events which change the intrauterine environment can significantly impact the developing fetus. One example was discussed in the section Atherosclerotic Vascular Disease; Tobacco smoke exposure. Maternal smoking can epigenetically modify placental genes and through this mechanism the nature (usually in a deleterious way) of the intrauterine environment. Mothers who smoke generally give birth to small for gestational age infants who are at increased risk for developing more serious "health" issues as adults. These health issues include a higher mean arterial pressure and evidence of more extensive atherosclerotic –type vascular remodeling.

Humans are a very social species. Most of us live in urbanized settings containing large numbers of people. As briefly reviewed in the beginning of this section on Hypertension, urbanization of rural populations, greater levels of acculturation and a developed nation- type lifestyle are associated with higher levels of arterial pressure. Recreating experimentally in animal studies the complex social interactions that occur within human society is essentially impossible. Hence animal experiments will give only a limited perspective on the cardiovascular effects of these (social) environmental cues. Never the less, these animal experiments do point out the link between social environment and social interactions and arterial pressure.

Coelho et al., (1991) looked at the effect of housing conditions on the arterial pressure of captive male baboons. Three housing conditions were used; subjects individually housed, subjects housed with two familiar companions, subjects housed with two unfamiliar companions. Arterial pressures and heart rates were continuously monitored with an indwelling arterial catheter. In general, the unfamiliar social (housing) environment was associated with the highest mean arterial pressure with the familiar companion housing associated with the lowest mean arterial pressure. The individual housing setup was associated with an intermediate value. These differences in mean arterial pressure were greatest between 6 pm and 5 am with an approximately 6 mmHg difference between the unfamiliar and familiar housing environments. Mean heart rate gave a similar pattern with again the largest differences being present over the night time period.

Fokkema et al., (1988) examined several types of social interactions on the cardiac physiology of an inbred strain of rats. Experimental male rats were housed individually with a sterilized female companion. Several social situations were created. The intruder test involved putting a non-territorial intruder rat into the experimental cage. In the defeat test, an experimental rat was introduced as an intruder into the territory of a trained fighter rat- the experimental rat showed clear signs of "defeat" after the confrontation. Psychosocial tests were conducted in which the experimental rat was again confronted with the same fighter rat by whom it was defeated but in this case direct physical contact was prevented. Arterial pressure was measured with an indwelling arterial catheter and a separate indwelling venous catheter was used for blood sampling. The greatest increase in mean arterial pressure (16 mmHg) was observed in the defeat test with the post defeat psychological test causing a significant but lesser increase (8 mmHg) in mean arterial pressure. Increases in plasma levels of epinephrine, norepinephrine and corticosterone showed a similar pattern; greatest increase with the defeat situation and a lesser increase in the post defeat confrontation test. The intruder test did not elicit any changes in mean arterial pressure or plasma levels of catecholamines or corticosterone above baseline.

The experimental observations of Fokkema et al., (1988) and Coelho et al., (1991) show a clear association between social environment/social interactions and mean arterial pressure. In addition, the data of Fokkema et al., (1988) demonstrate the involvement of the sympathetic system and adrenal gland in mediating this cardiovascular response. However, as discussed in the section Regulating mechanisms; there is an extremely complex interplay between the central nervous system, molecular clocks, renin angiotensin and dopaminergic systems and glucocorticoids with respect to regulating the function of the cardiovascular system. Social environment/social interactions intersect with this regulatory network at the level of the brain and as discussed in Atherosclerotic Vascular Disease; stress hormones, one such mechanistic example is that the nature of maternal care during a critical time window can set, through epigenetic mechanisms, the life- long stress responsiveness of the offspring.

The significant effects of environmental influences on cardiovascular physiology are illustrated by a comparison of the cardiovascular physiology of indigenous rural populations with comparable urbanized/industrialized populations. A review of data from four such observational studies follows.

Oliver et al., (1975) described cardiovascular variables in the Yanomamo Indians, an unacculturated tribe living in northern Brazil and southern Venezuela. The sample consisted of 500 males and females aged 10- 50+ years. Systolic/diastolic pressures were in the range of 100/60 mmHg and did not show any statistically significant increase with age. This population subsists on an extremely low sodium diet (mean 24 hour sodium excretion 1.02 mM) and as expected is characterized by extremely high levels of aldosterone excretion and plasma renin activity.

Pavan et al., (1999) compared the cardiovascular status of the Amondava population (30 males and females, age range 15-58 years), an isolated indigenous group living in Brazil, with age and sex matched samples from Venice (Italy), Gdansk (Poland) and Tanzanian Bantu. The Bantu lived a primitive farming- dominated life style. Mean systolic/diastolic pressures (mmHg) for these groups were; 110/69 (Amondava), 125/75 (Bantu), 125/75(Italy), 133/85 (Poland). Systolic pressure increased with age in the Polish and Italian groups but not in the Amondava or Bantu groups. The diet of the Amondava is rich in fibers and complex carbohydrates and low in salt (<3 gm/day). The Bantu diet is high in vegetable foods and low in animal fat and salt (< 4 g/day). The Polish group had a diet rich in meat and salt (> 9 g/day). The diet of the Italian sample is not specifically given but noted to be similar to that of the general Italian population. Mean BMIs (kg/m2) were; 20.9 (Amondava), 21.1 (Bantu), 22.1 (Italy) and 25.1 (Poland).

As a sub project of the INTERSALT study, Carvalho et al., (1989) measured arterial pressure in four remote population samples; Yanomamo and Xingu Indians of Brazil and rural populations in Kenya and Papua New Guinea. Each sample consisted of 200 males and females aged 20-59 years. Mean systolic/diastolic pressures (mmHg) in males were; 101/65 (Yanomano), 103/65 (Xingo), 109/64(Papua New Guinea) and 114/67 (Kenya). Mean pressures in females were about 7-10 mmHg lower in the Yanomamo and Xingu but similar to males in the samples from Papua New Guinea and Kenya. None of the four groups showed a significant increase in blood pressure with age. Mean daily salt intakes were; 0.05g (Yanomamo), 0.78 g (Xingu), 2.4 g (Papua New Guinea) and 3.6 g (Kenya).

Finally, Snodgrass et al., (2008) measured arterial pressure in three indigenous Siberian populations (Evenki, Buryat and Yakut). The Evenki were an indigenous population of reindeer herders who are still involved in this activity. The Buryat were traditionally cattle herders and hunters and the Yakut traditionally practiced a subsistence type of strategy. All three groups have had their life styles significantly altered by Russian contact and Soviet collectivization. The study populations were; Evenki, 63 males and females aged 16-53 years, Buryat, 135 males and females aged 16-74 years and Yakut, 123 males and females aged 18-56 years. Mean systolic/diastolic pressures (mmHg) for males were 126/81 (Evenki), 134/85 (Buryat) and 136/ 81 (Yakut). A similar pattern was seen for females. In the total combined sample (both sexes), age was positively correlated with systolic and diastolic pressure. Also in the total combined sample, mean BMI (kg/m2) was 24.2 for females and 22.9 for males. Since indigenous Siberians live in a circumpolar habitat, they have developed an elevated basal metabolic rate (relative to body mass, surface area and fat-free mass) as a physiological adaptation to chronic and severe cold stress. This higher basal metabolic rate (BMR) appears to be due to higher T4 levels. In a subset of the total combined sample, both males and females showed statistically elevated BMRs compared to values predicted on the basis of body mass and fat free mass. Using statistical modeling, Snodgrass et al., (2008) calculated that the (elevated) BMR was a significant predictor of systolic but not diastolic pressure.

The data from these observational studies indicate that indigenous, isolated populations have low levels of systolic and diastolic pressure which remain low throughout life. Common features for these groups include a simple subsistence -type life style with a social environment much less complex than that of urbanized groups and a diet characterized by a very low intake of salt. In addition, specific physiological adaptations can be layered on top of these common features in response to local environmental conditions. For example, the higher BMR characterizing groups living in circumpolar habitats which is adaptive with respect to thermoregulation, is associated with a higher arterial pressure.

As an approximation, the differences between these indigenous societies and modern urbanized societies encapsulate the social and environmental influences that have modified cardiovascular function and in particular levels of arterial pressure. The main influences appear to be degree of psychosocial stress, diet (particularly salt intake) and level of activity.

a) Psychosocial Stress

The topic of stress and its effects on the functioning of various body systems has been reviewed in a number of publications (McEwen, 1998, 2001). The autonomic nervous system and the hypothalamic-pituitary-adrenal axis are major players in the stress response. The stress hormones, cortisol (corticosterone in birds, rodents and reptiles) and aldosterone and their role in cardiovascular structural remodeling are discussed in the section Atherosclerotic

Vascular Disease; Stress hormones. The animal studies of Coelho et al., (1991) and Fokkema et al., (1988) indicate that certain housing, living arrangements and social interactions affect mean arterial pressure and that the stress response is the link between the environmental cue (social environment and social interactions) and the mean arterial pressure (phenotype). In the section Hypertension; Regulating mechanisms; the complex network regulating arterial pressure is discussed. This network comprises; the brain center(s) and interconnected molecular clocks which are the dominant regulator of the mean arterial pressure set point; the autonomic nervous system, renin angiotensin and dopaminergic systems which together comprise the effector mechanisms by which the mean arterial pressure level is maintained; glucocorticoids which function as gene transcriptional regulators in this network. Hence, glucocorticoids act as a bridge being both one of the chief mediators of the stress response and also the mechanistic link between the stress response and mean arterial pressure levels.

As discussed in the section Atherosclerotic Vascular Disease; Stress hormones; the stress phenotype i.e. the intensity of the stress response, of an animal is plastic and can be modified through epigenetic mechanisms by the nature of maternal care the animal received during a critical time period after birth. Hence, the intensity of an individual's (psychosocial) stress response to a given set of social environmental conditions will be determined by the nature of the maternal care received as a newborn as well as that individual's particular suite of genetic structural variations. As a result, the extent of the stress response will differ across individuals exposed to the same set of environmental stressors. A component of these differences in the stress response across individuals will be apparent as differences in the levels of mean arterial pressure elicited.

b) Salt Intake

Perhaps the most important dietary component with respect to arterial pressure levels is salt (NaCl). Quoting from the INTERSALT study (Stamler,1997); "Habitual high salt intake is one of the quantitatively important, preventable mass exposures causing the unfavorable population-wide blood pressure pattern that is a major risk factor for epidemic cardiovascular disease." Data from the INTERSALT study also indicated that the upward slope of systolic and diastolic blood pressure with age could be attributed to high salt intake. The history of salt intake is quite informative. The evidence is that early in our history, humans consumed a diet low in salt. Regular addition of salt to food occurred about 7000 years ago when in conjunction with the development of agriculture and animal husbandry, there was a need to have a reserve of food and hence to preserve food.

A very elegant set of experiments documenting the influence of chronic salt intake on arterial pressure were performed by Denton et al., (1995). Captive chimpanzees chronically fed a diet containing 6-12 gm of salt per day showed an age related increase in arterial pressure. Chimpanzees mature at an age of approximately 12-14 years. Mean arterial pressure (systolic/diastolic) in infant chimpanzees was 120/60 mmHg rising to a mean value of 180/110 mmHg in chimpanzees 30-40 years old. Denton and colleagues took a colony of 26 chimpanzees (ages 5-18 years) living in a number of long standing socially stable small groups. Two matched groups were "created" and the only experimental variable was a gradual increase in the salt added to the diet of one of the groups. No other changes were made to the diet of the experimental group and the social groupings of the primates were left undisturbed. The experimental period lasted 89 weeks and was followed by a six month follow up period in which extra salt was not added to the diet. Arterial pressure increased as salt was added to the diet of the experimental group. The maximum change in arterial pressure was achieved with the largest addition of salt, 15 g per day. Compared to the control group, average systolic, diastolic and mean arterial pressures were higher by 33 mmHg, 10mm Hg and 15 mmHg respectively. The control group showed a constant mean pressure of 120/50 mmHg over this entire period. Following the period of salt addition to the diet, arterial pressures in the experimental group gradually returned to baseline (and equal to those of the control group) by 20 weeks after cessation of salt addition. An additional observation made by Denton and his colleagues was that within the experimental group the arterial pressure response to the high salt intake was variable. Eight chimpanzees had a large rise in arterial pressure which reversed when the salt addition ceased whereas five chimpanzees had little change in arterial pressure with salt addition to the diet. This important observation underscores the biological variability of responses to environmental cues (in this case a change in salt intake) across individuals.

Salt appetite is based upon a very complex set of behavioral mechanisms (Morris et al., 2008). Salt appetite is a plastic behavior. Contreras and Kosten (1983) adapted three groups of female Sprague-Dawley rats to three different salt diets; low (0.12%), mid (1%) and high (3%). These diets were maintained during pregnancy and lactation and in the weaned offspring until age 30 days postpartum. The offspring were then fed a standard diet until age 90 days at which time their salt preferences were tested. The offspring were presented with salt solutions of varying concentration and the strength of the salt preferences of the offspring mirrored the strength of the salt diet given to their mothers during pregnancy and lactation and to them during the first 30 days postpartum. Offspring of mothers fed the high salt diet had the strongest salt preference while offspring of mothers fed the lowest salt diet had the weakest salt preference. Offspring of mothers fed the mid salt diet showed an intermediate salt preference. Although these observations indicate that salt appetite is a plastic behavior, what is not clear is whether the responsible environmental cue is the maternal level of salt intake during pregnancy or the level of salt intake of the offspring in the early postpartum period (30 days).

In a later study, Contreras (1989) studied the arterial pressure consequences of different perinatal salt intakes. Again three groups of female Sprague-Dawley rats were adapted to three different salt intakes; low (0.12%), mid (1%) and high (3%). These diets were maintained during pregnancy and lactation and in the weaned offspring until age 30 days postpartum. Thereafter, the offspring were maintained on a standard diet until age 102 days. At this age the arterial pressure and arterial responsiveness of the offspring to subcutaneously injected angiotensin II were measured. The mean arterial pressure was significantly higher (127.1 mmHg) in the offspring exposed to a high salt diet during pregnancy, lactation and until postpartum day 30 compared to offspring exposed to the mid salt diet (117.4 mmHg) or low salt diet (115.8 mmHg). In addition there was a significant diet effect on the pressor response elicited by angiotensin II. The "high salt diet" offspring had a significantly greater increase in mean arterial pressure following administration of angiotensin II than either the "mid salt diet" or "low salt diet" offspring. The latter two groups showed equivalent responses to angiotensin II. The previous study (Contreras and Kosten, 1983) demonstrated that salt appetite or preference is a plastic behavior that persists long after the responsible environmental cue (level of salt exposure during the intrauterine and early postpartum period) has been removed and the second study (Contreras, 1989) demonstrated that the plastic nature of this behavior has consequences with respect to the level of mean arterial pressure in adulthood.

Morris et al., (2008) have reviewed the evidence that sodium appetite is mediated by brain centers (particularly dopaminergic neurons) that are associated with reward based behaviors. Pleasurable activities, ingestion of palatable foods and drug abuse are associated with increased brain extracellular levels of dopamine. Rats depleted of sodium also show increased levels of brain extracellular dopamine following saline intake. These and other observations suggest that sodium appetite is associated with neurochemical changes in specific brain centers (e.g. nucleus accumbens) which underlie the craving of salt for its reward value (Morris eta l., 2008). However, most of these studies have been done in animals subjected to repeated episodes of salt depletion in order to induce sodium appetite. In contrast, Lucas et al., (2000) studied the neural basis of sodium appetite induced in Sprague-Dawley rats by chronic administration of the mineralcorticoid, deoxycorticosterone acetate (DOCA). An important feature of this protocol is that these rats are both sodium replete and sodium appetitive. Control rats were injected with vehicle only while experimental rats received injections of DOCA for eleven consecutive days. Sodium appetite was monitored as the amount of 2% saline ingested. Compared to vehicle-treated rats, DOCA treated rats showed a robust appetite for salt as these treated rats ingested much more 2% saline than control rats. At the termination of the experimental period, midbrain regions of the rat were tested for the presence of mRNA levels of endogenous opioids (dynorphin and enkephalin) and cholecystokinin (brain cholecystokinin is associated with hunger suppression and opioid tolerance). Midbrain sections were also tested for abundance of tyrosine hydroxylase, an enzyme involved in dopamine biosynthesis, and dopamine transporter ligand binding. DOCA treated rats with access to salt had higher mRNA levels of endogenous opioids , lower mRNA levels of cholecystokinin and reduced abundance of dopamine transporter ligand binding and tyrosine hydroxylase compared to control rats. These neurochemical changes are consistent with salt appetite being a reward- linked behavior; ingestion of salt is associated with higher levels of endogenous opioids and activation of the dopaminergic system. Hence in summary, salt appetite is a plastic behavior and the underlying neurochemical basis for this plasticity is based upon the observation that salt appetite is also a reward –seeking behavior.

Before leaving this topic of salt intake, it is important to review how an increase in salt intake actually results in an increase in mean arterial pressure. The complexity of the link between salt intake and arterial pressure is underscored by the following observation (Lifton, 2001). Chronic administration of the mineralocorticoid aldosterone initially elevates arterial pressure via increases in intravascular volume and cardiac output. However with time, despite the continued administration of aldosterone, plasma volume and cardiac output are restored to baseline values. An elevated arterial pressure persists, however, as a result of an increase in systemic vascular resistance. In other words, the link between salt intake and arterial pressure is not simply the result of changes in plasma volume since sodium balance and plasma volume will be restored by the renal pressure natriuresis mechanism. A key observation in defining this link between increased salt intake and an elevated arterial pressure was the finding of an endogenous oubain (EO) substance in the plasma of humans which functioned as a sodium pump inhibitor (Blaustein et al., 2006).

EO is synthesized in the adrenal cortex and its synthesis and secretion is stimulated by a high salt intake and by ACTH. The initial construct was as follows. EO inhibits activity of the sodium/potassium ATPase pump in vascular smooth muscle cells and this sodium pump inhibition leads to elevated intracellular sodium. Through the action of sodium/calcium exchangers, the elevated intracellular sodium concentration promotes influx of calcium into the smooth muscle cell. The rise in intracellular calcium augments smooth muscle contraction and hence would increase total peripheral resistance to flow and arterial pressure. Data obtained by Manunta et al., (2006) supported this construct. Thirteen normotensive subjects were studied during three, 5 day dietary periods; normal salt intake, high salt diet (normal salt diet plus 10 gm NaCl per day) and normal salt diet plus daily hydrochlorothiazide (a diuretic). Individuals developed high levels of plasma EO by day three of the high salt diet. Interestingly, salt depletion caused by the diuretic also led to elevated levels of plasma EO but of a much more modest increase than observed during the period of high salt intake. The other interesting observation was the marked individual variability to the same high salt diet in terms of the magnitude of the increase in plasma EO achieved.

Like most biological processes, what initially appears to be relatively simple turns out to be much more complex and this observation holds for the effects of EO as well. Hamlyn and Manunta (2011) have reviewed some of the more recent data with respect to endogenous oubain. The relationship between EO levels and acute changes in salt intake as described by Manunta et al., (2006) are transient and do not reflect the situation that occurs with chronic steady state changes in salt intake. In chronic settings, EO is stimulated by salt restriction and not salt excess. In addition, prolonged exposure to EO up regulates the expression of alpha 2 isoform of the sodium/potassium ATPase pumps as well as sodium/calcium exchangers. Hamlyn and Manunta (2011) appear to conclude that EO plays a permissive role in the genesis of hypertension; individuals with elevated levels of EO on a normal salt intake have an elevated arterial pressure related to modulation of EO biosynthesis, clearance or both.

Leenen (2010) has proposed a different construct to explain the link between salt intake and arterial pressure. In this construct the brain is the dominant site for the regulation of arterial pressure and the key parameter "monitored" by the brain is the cerebrospinal fluid (CSF) sodium concentration. CSF is formed by the choroid plexus and reabsorbed by the arachnoid granulations. Transporters such as epithelial sodium channels (ENaC) and sodium/potassium ATPase pumps in the plasma membrane of choroid plexus epithelial cells regulate the movement of sodium between plasma and CSF. Sodium transporters in the plasma membrane of ependymal cells (which line the ventricles) regulate the flow of sodium between CSF and brain parenchyma. Experimentally induced increases in CSF sodium concentration lead to a number of effects. Specific brain regions show an increase in sympathetic activity with an increase in arterial pressure and these effects can be prevented by central angiotensin II blockade or by angiotensin receptor antagonists. Increases in CSF sodium concentration are associated with increases in the hypothalamic content of aldosterone, corticosterone and endogenous oubain. Leenen has attempted to integrate the respective roles of the sympathetic nervous system, brain renin- angiotensin- aldosterone system and brain endogenous oubain in the production of an elevated mean arterial pressure in response to an increase in CSF sodium concentration.

It is clear that as discussed in the section; regulating mechanisms; b) brain; the central nervous system is most probably the primary site for regulation of mean arterial pressure but that the details of this regulatory mechanism are highly complex and currently poorly understood. The proposal that CSF sodium concentration is the key parameter monitored and that changes in sodium concentration are the primary "driver" for changes in arterial pressure is probably not correct. Most likely the key parameter monitored is some measure of blood flow or "nutrient" delivery to specific "sensor" brain regions.

c) Activity

There are a number of natural animal models available to study the impact of activity on the cardiovascular system. These natural models involve the concept of the "athletic" animal. As discussed in the section; Comparative biology of the cardiovascular system; phylogenetic determinants of arterial pressure include body mass, metabolic needs (e.g. thermoregulation) and habitat (water or land or air). However, even within a given phylum, there can be considerable variation in level of activity among species occupying the same habitat. Poupa and Ostadal (1969) reported the heart ratios (heart mass to body mass) of 42 species of fish classified as having a high, medium or low level of motility. Heart ratio was highest in the most active fish species and smallest in the least active fish species. A similar observation held for birds and mammals. Falcons have greater heart ratios than pigeons and hens and hares have higher heart ratios than tame rabbits. These higher heart ratios in animals with a more active behavioral phenotype are developmentally established. These more "athletic" animals clearly need a larger heart, higher arterial pressure and higher blood flows to meet the metabolic requirements of a more physically active life.

Poupa and Ostadal (1969) compared three groups of rats; wild rats (W), control albino rats (A) and albino rats with surgically induced aortic constriction (AAC). Heart ratios were equivalent in the athletic wild rats (W) and AAC rats and greater than the heart ratio for the A rats. However, the structural cardiac changes in the W and AAC rats were not equivalent. The increased heart size in the wild rats compared to control (A) rats was due to an increased number of myocytes with a corresponding increase in the density (growth) of capillaries. By contrast the increased heart size in the AAC rats compared to control rats was due to an increase in size not number of myocytes with an actual reduction in the density of capillaries. Hence, "athletic" animals have a developmentally set heart size that is larger than comparable animals with a less active behavioral phenotype.

How do these considerations apply to humans? As discussed by Bramble and Lieberman (2004) humans are athletic animals. Although humans are poor sprinters, they are biomechanically and energetically designed for endurance running which is defined as the capacity to run many kilometers over extended time periods using aerobic metabolism. No primates other than humans are capable of endurance running and the sustainable endurance running speeds of humans are surprisingly comparable in many respects to the trotting of specialized mammalian cursors such as dogs and horses. Bramble and Lieberman (2004) argue that the ability for endurance running in humans was not solely a by-product of selection for long distance walking and that it had a positive selection advantage of its own. However, the environmental pressures that selected for endurance running are not known. One speculation is that humans used endurance running to pursue and track down game for food prior to the invention of hunting technologies such as bows and arrows, spears and nets. Hence, for whatever reason, humans have evolved as an athletic animal and since the capacity for endurance running has been retained, this behavioral phenotype must have a positive selection value. Evolution is a conservative process that deals with compromises. The capacity for endurance running necessitates that other physiological and metabolic processes within the body be such as to support this activity.

The evolutionary importance of endurance running is substantiated by the observation that runners experience a neurobiological reward associated with endurance exercise. Raichlen et al., (2012) measured blood levels of two endocannabinoids (anandamide (AEA) and 2-arachidonylglycerol (2-AG)) in a group of recreational runners, mixed-breed dogs and ferrets before and after 30 minutes of treadmill running. Humans and dogs are cursorial species while ferrets are not. AEA blood levels were significantly elevated in humans and dogs following running compared to baseline values, but no increase in blood levels of AEA was seen in ferrets following 30 minutes of running. Walking in dogs and humans did not lead to an increase in AEA levels and 2-AG blood levels did not increase with exercise in humans, dogs or ferrets. Raichlen et al., (2012) also measured the psychological state (positive affect) of the human runners pre- and post-running using a standard questionnaire. They found a good correlation between the level of positive affect (difference between pre- and post-running scores) and the difference in blood AEA levels taken pre- and post-running. Hence, the physiological and metabolic capacity of humans to perform endurance running has been reinforced by the neurobiological rewards associated with this behavior.

There have been a number of studies which have examined the effects of endurance exercise on cardiovascular function and structure. Pyorala et al., (1967) compared a group of 61 male former endurance runners with a comparable control group. The age ranges were 40-79 years. What is not clear is how active the former endurance athletes were at the time of the study. Mean blood pressure values (systolic/diastolic) were higher in the control group compared to the former athletes; 147.1/92.4 mmHg versus 136.7/87.4 mmHg. Pollack et al., (1997) followed 21 older male track athletes for twenty years following initial recruitment into the study. Follow up examinations were done at years 10 and 20 after recruitment. At the 20 year time point the subjects ranged in age from 60-92 years and at this time point the participants were classified into high, medium and low intensity groups based upon level of activity. Maximum aerobic capacity (VO2 max) decreased in all three groups with age but the curves for the high and medium intensity groups always remained above published values for untrained healthy persons. In the low intensity group, VO2 max declined more steeply with age and at 70 years of age fell on the curve for untrained subjects. Resting heart rate was low in all three groups (46-56 beats per minute) and did not significantly change over the observational period. Portier et al., (2001) measured cardiovascular physiological parameters in 9 subjects (ages 29-35 years) who had engaged in endurance running for 15 years. The investigators compared two periods in these 9 athletes; a 3 week light training period and a 12 week period of intensive training in preparation for a competition. Subjects were tested at the end of the two periods. VO2 max and resting heart rate did not differ at the ends of the light and intensive training periods. However, systolic, diastolic and mean arterial pressures were lower (both in the decubitus and standing positions) at the end of the intensive period compared to the light training period. Laurent et al., (2011) compared two groups of subjects; 30 male endurance athletes of mean age 40.9 years and 30 matched males with a sedentary life style, mean age 40.6 years. BMI and resting heart rate were significantly lower in the endurance athletes. Arterial pressure differences between the two groups were as follows. Brachial artery systolic, diastolic and mean pressures were equivalent in the athletes and sedentary males. However, central (carotid artery) systolic pressure was higher in the male athletes (123 mmHg) than in the sedentary males (110 mmHg) although carotid artery diastolic pressure was the same in both groups (72 mmHg athletes, 76 mmHg sedentary males). VO2 max and indexed stroke volumes were significantly greater in the athletes but indexed systemic vascular resistance was similar in the two groups.

Wilson et al., (2010) recently reviewed the cardiovascular physiology and morphology of the veteran athlete. These investigators defined a veteran athlete as any individual greater than 50 years of age competing in endurance events. As already noted VO2 max falls with age in the veteran athlete due to a decline in both maximal heart rate and peak exercise stroke volume but the fall in VO2 max in the athlete is less than that of the untrained individual. Although resting left ventricular systolic function does not decrease with age, during exercise ejection fraction is significantly higher in veteran athletes than age matched control participants. A reduction in left ventricular diastolic function occurs with ageing, but this decline in left ventricular diastolic function is partially attenuated in the veteran athlete. With ageing, left ventricular wall thickness increases due to hypertrophy of cardiomyocytes and an increase in interstitial tissue. In the endurance athlete, left ventricular wall thickness is also increased and there are some data indicating that left ventricular cavity size is enlarged. More recent observations suggest that repetitive endurance exercise may result in fibrous replacement of the myocardium. However, as Wilson et al., (2010) point out, in the veteran athlete it is difficult to tease apart the structural cardiac changes that are due to ageing from those due to endurance exercise. In the arterial vasculature, exercise training enhances compliance in the larger vessels and also attenuates age- related wall thickening of peripheral arteries and decreases the wall thickness to lumen ratio of these arteries. Although, cerebral blood flow velocity decreases with age in both athletes and non-athletes, individuals engaged in regular physical activity show an approximately 17% greater cerebral flow velocity at all ages compared to sedentary individuals.

Even within a single species there can be significant variation in the athleticism of different strains. Among dogs, greyhounds are considered athletic animals and heart ratios in greyhounds are greater than those in mongrel dogs (Pape et al., 1986). Pape et al., (1986) studied cardiovascular function in a group of greyhounds trained to race compared to two control groups; greyhounds that had never been trained to race and a group of mixed-breed (mongrel) dogs. The untrained greyhounds and mongrel dogs had comparable mean aortic arterial pressures (117 mmHg and 115 mmHg respectively), similar left ventricular stroke volumes and similar systemic vascular resistances to flow. Mean heart weight to body weight ratio was significantly greater in the untrained greyhounds compared to the mixed-breed group. Trained greyhounds, untrained greyhounds and interestingly greyhound puppies all had similar mean heart weight to body weight ratios. However, trained and untrained greyhounds differed in terms of hemodynamic features. The trained greyhounds compared to the untrained group had a higher mean aortic arterial pressure (126 mmHg versus 117 mmHg), greater left ventricular stroke volume (67 ml versus 42 ml) and a significantly lower systemic vascular resistance to flow (2586 dynes.sec.cm-5 versus 7474 dynes.sec.cm-5).These observations indicate that although the cardiomegaly in greyhounds is developmental, exercise training can significantly alter cardiovascular physiological characteristics.

The data in the human and in the greyhound indicate that endurance training can significantly alter left ventricular function; VO2 max is increased as is maximum heart rate and peak systolic volume. The effects of endurance training on arterial pressure are variable as discussed in the preceding paragraph and the effects of endurance training on cardiac structure are still somewhat controversial. With ageing there are changes in cardiac and vessel wall structure as well as a decline in left ventricular diastolic function. VO2 max and cerebral blood flow both fall with age. Endurance training does not reverse these ageing trends in that the slopes of decline versus age are approximately equivalent in the untrained and endurance trained individual. However, although the slopes are parallel, VO2 max and cerebral blood flow both start from a higher level in the endurance trained subject compared to the sedentary individual. In this sense, endurance training attenuates the effects of the ageing process.

The studies done on the greyhound by Pape et al., (1986) give an additional important insight. Wild animal species engage in specific levels of activity that have been selected by different environmental pressures, such as habitat and food availability. The grey hound has been bred to race and as part of its "racing" phenotype it has developed cardiomegaly when compared to dogs that have not been bred to race. However, the greyhound's racing phenotype is plastic. Greyhounds that are not allowed to race have a lower arterial pressure, lower left ventricular stroke volume and higher total vascular resistance to flow than greyhounds that race. By analogy, when wild animal species are prevented from engaging in the level of activity that has been evolutionarily set for them as for example by being restricted in a zoo, their ageing pattern changes. As noted in the section Atherosclerotic Vascular Disease; Influence of social environment; zoo animals develop similar "health" problems as observed in humans.

Humans have evolved to engage in endurance running and this level of activity was selected by the environmental pressures faced by humans thousands of years ago. However, we as modern urbanized humans have strayed considerably from this evolutionary baseline. Modern urbanized humans, just like captive wild animals, cannot engage in their evolutionarily set level of activity and this reduction in natural activity is one factor that has shaped our modern day ageing pattern. Even though exercise has definite positive "health" benefits, the core problem is that the level of activity of modern humans is well below the level for which our body was designed.

Summary and Perspectives

The simplicity in the measurement of arterial pressure in a human belies the complexity inherit in the actual value obtained. Although we are beginning to clarify the multiple interacting biological systems underlying arterial pressure regulation, the finer details are still unknown. The arterial pressure level is determined by the integration of a number of signals (originating for example from molecular clocks and the renin angiotensin and dopaminergic systems) that input into the regulating center(s). The site of these center(s) is most likely the brain regions that control the autonomic nervous system. For a given species, arterial pressure range is developmentally set. Some of the developmental processes responsible may actually occur in the postnatal period such as the pressure changes that take place in the pulmonary and aortic circuits with the onset of respiration and the increase in the vertical distance between heart and brain that results from postnatal growth. Engrafted upon this phylogenetically based arterial pressure setting is the influence of various environmental cues which act at the level of the individual animal. Some of the most important environmental cues especially in humans include social environment, salt intake and level of activity. The genetic mechanisms underlying the link between an environmental cue and a specific biological process are poorly understood but presumably environmental cues "reset" arterial pressure through an effect on the brain regulating center(s). Social environment appears to "work" through the stress response and the multiple effects of the corticosteroid stress hormones.

The stress response itself is a plastic behavior and can be shaped in offspring by the nature of maternal-infant interactions in early life. Salt appetite is also a plastic behavior that can be modified by the pattern of early life maternal care. In addition, salt appetite is tied into the reward- associated set of behaviors. These two attributes of salt appetite, plasticity and reward seeking behavior result in a decoupling of salt intake from physiological need. As reviewed in the previous section, level of activity has important cardiovascular effects both developmentally and non- developmentally. Endurance training in cursorial mammals improves left ventricular systolic and diastolic function as well as increasing VO2 max. Endurance training, like salt appetite, is a reward seeking behavior. Two other observations need to be added to this biological mix.

First, no two individuals share the same genome and epigenome. There are significant variations across individuals with respect to both DNA sequences and patterns of epigenetic marks. This genetic variation means that individual responses to the same set of environmental cues will differ. Secondly, the systems involved in vascular remodeling (discussed in the section; Atherosclerotic Vascular Disease) such as molecular clocks and stress hormones are also operative in determining arterial pressure levels. Vascular remodeling as a repair process in response to changes in shear stress and vascular remodeling as a repair process initiated by changes in circumferential wall stress (pressure) are largely inseparable and intermixed. Given this complexity in the biology underlying arterial pressure levels, it is not surprising that it is difficult to establish so-called normal values for arterial pressures in humans.

The concept that (essential) hypertension is a disease has been based to a large extent upon the results of large scale epidemiological studies. Essentially these studies can be classified into two broad categories. In one set of studies, statistical associations are drawn between levels of arterial pressure and various cardiovascular endpoints such as deaths from cardiovascular causes. In another set of studies, statistical correlations between arterial pressure reduction by pharmacological agents and changes in the frequency of cardiovascular end points are examined. A wealth of both types of studies has been published in the literature so only three will be considered in this discussion.

Lewington et al., (2002) did a meta-analysis of 61 prospective observational studies that included data on age, arterial pressure and vascular endpoints. Subjects were considered to be free of clinical evidence of vascular disease at the time of enrollment in a study. The total number of participants in the meta-analysis was 958,074.The end points were death attributed to stroke, ischemic heart disease (IHD), other vascular causes and unknown cause. The date or age of death was available for all subjects during more than 5000 person-years of follow up. Participants were divided into 5 age ranges and 10 systolic blood pressure ranges and into 5 age ranges and 6 diastolic blood pressure ranges. The two core observations from this data are that the rates of mortality from stroke, IHD and other vascular causes are statistically associated with age and arterial pressure (systolic and diastolic). In the case of arterial pressure there was no break in the relationship between vascular (stroke, IHD or other vascular causes) mortality and arterial pressure down to values of 115 mmHg systolic and 75 mmHg diastolic. For example in the case of IHD, if subjects aged 40-49 years with a usual systolic pressure of 115 mmHg have an arbitrary mortality rate of 1 than by comparison subjects in the age decade 80-89 years have a mortality rate of 79. For the subjects in the age decade 40-49 years an increase in systolic pressure from 115 mmHg to 180 mmHg increases IHD mortality from 1 to approximately 12. Similar considerations apply to diastolic pressures and mortality rates due to stroke and other vascular causes. In the discussion section of this report, the authors make the following comments. “These relationships with vascular mortality continue steeply down at least as far as a usual systolic blood pressure of 115 mmHg and a usual diastolic blood pressure of 75 mmHg, below which there is little evidence. This refutes the recent suggestion that there might be a threshold level of systolic blood pressure at about 140-160 mmHg (depending on age), below which lower blood pressure levels are not associated with lower disease risks.” “Among people with no previous vascular disease recorded, the usual blood pressure is positively related to the risks of death from vascular disease not only among individuals who might be considered hypertensive , but also among those who would usually be considered normotensive (at least down to usual blood pressure levels of 115/75 mmHg).” The observation that these investigators were not able to demonstrate a break in the log-linear plot of mortality (due to vascular causes) versus arterial pressures down to a value of 115 mmHg systolic and 75 mmHg diastolic indicates that a so-called normal reference level for arterial pressure in humans cannot be defined.

However, the data of Lewington et al., (2002) are subject to a different interpretation. First, it is important to remember that a statistical association does not necessarily indicate a cause and effect relationship between the two correlated variables. In a population of humans there will be a range of arterial pressures. This variation in blood pressure is due to the uniqueness of each individual’s response to similar environmental cues and these cues include those that are operative in the intrauterine milieu and in early life. Variation in the genome and epigenome across individuals and the plasticity of behaviors such as those encompassing the stress response and sodium appetite underlie this uniqueness. Since the biological determinants of arterial pressure are the same biological processes involved in cardiovascular remodeling, it is not unreasonable to expect the two to be correlated. Individuals with higher arterial pressures would be expected to have more evidence of cardiovascular remodeling. This remodeling should be considered part of a repair process with the inciting vascular injuries being changes in shear stress and circumferential wall tension. Environmental cues act on the arterial pressure regulating brain center(s) but the mechanisms are unknown. In fact it is not known what are the critical parameter(s) monitored by these center(s). The higher arterial pressure of some individuals is due to their specific responses to their environmental circumstances and the data of Lewington et al., (2002) indicate that these individuals also manifest more extensive cardiovascular remodeling repair processes. The basis for the statistical association observed in their data is the commonality of the biological processes which underlie both the regulation of arterial pressure and the cardiovascular remodeling repair processes.

In a second category of epidemiological studies, the effects of antihypertensive drugs on cardiovascular endpoints are measured. Since the genome and epigenome of each individual human is unique, the resultant phenotypic variation across humans means that there is no natural control group for inclusion in such epidemiological studies. This situation places constraints on the design of these studies such that they must rely on statistical rather than biological end points. As a result, the interpretation of data from epidemiological studies becomes more difficult since end points that are statistically significant may not necessarily be biologically significant. The study design consists of comparing groups that have been statistically matched at baseline; either matched groups receive different drugs or one group receives a placebo and a matched group receives an active drug.

In a study reported by Staessen et al., (1997), a placebo group was compared to a group receiving three antihypertensive medications; nitrendipine (calcium channel blocker), enalapril (angiotensin converting enzyme inhibitor) and hydrochlorothiazide (diuretic). The mean age of each group was 70 years with a standard deviation of about 7 years. Hence the age range (using two standard deviations) was about 56-84 years. I will consider only one end point; fatal strokes. The placebo group had a rate of fatal strokes of 3.7 per 1000 patient-years. The treated group had a rate of 2.7 per 1000 patient-years. This was a non-statistically significant result. The mean arterial pressures in the treated group were 10 mmHg (systolic) and 5 mmHg (diastolic) lower than in the placebo group. It is interesting to return to the study by Lewington et al., (2002) already discussed. The rate of fatal strokes in those aged 50-89 years with arterial pressures ranging from 115-180mmHg systolic was 1.5 per 1000 patient-years. The Lewington et al., (2002) meta-analysis did not include treated patients. Hence the subjects in the Lewington et al., data set had a fatal stroke rate lower than the rate in the treated group of Staessen et al., (1997).

Wright et al., (2002) compared the effects of three different antihypertensive medications on cardiovascular endpoints. The three matched groups had an age range of 55-85 years using reported mean values and two standard deviations. One group received chlorthalidone (diuretic), one group amlodipine (calcium channel blocker) and the third group received lisinopril (angiotensin converting enzyme inhibitor). Mean arterial pressures were equivalent in the three groups. The rate of fatal strokes in the three groups (per 1000 patient-years) were 2.3 (chlorthalidone), 2.3 (amlodipine) and 2.7 (lisinopril). These three rates are statistically the same but higher than the rate of 1.5 per 1000 patient-years based on the data set of Lewington et al., (2002).

One other study worth considering is the so-called JUPITER trial reported by Ridker et al., (2008) even though this study did not include the use of an antihypertensive drug. In this study two groups were statistically matched; one group received a placebo and the other group received a cholesterol lowering drug rosuvastatin, a HMG-CoA reductase inhibitor. The age range was 60-71 years of age. To simplify the discussion, I will look at one end point; any death. The rate for any death was 10 per 1000 patient-years in the rosuvastatin group and 12.5 per 1000 patient-years in the placebo group; a statistically significant difference. The data set of Lewington et al., (2002) gives a different value. Subjects aged 60-69 years had an all cause death rate of 14.7 per 1000 person-years. The placebo group in the JUPITER trial had a lower death rate than the death rate of a comparably aged group reported by Lewington et al., (2002).

The problems with these studies are rooted in the underlying assumptions. A key assumption is that matching of groups statistically is equivalent to matching them biologically. However, this is not a valid assumption. The JUPITER trial, discussed in the previous paragraph, followed a number of cardiovascular outcomes in the study participants. One of the endpoints was a non-fatal or fatal stroke. Over the study period, the number of subjects experiencing any stroke was 33 in the rosuvastatin group (n= 8901) and 64 in the placebo group (n= 8901). Based upon the assumption that statistical matching is equivalent to biological matching, the extrapolation is made that in the rosuvastatin group, 64 subjects should also have suffered strokes over the study period. However, the rosuvastatin group had only 33 individuals who experienced a stroke and it is therefore assumed that this reduction in the number of strokes by 31 is due to the effect(s) of the rosuvastatin. Is this a valid assumption? Could this difference between these two statistically matched groups in the number of subjects who had a stroke simply reflect the biological variation between these two groups? In fact, the difference in number of strokes between these two groups (although statistically significant) does actually underscore the effect of biological variation. Consider the rosuvastatin group alone. If there were very little biological variation across the individuals in this group, then all of the subjects should have responded to the rosuvastatin, not just 31 out of the 8901 members of this group. The same argument holds for the other cardiovascular end points monitored in this study. Hence, statistical matching of populations is not the same as biological matching. The "statistically significant" effects in these studies reflect weak biological effects at best and these studies should be viewed as hypothesis generating only.

Since both the comparative biological data and the epidemiological data of Lewington et al.,(2002) indicate that a so called normal reference arterial pressure level cannot be defined in humans, then is there really a disease called "hypertension"? I believe the answer is no. The level of arterial pressure and the extent of cardiovascular remodeling (as a repair process) vary considerably from individual to individual. The underpinnings of this variation across individuals are the uniqueness of individual genomes and epigenomes and the differences in individual responses to the same environmental cues. Ageing or more precisely the age-related decline in effectiveness of repair processes also varies between individuals. The apparent association between the height of the arterial pressure and the extent of organ dysfunction is not a cause and effect relationship. These two variables are linked because a common set of biological processes are instrumental in both determining the arterial pressure and in fashioning the structural remodeling of the heart and vascular tree. The data of Lewington et al., (2002) simply indicate that changes in arterial pressure and cardiovascular remodeling vary in tandem; higher levels of arterial pressure appear to be associated with more extensive remodeling. Given these considerations, our current focus on specific arterial pressure levels and our preoccupation with pharmacologically reducing these levels are not justified.

Chapter IV

Diabetes Mellitus (Type 2)

(This discussion will be limited to type 2 Diabetes Mellitus.)

Diabetes has been defined as a disease characterized by abnormal metabolism, most notably hyperglycemia, and an associated increased risk for long term complications affecting the eyes, kidney and nervous system (Nathan, 2009). Three measures of glucose plasma levels are used to define this "disease"; fasting plasma glucose concentration (FPG), 2 hour (post 75 gram oral glucose load) plasma glucose concentration (2 hour glucose) and percent glycated hemoglobin (HbA1C). Unlike arterial pressure levels which demonstrate no break or threshold value when plotted against the rate of mortality from vascular causes (section Hypertension; Summary and perspectives), plasma glucose values do demonstrate a break or threshold value when plotted against the prevalence of retinopathy (Nathan et al., 2009). This threshold value appears to be at a FPG of about 6.0 mM, a 2 hour glucose of about 8.3 mM or a HbA1C of about 6.5%. Above this threshold value, increasing plasma glucose concentrations are associated with a progressive rise in the prevalence of retinopathy. This threshold holds for both cross-sectional and longitudinal studies.

Engelgau et al., (1997) did a cross-sectional study of 1018 individuals in Egypt (Cairo and three rural areas) comparing tests for the diagnosis of diabetes. The test results were compared to the prevalence of retinopathy. All three measures of blood glucose (FPG, 2 hour glucose and HbA1C) showed a break when plotted against the prevalence of retinopathy. Below levels of FPG of 5.6 mM, 2 hour glucose of 9.7 mM and HbA1c 6.5 %, the prevalence of retinopathy was low (about 5%) whereas above the threshold there was a progressive increase in the prevalence of retinopathy reaching a value of approximately 50% at a FPG of 22 mM or a 2 hour glucose of 27.7 mM or a HbA1C of 13%.

McCance et al., (1994) did both a longitudinal and cross-sectional study on tests for diabetes in a population of Pima Indians in Arizona. The cross-sectional study involved 960 males and females, 25 years of age and older. The threshold values were FPG 9.3 mM, 2 hour glucose 12.6 mM, HbA1C 7.8 %. Below these values the prevalence of retinopathy was 0.5-1.3 % and above these values the prevalence was 13.3-16.3 %. The longitudinal study involved 927 subjects free of retinopathy at baseline who were followed for 5 years. The five year cumulative incidence of retinopathy confirmed the utility of these thresholds. Below the threshold values the cumulative incidence of retinopathy was essentially zero. Above the threshold values there was a progressive rise in cumulative incidence of retinopathy reaching a level of about 20% at values of FPG 10.2 mM, 2 hour glucose 18.1 mM and HbA1C 9.1%.

In 1993, the Diabetes Control and Complications Trial Research Group published a study comparing conventional versus intensive insulin therapy in insulin dependent diabetics of 1-5 years duration, age range 13-39 years, who were free of retinopathy at the time of study enrollment. The range of follow up was 3-9 years. The conventional treatment group had a mean HbA1C of 9% while the intensive treatment group had a mean HbA1C of 7%. For the first 3 years of follow up the cumulative incidence of retinopathy was equivalent in the two groups, about 5%. At the three year mark the two groups began to diverge and for the cohort followed for a full 9 years the cumulative incidence of retinopathy was about 50% in the conventional group and about 10% in the intensive treatment group.

An important point to note, however, is that not all individuals with chronically elevated blood glucose concentrations above the threshold value develop retinopathy. As will be discussed in subsequent sections, this observation implies that the diabetic state is not a single phenotype but a collection of phenotypes.

In human populations, the frequency distributions of plasma glucose concentrations have been reported as being bimodal (Loo et al., 1993; McCance et al., 1994; Engelgau et al., 1997; Lim et al., 2002; Fan et al., 2005). This bimodal pattern has been interpreted as indicating that populations naturally segregate into two groups; a normal non-diabetic group and a diabetic group (Lim et al., 2002). In addition, the bimodal pattern has been used as evidence for the existence of two different genotypes; one without and one with diabetes. There are a number of reasons why the finding of a bimodal distribution for blood glucose values within a population is difficult to rationalize physiologically. In the reports cited above, the raw blood glucose concentrations have been log-transformed which reduces the skewness (particularly right sided skewness) one would expect. Statistical modeling was then performed using these transformed values. In fact, if one examines the frequency histograms illustrated in the report by Fan et al., (2005) which contain glucose concentrations in a linear (non log transformed) scale, these distributions conform to a unimodal pattern with right sided skewness. As pointed out by Cochrane (1972), quantitative traits in populations always show a unimodal distribution although usually skewed in some way. Physiologically one would expect that blood glucose concentrations within a population should be unimodal with right sided skewness. The argument underlying this expectation is similar to the one advanced by Gould (1996) to explain why evolution appears to have proceeded in the direction of increasing complexity. The distribution of blood glucose concentrations within a population is squeezed up next to the left wall of metabolically permissible low blood glucose values. If the mean blood glucose concentration is approximately 4 mM, then the blood glucose concentration cannot fall much lower without leading to life- threatening hypoglycemia. Hence the left side of the distribution curve will be steep. Diversity among humans, in terms of blood glucose values, can only be expressed in one direction; increasing values. Hence one would expect the curve to be skewed to the right, as it is (Fan et al., 2005). In addition, since humans evolved in an environment of food scarcity, our metabolic homeostatic mechanisms are designed to defend against energy deficiency rather than energy surfeit as exists in today's environment of food abundance. Hence one would expect behaviors such as excessive intake of high fat and sugar diets and the increase in glycemic levels that occurs with "normal" ageing (Pani et al., 2008) to result in additional skewing of the glucose distribution curve to the right. As expected, the right sided skew is much more pronounced in older populations

(Loo et al., 1993; Fan et al., 2005). Hence, it is much more plausible to expect population blood glucose values to be unimodal in distribution with a pronounced right sided skew.

The data relating blood glucose values in humans with the prevalence of retinopathy suggests that the human at least, is designed to have a blood glucose concentration below a certain value; higher values are associated with micro vascular changes in the retina. The occurrence of micro vascular retinal changes appears to be a function of both the height of the glucose concentration and its duration. What is known about blood glucose concentrations in other species of mammals and in other vertebrates?

Comparative Blood Glucose Values

Polakof et al., (2011) have reported blood glucose values for fish, amphibians, reptiles, birds and mammals. The number of species in the data set ranged from 19 species of amphibians to 511 species of birds. Mean values for blood glucose concentrations (mM) were; fish 3.55, amphibians 2.7, reptiles 5.4, birds 15.6, mammals 7.0. What follows are a few brief comments with respect to blood glucose values in birds, fish and mammals.

Birds have higher blood glucose concentrations than mammals of similar mass (Singer, 2007). The relationship between plasma glucose concentration and log body mass based on a data set of 97 bird species and 162 mammalian species describes two distinct parallel lines with y intercepts of 15.3 mM for birds and 7.6 mM for mammals (Braun and Sweazea, 2008). Published values for individual species vary from 12.1 mM in the chicken to 23 mM in the prairie falcon. These levels are higher than the threshold values in humans diagnostic of diabetes (discussed in the previous paragraph). Nectarivorous birds have extremely high post feeding blood glucose values and levels as high as 42 mM have been measured in Anna's hummingbird after feeding (Singer, 2007).

Fish tend to have low blood glucose concentrations. Soivio et al., (1975) measured arterial blood glucose concentrations in rainbow trout and documented values ranging from 2.5 mM to 3.8 mM. Chavin and Young (1970) measured serum glucose levels in 300 goldfish and the values ranged from 0.71 mM to 5.1 mM with a mean value of 1.6mM. Moon (2001) has pointed out that teleost fish are characterized by glucose intolerance defined as the inability of an organism to rapidly deal with a glucose load. However the time period of hyperglycemia following a glucose load is species and condition dependent. For example, the more carnivorous is the species, the longer the time needed to clear a glucose load. There is some suggestion that marine species are more tolerant of a glucose load than fresh water species. The mechanisms underlying the glucose intolerance in teleosts appear to be multi factorial (Moon, 2001); low metabolic rate in fish compared to mammals, the absence of a detectable (insulin responsive) glucose transport protein in skeletal muscle, undefined interactions in the fish between insulin, glucagon and glucagon- like peptide to cite a few possible factors.

Blood glucose concentrations are quite variable across different mammalian species. The nectarivorous bat, unlike the nectarivarous bird, has a fasting blood glucose concentration of 1.4 mM (Singer, 2007). The long lived naked mole rat, which shows negligible senescence, has a mean fasting glucose concentration of 4mM but displays an abnormal response to the intraperitoneal injection of glucose (2g per kg body weight). The pattern is one of glucose intolerance. Compared to the pattern observed in control mice, the blood glucose concentration in the naked mole rat rises more slowly after the injection and remains higher for a longer time (Buffenstein and Pinto, 2009). For example, at 1 hour post injection, control mice had a mean blood glucose concentration similar to baseline while the naked mole rat still had a mean glucose value of 14 mM. Unlike teleost fish which display glucose intolerance but have adequate insulin levels, the naked mole rat has undetectable insulin levels in the fasting state (Buffenstein et al., 2007). In non-human primates, fasting glucose concentrations are in the range of 3.1-3.6 mM (Wagner et al., 2006).

Even though this sampling of blood glucose concentrations in various animal groups is limited, it is clear that as a group birds have the highest blood glucose values and amphibians the lowest. Two general trends that have been noted are a positive correlation between blood glucose concentration and metabolic rate and a negative correlation between blood glucose concentration and log body mass (Polakof et al., 2011). The wide range of blood glucose concentrations across vertebrate groups are in reality a reflection of differing energy homeostatic systems across these same vertebrate groups i.e. glucose regulation is a component of overall energy balance. The answer to why, for example, a high blood glucose concentration is adaptive for a bird but not a primate will require a much more detailed understanding of energy homeostasis in these two animal groups.

Natural Animal Models of Diabetes

Birds

Birds are clearly natural animal models for diabetes given that high blood glucose concentrations are one of their metabolic characteristics. This hyperglycemia does not lead to any adverse consequences since birds do not experience any micro vascular changes in their kidneys or eyes and the maximum life span of a bird is approximately two and a half times longer than that of a mammal of equivalent mass (Singer, 2007). Glucose regulation in birds has recently been reviewed by Braun and Sweazea (2008) and there are no major differences compared to mammals that might explain the ability of the bird to sustain such high blood glucose levels without developing tissue damage. The structure of the insulin receptor in chicken tissues is very similar to that described in mammals (Dupont et al., 2009). However, insulin signaling in chicken skeletal muscle appears to differ from that of mammals. Chicken skeletal muscle has about thirty fold greater PI3K (phosphatidylinositol 3- kinase) activity than rat skeletal muscle (Dupont et al., 2009). The significance of this observation is unknown. The insulin responsive glucose transporter (GLUT4) has not been detected in avian adipose tissue and it is still controversial whether GLUT 4 is expressed in avian skeletal muscle. In fact no DNA sequence coding for GLUT 4 has been identified in the chicken genome (Dupont et al., 2009). HbA1C levels are low in birds compared to mammals but this low value is probably a function of the shorter lifespan and lower glucose permeability of avian erythrocytes compared to those of mammals (Singer, 2007). In contrast, levels of glycosylated albumin are much higher in birds compared to mammals. Rendell et al., (1985) reported mean glycosylated albumin levels of 2.85% in 3 species of birds and 1.06% in 7 species of mammals including humans. Hence, even though the bird does not have tissue damage from high glucose levels, tissue proteins in this vertebrate are more extensively glycated as a result of exposure to the increased glucose levels.

Overt diabetes mellitus has been observed in birds but this is an unusual occurrence and generally occurs in pet (captive) birds. Pilny and Luong (2005) described diabetes in a captive Chestnut-fronted Macaw. On presentation the blood glucose concentration was 54.8 mM. Insulin administration failed to lower the blood glucose level. At autopsy, the pancreas showed diffuse vacuolar cellular degeneration with infiltration by lymphocytes and plasma cells and the absence of insulin by immunostaining.

Hence, much could be learned by defining the nature of the physiological and metabolic features of the bird that "protect" this vertebrate from the chronic hyperglycemia-induced micro vascular tissue damage as observed in mammals. The bird has clearly been under-utilized as a natural animal model for exploring links between chronically high blood glucose concentrations and changes in the structure and function of the microvasculature.

Fish

By human standards fish display an abnormal response to a glucose load as noted in the previous section (Comparative blood glucose values). Moon (2001) summarized the results of glucose tolerance tests in teleost fish and all species examined showed persistent hyperglycemia following a glucose load although how long the hyperglycemia persisted following the glucose challenge was species and experimental- condition dependent. Since the structure of insulin and its receptor are well conserved across vertebrates including fish, a possible lack of insulin in teleosts does not appear to be the mechanism responsible for the glucose intolerance (Moon, 2001). Moon (2001) notes that insulin receptors do exist in fish skeletal muscle and that hyperinsulinemia down regulates receptor numbers. Apparently a glucose transporter homologue has been detected in trout skeletal muscle but whether it is insulin responsive is unknown.

The zebra fish is emerging as an important natural animal model in a number of fields including endocrinology. Its popularity as a natural model is based on a number of attributes one of which is that its genome has been sequenced (McGonnell and Fowkes, 2006). For example, the pancreas of the zebra fish consists of both an endocrine and exocrine component. Zebra fish genes for glucagons, insulin and somatostatin have been cloned and there is a high level of sequence conservation with the mammalian genes (McGonnell and Fowkes, 2006).

Since the endocrine system of the fish shares many common features with those of other vertebrates, disentangling the factors responsible for the glucose intolerance in fish, which is a natural metabolic feature of this vertebrate group, could help clarify mechanisms underlying insulin "resistance" in other animal groups e.g. mammals.

Naked Mole Rat

The naked mole rat is an extremely long-lived rodent displaying negligible senescence (Edrey et al., 2011a). The unusual features of glucose regulation in this mammal have been noted in the section; Comparative blood glucose values. Briefly, the naked mole rat has a low normal fasting blood glucose concentration, undetectable fasting insulin levels and like fish, a prolonged elevated blood glucose concentration following a glucose load. In addition this mammal shows no age- associated changes in blood glucose concentrations or glucose tolerance test results from ages two to twenty four years (Edrey et al., 2011b). Glycated hemoglobin levels remain low at both ages. Autopsy findings for two females that died at ages 29 and 30 years included; degeneration of the retina and focal interstitial fibrosis in the kidney with some periglomerular fibrosis and increased mesangial tissue within the glomerulus.

There has been speculation that there is a relationship between the extremely long life span of this mammal and its apparent insulin deficiency state (Edrey et al., 2011a). In fact, mutations in many genes in the insulin/insulin-like growth factor-1 signaling pathway can prolong lifespan in model animals (Russell and Kahn, 2007). This relationship between glucose homeostasis and lifespan/ageing is discussed in a subsequent section.

Non-human Primates

Diabetes (generally type 2) has been described in non-human primates (Wagner et al., 2006) although the qualification is that these are captive animals. In one study, Wagner and colleagues fed a group of cynomolgus monkeys a high carbohydrate low cholesterol diet and then characterized their glucose regulatory mechanisms on the basis of an intravenous glucose tolerance test. Out of a total of 35 monkeys, twelve were classified as normal (N), eight showed hyperinsulinemia (HI), ten displayed impaired glucose tolerance (IGT) and five had a combination of hyperinsulinemia and impaired glucose tolerance (HI + IGT). Some of the mean biochemical values for the four groups were; fasting glucose concentration (mM) N= 3.1, HI =3.8, IGT= 3.4, HI + IGT = 4.9; fasting insulin levels (u IU/ml) N= 12.8, HI= 56.5, IGT = 15.1, HI + IGT= 62.7; glucose clearance based on intravenous glucose test (a higher number indicates faster glucose disappearance) N= 5.2, HI= 4.5, IGT= 2.1, HI + IGT= 1.5. Body weight was highest in the HI and HI + IGT groups. Within a year of the study one of the ten monkeys in the IGT group and three of the five monkeys in the HI + IGT group became overtly diabetic. Histological sections of pancreases from diabetic monkeys showed deposits of amyloid in the islets and reduced insulin immunostaining. The extent of these changes depended upon the duration of the diabetes. Interestingly, Wagner and colleagues found that young African green and patas monkeys living under crowded social conditions were more likely to have impaired glucose tolerance than non-crowded controls. However, experimental details for this particular study are not given.

Wagner et al., (2006) summarized the stages in the progression of glucose metabolic impairments in cynomolgus monkeys. The initial stage appears to be one of insulin resistance with compensatory hyperinsulinemia. Glucose clearance falls and then hyperglycemia follows.

The group of cynomolgus monkeys studied by Wagner and colleagues were captive and part of a breeding colony maintained at the Wake Forest University School of Medicine (Wagner et al., 2001). Diabetes occurred spontaneously in this population although Wagner et al., (2001) were not able to estimate the prevalence. Diabetes was initially diagnosed based upon a fasting blood glucose concentration in excess of 7.0 mM. However, approximately

30% of monkeys older than 15 years of age had basal hyperinsulinemia and/or post prandial hyperinsulinemia.

Glucose regulatory mechanisms have been studied in free-ranging monkeys by Howard and co-investigators (1986, 1990). Rhesus macaques from India were introduced onto the island of Cayo Santiago Puerto Rico in 1938. The colony has been maintained through births only, with no new stock being added. By 1976, the colony had become organized into five matrilineal social groups. Animals were provisioned daily with commercial chow although the monkeys were free to forage. Study animals were removed from the colony and transported to the primate research center near San Juan. In 1986, Howard and colleagues reported the results of a study of 150 Rhesus macaques (Macaca mulatta) housed at the primate center. The metabolic parameters measured included; fasting glucose and insulin levels, glucose and insulin levels following a glucose load and a calculated glucose clearance. Morphometric measurements were made for all of the study monkeys. Based on these measured parameters the following impairments were defined; elevated fasting glucose concentration, reduced glucose clearance, altered fasting levels of insulin and altered insulin secretory response to a glucose challenge. Thirty one percent of the studied monkeys displayed one or more impairment of glucose regulation. All of the monkeys were more than six years old but age itself did not correlate with the prevalence of impairments. Body mass and weight were greater in the impaired- compared to the non-impaired monkeys.

In a subsequent report, Howard et al., (1990) compared macaques that had been free ranging on Cayo Santiago Island to macaques housed in corrals or gang cages at the research center. The sample sizes were 127 free ranging monkeys and 173 monkeys at the research center. The prevalence of glucose regulatory impairments was similar in the two groups; 34% of the free ranging monkeys and 28% of the monkeys from the research center.

Although the macaques on Cayo Santiago Island were free ranging, they were not wild. These macaques comprised a dense population and were fed on commercial monkey chow. In contrast, Dunaif and Tattersall (1987) studied a wild population of long tailed macaques (Macaca fascicularis) on the island of Mauritius. This population had existed on the western part of the island for about 400 years. They were highly active and consumed a high- fiber complex carbohydrate diet. The study group consisted of thirty animals that were trapped and tested for impairments in glucose regulation. The prevalence of animals with impairments was 13%; four animals. All four animals showed glucose intolerance and abnormal insulin secretory responses to a glucose challenge. These four macaques were young and not obese.

In the studies performed by Wagner et al., Howard et al., and Dunaif and Tattersall, parameters of glucose regulation were measured in the fasting state and after a glucose challenge. Normal values were then established by calculating means and standard deviations from the data set of measured values. An abnormal value or impairment was defined as a value different from the mean by an arbitrary number of standard deviations. Standard deviation does give an indication of the variance or splay of a measured value across the study group of animals, but the statistical mean has no actual biological reality. The mean represents the average value for a measured parameter in the total group, but no one particular animal is characterized by a parameter with this mean value. In reality, the parameters used to characterize glucose regulation should be considered as comprising a "glucose metabolic" phenotype. Each animal has a unique genome and epigenome and this genetic variation across animals within the population will be expressed as phenotypic variation across these same animals. For example, in the study by Dunaif and Tattersall (1987), there is no biological justification for labeling four animals of the study group as suffering from metabolic impairments. These four animals were simply displaying more extensive phenotypic variation and in a statistical sense were residing at one end of the bell curve distribution.

Individual patterns for glucose and insulin levels following an intravenous glucose test are presented in the reports by Howard et al., (1986) and Dunaif and Tattersall (1987). The patterns are different for each individual even though some individuals have been lumped together as having the same glucose regulatory impairment. These differences in individual patterns underscore the importance of recognizing the significant individual variation that characterizes biological processes.

The influence of environmental cues, particularly social environment, is underscored by comparing the observations of Dunaif and Tattersall (1987) with those of Howard et al., (1986, 1990). The macaques living on Cayo Santiago Island were not wild and had a much different social environment (including food source) than the wild macaques on the island of Mauritius. The pattern of phenotypic variation between these two macaque populations was different. The wild macaque group contained fewer individuals with a phenotype that the investigators labeled as abnormal.

The influences of social environment on arterial repair/remodeling and arterial pressure regulation, were discussed in previous sections; Atherosclerotic Vascular Disease and Hypertension. The non-human primate has been used as a model to examine the effects of social environment on the complex relationships between metabolic characteristics (glucose regulatory mechanisms), obesity, arterial remodeling and arterial pressure regulation. Shively et al., (2009) described a study using female cynomolgus monkeys that were part of a breeding colony maintained at Wake Forest University Primate Centre. The study animals were put in social groups comprising three to five animals and consumed a "typical" North American diet. Female cynomolgus monkeys when placed in a group, organize themselves into social status hierarchies. Within this social hierarchy, subordinate monkeys experience more hostility and have less positive social experiences than dominant monkeys. Subordinate monkeys had a more extensive response to a standard stressor challenge and had higher basal cortisol levels than dominant monkeys. Subordinate monkeys had a higher prevalence of central fat deposition (presumably due to the sustained increase in cortisol production) than dominant monkeys and excessive central fat deposition was found to statistically correlate with higher systolic and mean arterial pressures and with more extensive coronary artery plaque formation.

As discussed in previous sections, these observations of Shively et al., (2009) are consistent with the proposal that the phenotypic effects of an animal's social environment are due to the associated chronic stress with the secretion of increased corticosteroid hormones. Alterations in social interactions that occur for example, in zoo populations (compared to wild animals), animal groups in which their breeding grounds have become contracted or in indigenous rural human populations that are subjected to urbanization, induce phenotypic changes that are engrafted onto the existing phenotype. The details by which the social environment leads to phenotypic changes are unknown but the mechanisms appear to involve stress hormones and the establishment of epigenetic marks that alter gene expression profiles. A number of phenotypic changes appear to be bundled together. This bundling is most likely because there is involved a common set of underlying biological processes. In general, the phenotypic changes induced by social environmental stresses appear to be in a direction that involves for example; more extensive vascular repair and remodeling, an upward resetting of mean arterial pressure, increases in blood glucose concentrations, changes in body fat distribution to name but a few. However, there are exceptions to this generalization and one glaring exception is the naked mole rat. This subterranean rodent is very social and lives in colonies of up to 295 individuals. Male and female naked mole rats carry out communal tasks while reproduction is generally restricted to one breeding female and several breeding males (Edrey et al., 2011a). Yet the naked mole rat has an exceptionally long maximum life span and displays negligible senescence during most of its life.

Biology of Glucose Regulating Mechanisms

Glucose Sensing Mechanisms

Glucose sensing mechanisms have been described in a variety of sites including pancreas, brain, liver, hepatoportal system, carotid body and probably muscle and adipose tissue (Herman and Kahn, 2006; Routh, 2003; Levin et al., 2004). The pancreas and brain have been the sites most thoroughly studied and in general, the models developed have been based on studies done in mammals.

a) Pancreas

Pancreatic B- cells express GLUT 2 glucose transporters and with a rise in extracellular glucose, these transporters facilitate trans membrane movement of glucose into the cell. Within the B-cell, glucokinase (GK) catalyzes the phosphorylation of glucose; there is an increase in glycolytic flux and activation of mitochondrial glucose oxidation. The ratio of cellular ATP to ADP is increased and this leads to closure of ATP sensitive potassium channels. The closure of these channels causes membrane depolarization, opening of voltage dependent calcium channels, influx of calcium and release (exocytosis) of insulin (Schuit et al., 2001). A second glucose sensing signaling pathway independent of ATP sensitive potassium channels has been described but the details are not as well understood (Schuit et al., 2001).For both pathways, glucose entry into the cell is not the rate limiting step for glucose stimulated insulin secretion since the B-cell membrane contains GLUT2 transporters. Glucose phosphorylation by GK is the rate-controlling step (Polakof et al., 2011). GK gene transcription is affected by a number of factors including insulin and GK activity is regulated at the post translational stage mainly by glucose (Polakof et al., 2011).

In contrast to the B-cell, the pancreatic glucagon secreting A-cells are inhibited by an increase in extracellular glucose concentration. The mechanisms underlying this glucose induced inhibition are unknown but possibilities include; inhibition by locally produced substances such as somatostatin and glucose suppression of islet sympathetic nerves which directly activate islet glucagon release through norepinephrine and galanin (a neuropeptide) (Schuit et al., 2001).

The pancreas, specifically B and A cells, represents a well-defined glucose sensor with insulin and glucagon being the effector molecules that act to regulate glucose concentrations.

b) Brain

Approximately fifty years ago glucose sensing neurons were described in the rat brain and were characterized as being either glucose-excited (GE) or glucose inhibited (GI) depending upon whether a rise in extracellular glucose increased or decreased neuronal activity (Levin et al., 2004). Glucose sensing neurons are found within the hypothalamic arcuate nucleus (ARC), ventromedial hypothalamic nucleus (VMN) and the hindbrain nucleus tractus solitarius. The mechanism underlying glucose sensing in GE neurons is similar to that of pancreatic B-cells (Levin et al., 2004). The primary trans membrane glucose transporters in these neurons are GLUT 3 and GLUT 2. Glucose transported into the cell is phosphorylated by hexokinase I and GK. Mitochondrial oxidation of glucose increases the ATP/ADP ratio. ATP binds to the ATP sensitive potassium channel leading to its closure. The cell membrane is depolarized, voltage sensitive calcium channels open and there occurs an influx of calcium. The result is an increase in action potential frequency and neurotransmitter secretion. There are most likely other glucose sensing mechanisms in GE neurons since the ATP sensitive potassium channel is present in non-glucose sensing neurons as well. With respect to the glucose sensing mechanism in GI neurons much less is known (Levin et al., 2004). In one possible mechanism, the rise in extracellular glucose and subsequent increase in the ATP/ADP ratio increases Na, K –ATPase activity and/or the opening of ATP regulated chloride channels (Polakof et al., 2011). These changes would hyperpolarize the GI neuronal membrane and action potential firing would be suppressed.

Although a consensus on the physiological role of neuronal glucose sensing has not been achieved (Levin, 2007; Levin et al., 2004), there is accumulating evidence that nutrient homeostasis is regulated by a complex network involving neurons and endocrine cells (Schuit et al., 2001). One physiological mechanism involving these neurons is the so-called counter-regulatory mechanism in response to hypoglycemia (Routh, 2003). Glucose sensing neurons in the ARC and VMN project directly to the sympathetic preganglionic cell bodies in the spinal cord and parasympathetic (vagal) nuclei in the brain stem. The counter-regulating response to hypoglycemia involves the release of glucagon and glucocorticoids as well as the release of epinephrine from the adrenal medulla. Hence glucose sensing neurons are well situated to integrate and coordinate input signals with a sympatho-adrenal output response.

A number of observations indicate that glucose sensing neurons should really be considered metabolic sensing neurons since they are involved in a much broader range of physiological processes than just glucose homeostasis. The ARC contains two important populations of neurons that are involved in energy homeostasis. One population consists of appetite stimulating cells that express two peptides; neuropeptide Y (NPY) and Agouti-related protein (AgRP), an antagonist of melanocortin receptors 3 and 4 (MC-3 R and MC-4 R) (Schuit et al., 2001; Cowley et al., 1999). Some of these cells also express GLUT 2 and glucokinase (GK) and so qualify as glucose sensing cells. Injection of NPY into the hypothalamus stimulates feeding, regulates peripheral energy metabolism, increases plasma insulin levels and decreases sympathetic nerve activity in brown adipose tissue (Cowley et al., 1999). A second population of ARC neurons (POMC neurons) transcribes the pro-opiomelanocortin gene which codes for the precursor of A-melanocyte-stimulating hormone (MSH), an appetite suppressing peptide. An obesity syndrome has been described in families with a rare mutation in the pro-opiomelanocortin gene (Cowley et al., 1999). These two populations of neurons send projections to the paraventricular nucleus of the hypothalamus (PVN) and Cowley et al., (1999) demonstrated co-localization of NPY and AgRP in the same neuronal processes in the PVN, but no co-localization of NPY and A-MSH within the same neuronal processes in the PVN. However, these studies demonstrated that neurons containing the peptides NPY, AgRP and A-MSH are closely located within the same anatomical area, a feature that would facilitate functional integration of orexigenic and anorexigenic behaviors in response to information as to the animal's nutrient state (Cowley et al., 1999).

Parton et al., (2007) examined the consequences of impaired glucose sensing in POMC neurons. These investigators created transgenic mice with a mutation in a subunit of the ATP sensitive potassium channel in POMC neurons. In hypothalamic slices from wild mice, a reduction in extracellular glucose concentration decreased neuronal firing rate in 50% of tested POMC neurons. (Only a subpopulation of POMC neurons is glucose sensing). In hypothalamic slices from transgenic mice, none of the tested POMC neurons showed a change in activity with a decrease in extracellular glucose concentration. In hypothalamic slices from wild mice, an increasing extracellular glucose concentration resulted in an increase in A-MSH secretion whereas in hypothalamic slices from transgenic mice, an increase in extracellular glucose concentration did not result in a stimulation of A-MSH release. Consistent with these in vitro observations, transgenic mice showed impaired glucose tolerance following a glucose challenge. In an additional study, wild mice were made obese by being fed a high fat diet for 20 weeks. Hypothalamic slices from these obese wild mice were tested for glucose sensing; POMC neurons from these mice did not respond to glucose with an increase in A-MSH secretion. These observations indicate that glucose sensing POMC neurons are involved in systemic glucose homeostasis and that obesity, linked to a high fat diet, can impair glucose sensing in POMC neurons. As pointed out by these investigators, POMC neurons represent only a fraction of glucose sensing neurons. In keeping with the concept that glucose sensing neurons should actually be considered metabolic sensors, these neurons also express receptors for ligands such as leptin and insulin (Levin et al., 2004).These observations underscore the complex interplay between glucose sensing neurons, obesity, and impaired glucose tolerance.

The experimental observations on glucose sensing mechanisms discussed in the previous paragraphs apply primarily to mammals and were obtained almost exclusively in rodent models. However, there is a limited amount of data about glucose sensing mechanisms in other vertebrate groups (Polakof et al., 2007; Polakof et al., 2011). The vertebrate group best studied next to the mammal is fish and in particular teleost fish. In teleosts, there is good experimental evidence for glucose sensing mechanisms in both peripheral B-islet cells/Brockmann bodies and the brain. In addition, the experimental data are most consistent with mechanisms similar to those described in mammals. In amphibians and reptiles there is evidence for pancreatic glucose sensors but no data as to the presence or absence of brain glucose sensing mechanisms. With respect to birds, there are features of pancreatic function that imply the presence of glucose sensors but the high glucose concentrations characteristic of birds makes interpretation of the experimental data difficult. Currently there are no data as to whether brain glucose sensors are present in the bird. As noted by Polakof et al., (2011), the presence and features of glucose sensing mechanisms in a given species might be directly related to the importance of glucose as a metabolic substrate in that particular species. A better understanding of glucose sensing mechanisms in non-mammalian vertebrates would give a broader picture as to the evolutionary history of these sensing mechanisms, at what stage glucose sensing mechanisms and mechanisms sensing the status of other nutrients became localized to the same neurons and what were the environmental pressures driving this evolution.

Insulin/Insulin-like Growth Factor Signaling Pathway (Insulin/IGF Pathway)

The insulin/IGF pathway is a highly conserved signaling pathway with similar key elements in invertebrates and vertebrates (Russell and Kahn, 2007; Taniguchi et al., 2006). The insulin gene superfamily includes three distinct genes for insulin and insulin like growth factors I and II (IGF I and IGF II) (Chan and Steiner, 2000). Structurally, insulin has comparable features across vertebrate groups and for example, hagfish and human insulins share 61% amino acid identity (Chan and Steiner, 2000). IGF I and II are about 70% identical to one another and these factors share about 50% identity with human insulin (Stewart and Rotwein, 1996). Insulin is produced by the B cells of the pancreas and most of the circulating IGF I and II is produced in the liver. Insulin and IGF I and II exert their effects by first interacting with specific receptors. The insulin receptor (IR) and the IGF I receptor (IGF IR) belong to a subfamily of receptor tyrosine kinases and in humans, are widely expressed on normal tissues. Both types of receptors have tetrameric structures containing two predominantly extracellular A chains involved in ligand binding and two predominantly intracellular B chains which contain the tyrosine kinase domain. These receptors function in trans membrane signaling; ligand binding triggers a conformational change that leads to activation of the kinase activity of the B chains. The IGF II receptor is a single chain membrane spanning glycoprotein that does not appear to have signaling properties (Hernandez-Sanchez et al., 2008). In general, in vertebrates, the function of IGF I and II are restricted to regulation of cellular growth (IGF I post natal growth and IGF II fetal growth) whereas insulin has become a metabolic regulatory hormone controlling homeostasis of different metabolites but most prominently glucose (Hernandez-Sanchez et al., 2008).

The insulin/IGF I signaling pathway has been well studied but many details still remain unknown. The IR has two splice isoforms which are usually co-expressed in cells that also express the highly related IGF I R (Taniguchi et al., 2006). There is considerable evidence that the receptors (IR and IGF I R) and not the growth factors (ligands) mediate the pleiotropic cellular responses that follow ligand receptor binding (Schlessinger and Lemmon, 2006). There are many similarities in the signaling pathways encountered downstream of the IR and IGF I R which make it difficult to delineate the basis for the different physiological effects of insulin (metabolic/carbohydrate regulation) and IGF I (predominantly cellular proliferation/growth control) (Pollak, 2008).

Binding of IGF I and insulin to their respective tyrosine kinase receptors leads to phosphorylation of intracellular proteins known as insulin receptor substrate proteins (IRS) (Saltiel and Kahn, 2001). The phosphorylated tyrosines in the IRS act as docking sites for other proteins. There are six IRS proteins and they do not all have the same tissue distribution; IRS 1 and 2 are widely distributed, IRS 3 is largely limited to brain and adipocytes, IRS 4 is expressed in embryonic tissue and IRS 5 and 6 have a limited tissue distribution (Taniguchi et al., 2006). The different tissue distributions of the IRS proteins is probably one factor explaining different cellular effects in different tissues following insulin/IGF 1 receptor binding (Saltiel and Kahn, 2001). The physiological effects mediated by the different IRS proteins are reviewed by Taniguchi et al., (2006). An important protein that interacts with phosphorylated domains in IRS proteins is phosphatidylinositol 3- kinase (PI3K) and this interaction activates PI3K. This enzyme plays a pivotal role in the metabolic effects of insulin including insulin stimulated glucose uptake (via GLUT 4) in skeletal muscle and adipose tissue (Taniguchi et al., 2006). Fuller descriptions of the insulin/IGF I signaling pathway are given by Taniguchi et al., (2006) and Saltiel and Kahn, 2001).

Signaling pathways are no longer viewed as simple linear cascades but rather as complex networks containing critical nodes that participate in cross talk with other signaling networks. Taniguchi et al., (2006) discuss the organization of the insulin/IGF I pathway in terms of three critical nodes; one is the IRS complex of proteins, a second node comprises PI3K kinase and its interactions and a third node is centered around AKT, also known as protein kinase B (PKB), a serine/threonine kinase that is a downstream target of PI3K signaling. PI3K signaling is also central to insulin stimulated glucose uptake via GLUT 4 translocation, in muscle cells and adipocytes. As emphasized by Taniguchi et al., (2006), these nodes represent junctions that allow for cross talk between the insulin/IGF I network and a number of other signaling networks, one example being the mTOR; mammalian (or mechanistic) target of rapamycin network.

The mTOR pathway is a "nutrient" signaling network that senses amino acid levels and energy stores and integrates this information in the regulation of cell growth, protein synthesis and metabolic functions (Stanfel et al., 2009; Zinzalla et al., 2011). mTOR is a serine/threonine kinase, a member of the PI3K related kinase protein family, which forms two complexes by binding to accessory proteins; mTORC1 which contains mTOR and raptor (regulatory associated protein of mTOR) and mTORC2 which contains mTOR and rictor (rapamycin insensitive companion of mTOR) (Stanfel et al., 2009). mTORC1 is activated by AKT/PKB (through a multi-step phosphorylation mechanism)in response to insulin, IGF 1 and other growth factors (Zinzalla et al., 2011).The regulation of mTORC2 is less well understood but growth factors such as insulin, IGF 1 and other receptor tyrosine kinases are involved. Downstream targets of mTORC1 include; 4E- BP (eukaryotic initiation factor 4E binding protein) and S6 kinase 1. Non phosphorylated 4E-BP binds to a translation initiation factor which prevents recruitment of mRNAs to the ribosome. Phosphorylation of 4E-BP by mTORC1 releases 4E-BP from the initiation factor allowing translation to proceed (Schrufer et al., 2010). The S6 kinase 1 is also involved in regulating protein synthesis. Downstream targets of mTORC2 include; PKC alpha, AKT/PKB, SGK1 (serum and glucocorticoid inducible kinase 1) and NDRG 1 (N-myc downstream regulated 1; a protein involved in stress and hormone responses, cell growth and differentiation) (Lamming et al., 2012; Zinzalla et al., 2011). In a recent publication, Lamming et al., (2012), using a mouse model, were able to decouple the functions of mTORC1 and mTORC2 signaling. Basically, disruption of mTORC1 signaling resulted in life- span extension with normal glucose homeostasis, while disruption of mTORC2 signaling resulted in a state of hepatic insulin resistance, impaired ability to suppress hepatic gluconeogenesis, but normal glucose uptake into skeletal muscle and adipose tissue.

Another example of cross talk is underscored by the observation that endothelial cells secrete platelet-derived growth factor (PDGF) which through binding to its receptor increases AKT/PKB activity (the third node of the insulin/IGF1 pathway). AKT/PKB signaling is involved in the recruitment and maintenance of retinal pericytes (discussed in the section; tissue damage).

An interesting question relates to the mechanisms that underlie the different physiological and metabolic effects of insulin and IGF I given that both of these factors appear to feed into the same highly conserved signaling pathway. In vertebrates this pathway is highly complex with both insulin and IGF I having acquired important and diversified metabolic functions beyond their original growth-stimulating role in invertebrates. Invertebrates have only a single receptor which can be considered the orthologue of the mammalian insulin and IGF I receptors (Russell and Kahn, 2007; Wu and Brown, 2006). This single invertebrate receptor binds multiple insulin-like peptides.

Insulin signaling acts primarily to regulate glucose and lipid metabolism by controlling glucose output from the liver , glucose uptake by fat and muscle tissue, and lipogenesis and lipolysis (Saltiel and Kahn, 2001). Insulin, however, also has anabolic functions and can stimulate protein synthesis and cell growth. In contrast, IGF I signaling functions to primarily regulate cell growth, reproductive function and longevity (Dantzer and Swanson, 2012). Insulin is produced in the pancreas whereas IGF I is made predominantly in the liver. As discussed by Dantzer and Swanson (2012), IGF I appears to be an important regulator, across vertebrate groups, of trade- offs involving the life history traits; body size and growth, reproductive timing and output, and lifespan. For example, high growth rates, early age of maturity and high reproductive rates tend to be associated with shortened lifespan. What are the mechanisms that allow IGF I and insulin to elicit such different responses?

A piece of the puzzle lies at the level of the insulin and IGF I receptors. The insulin receptor (IR) and IGF I receptor (IGF IR) were apparently formed by gene duplications from a common ancestor (Hernandez-Sanchez et al., 2008). The structures of human IR and IGF IR were compared by Ullrich et al., (1986) and both receptors were found to have a comparable tetrameric topology. However, there were amino acid differences in both the ligand binding and tyrosine kinase domains. In vitro cell studies appear to point to the cytoplasmic tyrosine kinase domain as mediating mitogenic responses in the case of the IGF IR and metabolic responses e.g. glucose transport, in the case of the IR (Lammers et al., 1989).

A second piece of the puzzle involves the insulin receptor substrate (IRS) proteins. As already noted, the different IRS proteins have different tissue distributions which may help to explain part of the specificity of IR and IGF IR mediated responses. Another part of the puzzle relates to different functions for different IRS proteins, revealed by experiments in mice with targeted IRS gene disruptions. Withers et al., (1998) created mice with a deletion of the IRS 2 gene. Heterozygous mice were normal whereas homozygous mice developed severe fasting hyperglycemia, elevated fasting insulin levels and severe insulin resistance in liver and skeletal muscle. Mice homozygous for the IRS 2 gene deletion showed less insulin stimulated IRS 1 (IRS 2 is absent) activation of PI3K in muscle and liver tissue than wild mice; PI3K is involved in regulating the metabolic actions of insulin. A different phenotype is observed in mice homozygous for the IRS 1 gene deletion (Araki et al., 1994). These mice demonstrated reduced intrauterine growth with birth weights of about 40-60% of that of wild type littermates but normal post natal growth rates. In addition to reduced fetal growth, mice homozygous for the IRS 1 deletion showed a number of metabolic abnormalities when compared to wild type mice; normal fasting blood glucose concentration, high fasting plasma insulin levels , impaired glucose tolerance, reduced insulin stimulated glucose uptake by adipocytes and reduced hypoglycemic response to insulin or IGF I. In contrast to mice deficient in IRS 2, mice deficient in IRS 1 showed enhanced insulin stimulated IRS 2 (IRS 1 is absent) activation PI3K activity in muscle and liver. In summary, mice missing IRS 2 show severe metabolic abnormalities whereas mice missing IRS 1 show a combination of reduced intrauterine growth and metabolic abnormalities that are less profound than those of IRS 2 deficient mice.

The insulin/IGF 1 signaling pathway is one of the better studied intracellular signaling pathways and yet there are still many unknown details. Perhaps the most notable unknown is what mechanisms regulate the differential effects of insulin and IGF 1 given the homology between insulin, IGF 1 and their receptors.

In fact, this question as to how different receptors which appear to share the same signaling machinery produce different phenotypes has been addressed by Miller-Jensen et a l., (2007) and Gordus et al., (2009).

Miller-Jensen et al., (2007) looked at the actions of tumor necrosis factor (TNF) in several cell lines. Their observations were consistent with the following model. The cell specific actions of a cytokine such as TNF originate from the differential upstream activation events induced by the stimulus (e.g. TNF) on its receptor and the receptor associated kinases and transducers. Effector proteins downstream from these receptor associated events could be common to both different cell types and to more than one ligand receptor pair but yet the model still predicted resultant phenotypes which were both cell specific and ligand specific.

Gordus et al., (2009) examined the cellular effects of six different receptor tyrosine kinases (RTK). An individual RTK can induce different phenotypes in different cell types. For example fibroblast growth factor receptor 1 (FGFR 1) induces differentiation in neurons but induces proliferation in fibroblasts. Does this observation indicate that the signaling pathways for FGFR 1 are different in these two specific cell types? Gordus et al., (2009) examined how these six different RTKs behaved when placed in the same cellular context. These six RTKs shared many of the same signaling proteins. However, upstream events involving the recruitment of signaling proteins to the receptor and the number and affinities of available docking sites on the receptor appear to be the major factors conveying the specificity of the phenotype induced by the ligand- receptor interaction. Gordus et al., (2009) reported that despite activating many of the same signaling proteins, the specificity of these RTKs resides in the degree to which they differentially activate upstream signaling proteins. They also noted that the two most important upstream signaling proteins in their model were PI3K and Shc. Shc is an adapter protein involved mainly in growth factor and mitogenic signaling (Ravichandran, 2001). However, Shc probably has other signaling roles since this protein is recruited and targeted for phosphorylation by many different types of receptors (Ravichandran, 2001).

The observations that different receptors share a number of signaling molecules and that a specific receptor uses similar sets of signaling proteins in different cells underscore the principle that evolution is a very economical process. Despite using common sets of signaling proteins, specific receptors can still induce different phenotypes in different cell types and multiple receptors can each induce a different phenotype in the same cell type. Specificity appears to reside primarily in the upstream activation events resulting from the ligand-receptor interaction.

One final note; as reviewed by Pollak (2008) and Nicolucci (2010), there are both laboratory and epidemiological evidence that insulin and IGFs I and II are involved in the process of neoplastic transformation of cells. The initial link between insulin and IGFs with cancer was based on the known capacity of these factors to stimulate cell growth as discussed in the previous paragraphs. Hence, the insulin/IGF I signaling pathway appears to play a pivotal role in seemingly diverse phenotypes; metabolic (particularly glucose) homeostasis, growth, longevity and cancer. In addition, there are also data that dysregulation of mTOR signaling is also involved in carcinogenesis (Hosking, 2012).

Insulin Resistance

Insulin resistance is a key feature underlying type 2 Diabetes Mellitus and this phenotype can be defined as dysregulation of glucose homeostasis due to either ineffective action of insulin or to a faulty insulin secretory pattern. Both possibilities have been included in the definition since experimental results do not always allow discrimination between the two. Alterations in the functioning of the insulin/IGF I signaling pathway have been implicated in the genesis of insulin resistance (Pessin and Saltiel, 2000). One site that has been associated with insulin resistance is the IR itself. Several rare mutations have been described in the IR gene and such mutations have been associated with insulin resistance (Pessin and Saltiel, 2000). A group of proteins known as suppressor of cytokine signaling (SOCS) proteins down regulate IR kinase activity by inhibiting tyrosine phosphorylation of IRS proteins Taniguichi et al., 2006). SOCS proteins have been shown to be up regulated in the insulin resistance observed in obese animals. As discussed by Samuel and Shulman (2012), insulin resistance within skeletal muscle and liver is tied to (ectopic) lipid accumulation within these tissues. Lipid accumulation within muscle cells is associated with accumulation of diacylglycerols (DAGs) and the increased amount of DAGs limits translocation of GLUT 4- containing storage vesicles to the plasma membrane. This effect would be manifest as reduced insulin stimulated glucose uptake by muscle or insulin resistance. Ectopic lipid accumulation within the liver can result in hepatic insulin resistance. The resulting altered hepatic insulin signaling impairs the effectiveness of insulin to promote glycogen synthesis and suppress gluconeogenesis.

Samuel and Shulman (2012) also discuss a possible role of the unfolded protein response (UPR) in mediating hepatic insulin resistance. The UPR is discussed more fully in the section; Dementia. In brief, the UPR is a highly conserved response that is activated in response to an accumulation of unfolded or misfolded proteins in the lumen of the endoplasmic reticulum. The UPR halts protein translation and increases the production of molecular chaperones involved in protein folding. If the situation cannot be rectified, apoptosis occurs. Samuel and Shulman (2012) conclude that there is currently insufficient data to directly implicate the UPR in impairing insulin signaling. However, since UPR appears to be involved in neurodegenerative diseases, impairment in this response could represent a common link between “diabetes” and neuronal “diseases”.

Ultimately, insulin resistance must reside in dysregulation of the insulin/IGF 1 signaling network and its “cross talk” with other signaling networks. However, the underlying mechanistic links between specific experimental models and the insulin/IGF 1 signaling cascade are not always clear. Examples of experimental models associated with insulin resistance include; mice with impaired glucose sensing POMC neurons, disruption of the mTORC 2 signaling network, offspring of mothers fed a diet with reduced nutrient quality during pregnancy, leptin deficiency, adiponectin deficiency, overexpression of Neuropeptide Y and its receptor in adipose tissue, impaired regulation of fibroblast growth factor 1 (FGF 1) by the nuclear receptor peroxisome proliferator-activated receptor gamma (PPAR-g), abnormal signaling from gut microbiota to the host in mice deficient in Toll like receptor 5. The important point is that there are numerous and diverse molecular mechanisms underlying insulin resistance and two individuals with insulin resistance will not necessarily share the same underlying molecular phenotype.

Recently several other mechanisms underlying "insulin resistance" have been described by Greuter et al., (2012), Talchai et al., (2012) and Marcheva et al., (2010).

Greuter et al., (2012) examined the relationship between obesity, impaired glucose tolerance and cardiac regulation of whole body energy homeostasis. A short background digression is necessary to give a framework for the observations of Grueter et al., (2012). Micro RNA 208a (MiR 208a) is a cardiac specific micro RNA coded by an intron of the cardiac specific A-myosin heavy chain gene. Micro RNAs bind to the 3' untranslated regions of mRNAs resulting in repression of mRNA mediated protein translation. One of the targets of MiR 208a is a component of the mediator complex. The mediator multiprotein complex acts as a bridge between DNA bound transcription factors and RNA polymerase II which mediates mRNA transcription. The activity of the mediator complex is modulated by a regulatory unit containing several proteins one of which is MED 13. This regulatory unit interferes with the association of the mediator complex with polymerase II. Med 13 appears to be a target for MiR 208a. Within this framework, inhibition of MiR 208a would lead to overexpression of MED 13.

The experimental observations of Greutner et al., (2012), using the mouse as the study animal, were as follows. Inhibition of MiR 208a reduced fat weight gain in mice ingesting a high fat diet. Whereas the high fat diet- induced obese wild mice had impaired glucose tolerance, high fat diet MiR 208a-inhibited mice had normal glucose tolerance and had lower fasting levels of insulin and leptin then the obese wild mice. Mice overexpressing MED 13 were resistant to obesity when ingesting a high fat diet and this resistance was due to an increase in systemic energy consumption (reflected in an increase in oxygen consumption and carbon dioxide production). Overexpression of MED 13 down regulated a number of genes regulated by nuclear receptors (and in particular thyroid hormone receptor) that are involved in metabolism and energy balance. To summarize, in the heart, MED 13 by hindering the association between the mediator complex and RNA polymerase II down regulates the transcriptional activity of nuclear receptor (and in particular thyroid hormone receptor) target genes involved in energy balance. In addition MED 13 is regulated by the action of MiR 208a through the action of Mir 208a on (MED 13) mRNA translation. Hence, regulation of specific nuclear receptor (and in particular thyroid hormone receptor) target genes by MiR 208a and MED 13 within the heart appears to be part of the complex mix that can result in obesity and impaired glucose tolerance phenotypes.

One of the downstream targets of the insulin/IGF 1 signaling network is the forkhead (FOX) class of transcription factors (Taniguchi et al., 2006).The FOX family contains over 100 members and several of these (e.g. FOX01) are crucial for the actions of insulin. Talchai et al., (2012) developed a mouse strain with a somatic deletion of the FOX01 gene in pancreatic B cells. Metabolic stress in this mouse model induced by pregnancy or senescence led to dedifferentiation of islet B cells and the development of diabetes. In this mouse, diabetes occurred not because of B cell death but by regression of B cells to an endocrine progenitor like stage. A small subset of these dedifferentiated cells underwent conversion to other endocrine cells such as glucagon secreting A cells. The investigators postulated that the dedifferentiation was a "survival" mechanism for these islet B cells that occurred when

FOX01 expression was low or absent. These observations suggest that reduced insulin production in the course of diabetes may not be due to B cell apoptosis but rather to dedifferentiation of B cells with loss of insulin production.

Marcheva et al., (2010) examined the role of molecular clocks in glucose regulation. In one set of experiments, parameters of glucose homeostasis were measured in mice with a (whole body) mutation of the Clock gene. These mice were characterized by elevated blood glucose levels as well as an abnormal glucose tolerance test. Following a glucose challenge, these mice showed a very subnormal insulin response with about a 50% reduction in insulin levels as observed in wild-type mice. Further experimental testing using a number of insulin secretagogues confirmed a defect in insulin release from the pancreas. These Clock gene mutant mice showed other phenotypic changes including obesity and hyperlipidemia. In a second set of experiments, these investigators measured glucose regulation in mice with a defect only in the pancreatic molecular clock; a specific Bmal 1 gene mutation in pancreatic tissue. These mice displayed a more pronounced elevation of blood glucose levels and a more abnormal glucose tolerance test than that observed in the Clock gene mutant mice. The underlying defect in the pancreatic Bmal 1 mutant mice was a diminished glucose stimulated insulin release as observed in the Clock gene mutant mice. Hence, both global (multi-tissue) and tissue –specific (pancreas) molecular clocks are important regulators of pancreatic insulin secretion.

Hence, many mechanisms have been implicated in the genesis of insulin resistance and it is difficult to integrate these mechanisms into a single model. In fact, given the complexity of the insulin/IGF I signaling network, its multiple regulators and its cross-talk with other networks, it is highly probable that multiple mechanisms will underlie insulin resistance in any given individual and that the mix of operative mechanisms will vary from individual to individual.

Other Glucose Regulating Factors

Other factors known to be involved in glucose homeostasis include glucagon, glucagon like peptides and glucose dependent insulinotropic polypeptide (GIP). Most of the data related to the properties of these peptides have come from studies done in mammals.

The vertebrate proglucagon gene encodes three peptides all derived from a common ancestral sequence; glucagon, glucagon-like peptide 1 (GLP 1) and glucagon-like peptide 2 (GLP 2) (Irwin and Wong, 2005). Mammals possess a single proglucagon gene that expresses a single mRNA encoding a single precursor protein that contains glucagon, GLP 1 and GLP 2. Post translational processing of this proglucagon protein in the pancreas gives rise to glucagon and post translational processing in the intestine and brain gives rise to GLP 1 and GLP 2 (Baggio and Drucker, 2007). Glucagon, which is produced by the A cells of the pancreatic islets, is the counter-regulatory hormone to insulin. GLP 1 and 2 are secreted in the mammal by intestinal L cells. In mammals, GLP 1 functions as an incretin, potentiating the release of insulin from pancreatic B cells (Irwin and Wong, 2005). In fish, GLP 1 is secreted from both intestinal and pancreatic cells and has biological activities like that of glucagon. There is much less known about GLP 2 which in mammals appears to act as an intestinal growth factor.

Irwin and Wong (2005) carried out a phylogenetic analysis of proglucagon- derived peptide receptors which are G –protein coupled receptors. In vertebrates, the ancestor to fish and mammals had genes encoding for glucagon and GLP 1 receptors, but the fish lineage when it diverged lost the gene encoding for the GLP 1 receptor. In fish, the glucagon and GLP 1 receptors are duplicates of an ancestral glucagon receptor. Hence in fish, GLP 1 acts like glucagon since its receptor is closely related to the glucagon receptor.

Glucagon receptors have been identified in multiple tissues (liver, brain, pancreas, kidney, intestine, adipose tissue) but from a glucose homeostasis perspective, the important tissue is liver (Jiang and Zhang, 2003). Glucagon is released into the circulation when blood glucose is low. In the liver, glucagon binds to its unique seven- trans membrane G-protein coupled receptor. The binding of glucagon to the receptor activates the coupled G proteins and through a series of steps activates protein kinase A (PKA), a downstream target of the signal pathway. PKA appears to play a pivotal role in the major actions of glucagon which lead to an increase in hepatic glucose output. These actions include; potentiation of glycogenolysis and gluconeogenesis and inhibition of glycolysis and glycogenesis (Jiang and Zhang, 2003).

GLP1 and GIP are known as incretins; these gastrointestinal hormones increase the release of insulin from the B cells of the pancreas. As already noted, GLP 1 is encoded by the proglucagon gene in intestinal L cells, while GIP is produced in intestinal K cells by its own gene (Irwin, 2009). The strong conservation of glucagon across vertebrates is consistent with the notion that glucagon is the primary counter-regulatory hormone to insulin. GLP 1 and GIP show more variation across vertebrates than glucagon implying that these peptides are subject to fewer functional constraints than glucagon; these two hormones (GLP 1and GIP) would appear to be more likely to evolve species-specific functions (Irwin, 2009).

In mammals, GLP 1 has a number of actions (Baggio and Drucker, 2007). In the pancreatic B cells, GLP 1 binds to its receptor and through a series of signaling steps stimulates glucose-dependent insulin secretion; the mechanisms leading to insulin secretion are similar to those outlined in the section, Glucose sensing mechanisms, a) pancreas. GLP 1 also inhibits glucagon secretion from pancreatic A cells. GLP 1 has actions on a number of peripheral tissues as well including the heart, adipose tissue and the brain (Baggio and Drucker, 2007). GLP 1, through a neural mechanism, inhibits food intake and in the stomach, GLP 1 inhibits gastric emptying and acid secretion. The other incretin hormone is GIP. This hormone is encoded by its own gene which is expressed in the stomach and intestinal K cells. The GIP R is a G-protein coupled receptor in the same family as the glucagon and GLP 1and 2 receptors (Irwin and Wong, 2005) and has a wide tissue distribution (Baggio and Drucker, 2007). GIP has a number of biological actions which include; stimulation of glucose – dependent insulin secretion from the pancreas, promotion of neurogenesis in the hippocampus and osteoblast activity in bone tissue.

Although glucose regulation in mammals appears to be reasonably uniform, at least one mammal appears to have very unusual features with respect to glucose regulating hormones; the naked mole rat. The characteristics of glucose regulation in this mammal were noted in the section; Comparative blood glucose values. Briefly, the naked mole rat has a normal fasting blood glucose level but an undetectable fasting insulin level. This mammal also displays an abnormal glucose tolerance test with a prolonged period of hyperglycemia following a glucose challenge. Naked mole rats belong to the suborder hystricognathi in the order Rodentia; a suborder that includes guinea pigs and porcupines among others. Insulin and glucagon peptides have been examined in members of this suborder and have been noted to have unusual properties.

Irwin (2009) looked at the characteristics of glucagon peptides in a variety of vertebrates, two of which (guinea pig and degu) belonged to the suborder hystricognathi. Compared to human glucagon, guinea pig and degu glucagon showed five amino acid differences. This was the largest difference Irwin noted between glucagon sequences from different animals. The second largest difference was of four amino acids between the shrew and zebra finch glucagons. GLP 1 sequences were the same in the guinea pig, degu and human whereas GLP 2 had one amino acid different in the guinea pig and two in the degu compared to human GLP 2.

Hystricognathi insulins have a variable number of amino acid substitutions compared to other mammalian insulins. Referenced to human insulin, guinea pig insulin differs by eighteen amino acids, chinchilla by seven and casiragua by twenty (Conlon, 2001). However, there is no particular amino acid replacement pattern in the hystricognathi rodent insulins that is characteristic of this suborder (Beintema and Campagne, 1987). Zimmerman et al., (1974) reported on the biological activity of guinea pig insulin compared to bovine insulin using fat cells from rats and guinea pigs. Guinea pig insulin was about one tenth as active as bovine insulin in this in vitro system, but interestingly guinea pig insulin had almost 40% the potency of bovine insulin in lowering blood glucose concentration in guinea pigs. Horuk et al., (1979) looked at insulin and insulin receptors in several rodents belonging to the hystricognathi suborder; casiragua, coypu, guinea pig, and chinchilla. Horuk et al., (1979) noted that bovine insulin had a much greater binding affinity to casiragua liver plasma membranes and guinea pig liver plasma membranes than did casiragua and guinea pig insulins themselves. In addition, these investigators used an in vitro fat cell preparation to measure insulin stimulated glucose uptake and conversion into fat. Hystricognathi rodent insulins (casiragua and guinea pig) had less than 10% the biological activity of bovine insulin in a fat cell preparation of their own (casiragua or guinea pig) cells. Hence, bovine insulin binds more strongly to hysticognathi insulin receptors and stimulates more biological activity than hystricognathi rodent insulins themselves.

The amino acid substitutions in the hystricognathi insulins have rendered these insulins incapable of binding zinc and forming hexamers (Beintema and Campagne, 1987; Horuk et al., 1980). Hexamer formation is a characteristic property of most mammalian insulins. The hexamers are stabilized by hydrophobic interactions between surface residues of the monomers and coordination of two zinc atoms by histidine residues occurring at position 10 of the insulin B chain. Hexamers are the storage form of insulin in the storage granules of the pancreatic B cells.

In summary, hystricognathi rodent insulins have much less biological activity (specifically metabolic effects) than most other mammalian insulins and have also lost the capacity to self-associate. The naked mole rat is a member of the hystricognathi suborder but unfortunately its insulin has not been sequenced nor has its biological potency been specifically measured. However, one would predict that the insulin from the naked mole rat would have less biological potency than bovine insulin and probably is incapable of self-association. Edrey et al., (2011b) have reported several properties of insulin in the naked mole rat in agreement with these predictions. First the pancreas of the naked mole rat contains abundant insulin secreting B cells in the islets; hence the abnormal glucose tolerance test in this mammal is not due to non-availability of insulin. Secondly, the naked mole rat is extremely sensitive to exogenous insulin; this observation is consistent with the finding that bovine insulin has greater biological activity in hystricognathi rodents than their own insulins. Assuming that the insulin of the naked mole rat has properties similar to that of other hystricognathi rodents, the relationship between these properties and the unusual glucose homeostasis and negligible senescence of this mammal is clearly a research question that needs to be explored.

Although most of our knowledge of the biology of glucagon and the incretin hormones comes from studies in mammals and in particular rodent models, there are data from non-mammalian studies. Richards and McMurtry (2009) reviewed the characteristics of the proglucagon system in birds, although most of the data come from studies using a single species; the chicken. The avian and mammalian glucagon and incretin hormone systems appear to be quite similar but there are some specific differences. In mammals, the proglucagon gene expresses a single mRNA transcript which gives rise to a single precursor protein. Post translational processing of this single protein yields the glucagon, GLP1 and GLP 2 peptides. The chicken proglucagon gene expresses multiple mRNA transcripts. Two classes of mRNA transcripts have been identified which give rise to two different precursor proteins. Post translational processing of these two precursor proteins yields the peptides glucagon and GLP 1 from the one protein and glucagon, GLP 1 and GLP 2 from the other. These peptides (glucagon, GLP 1 and GLP 2 are produced in high levels in the pancreas and proventriculus. The chicken glucagon, GLP 1 and GLP 2 receptors share 70%, 78% and 65% amino acid identity with the human counterparts respectively. The tissue distributions of these receptors are somewhat different in the chicken compared to the mammal. Glucagon appears to have similar biological actions in the chicken and mammal; increases hepatic glycogenolysis, lipolysis and gluconeogenesis. Glucagon levels are in general much higher in birds than mammals. GLP 1 in chickens inhibits gastric emptying and acid secretion and also suppresses appetite and food intake. Although GLP 1 receptor mRNA has been detected in the chicken pancreas, an incretin effect (stimulation of glucose dependent insulin secretion) has not been experimentally demonstrated in the chicken. GLP 2 receptors are present in the chicken but a physiological role for GLP 2 has only been determined in mammals. How these differences between the avian and mammalian glucagon and incretin hormone systems relate to the higher blood glucose values characteristic of birds as compared to mammals is presently unknown.

The glucose dependent insulinotropic polypeptide (GIP) has been identified as a mammalian incretin hormone. Musson et al., (2009) examined the pattern of GIP in a model fish species, the zebra fish. In contrast to mammals in which GIP is principally expressed in the intestine, in zebra fish, GIP (zfGIP) is expressed chiefly in the pancreas where it co-localizes with insulin. The zebra fish and mammalian GIP peptides share a 36% identity in amino acid sequences; sufficient identity that zfGIP can activate mammalian GIP R. However a specific zfGIP R has not been identified. What was initially thought to be a GIP R in the zebra fish was actually more similar to a glucagon receptor. There is no evidence that GIP functions as an incretin hormone in the zebra fish; more likely GIP acts as a glucagon mimetic. In fish, GLP 1and GIP both function as glucagons since specific GLP 1 and GIP receptors did not evolve until after the divergence of fish and mammals.

Phylogenetic analyses can give valuable insights into the biological functions of the peptide hormones regulating glucose homeostasis. Fish possess the peptides glucagon, GLP 1 and GIP, but express essentially a single glucagon-type receptor. In the fish all three peptides appear to have similar glucagon-like actions. This functional pattern of peptides fits with the observation that fish are considered glucose intolerant and that insulin secretion is regulated more by amino acid secretogogues than by glucose (Musson et al., 2009). Birds produce glucagon, GLP 1, GLP 2 and GIP (Irwin, 2009). The bird has evolved specific receptors for glucagon and GLP 1 but an incretin role for GLP 1 has not been demonstrated in the bird. As far as I am aware, an avian GIP receptor has yet to be identified. The bird is characterized by high blood glucose values and presumably this functional pattern of peptides is consistent with its lack of "tight" glucose control. In mammals, glucose homeostasis is regulated by a complex interplay between insulin, glucagon and the incretin hormones GLP 1, GLP 2 and GIP. These ligands bind to their respective specific receptors which mediate the differential effects of each ligand. This complex system in the mammal fits with the observation that in general glucose is highly regulated in the mammal.

Stress Hormones

Corticosteroids represent the major stress hormones and the biological effects of these hormones on vascular repair/remodeling and arterial pressure regulation have been discussed in the sections; Atherosclerotic Vascular Disease and Hypertension. Glucocorticoids also have a number of metabolic effects e.g. promoting hepatic gluconeogenesis, which result in an increase in blood sugar concentration. The metabolic actions of glucocorticoids are partly mediated through serum and glucocorticoid inducible kinases (SGK) (Lang et al., 2006). Three SGK isoforms have been identified, SGK 1, SGK 2 and SKG 3, with the SGK 1 isoform being the best studied with respect to physiological functions. SGK1 is one of the downstream targets of mTORC2 (Zinzalla et al., 2011). SGKs are expressed in a wide variety of species and in mammals in virtually all tissues that have been tested. SGKs appear to be important regulators of ion channel activity, transport and gene transcription. The promoter for the mammalian gene for SGK 1 contains a number of transcription binding sites including one for the glucocorticoid receptor and one for the mineralocorticoid receptor. SGK 1 has been shown to increase the activity of the Na-glucose cotransporter (SGLT 1) and the glucose transporter GLUT 1 (Lang et al., 2006). The acute inhibitory effect of glucocorticoids on insulin release from pancreatic B cells is mediated by glucocorticoid up regulation of SGK 1 (Lang et al., 2006). The metabolic effects of glucocorticoids on glucose regulation have been well studied. However, experimental observations can sometimes be quite difficult to interpret.

Trenzado et al., (2003) examined the metabolic effects of acute confinement stress on two strains of rainbow trout (created by selective breeding) with divergent cortisol responses to standardized stressors; high (HR) and low (LR) responses. (These two strains of rainbow trout were previously described in the section; Atherosclerotic Vascular Disease; Stress hormones.) In these experiments, HR and LR fish were stressed by being transferred from a holding to a confinement tank and then being held in the confinement tank; stocking density of approximately three times that of the holding tank. Tissue and blood samples were obtained at 2, 6, 24, 168 and 336 hours of confinement and assay values were compared between HR and LR fish as well as with control fish. HR fish had a brisker cortisol response than LR fish with plasma cortisol levels being about three times higher at 2 hours in HR compared to LR fish. By 24 hours plasma cortisol levels were equal in both strains and by 168 hours of confinement cortisol levels were back to near baseline in both groups. Both HR and LR fish demonstrated a rise in plasma glucose concentration which peaked at the 24 hour time point. However, the peak value was higher in LR (18 mM) than in HR fish (9 mM). Plasma lactate and amino acid levels increased during confinement with the peak values occurring at time points 2 hours and 24 hours into confinement. LR fish had greater lactate and amino acid responses than HR fish. At 24 hours into confinement, the abundance of hepatic cortisol receptors was significantly reduced in HR and LR fish compared to controls but equal in both the HR and LR groups. These experimental observations demonstrate a definite metabolic response of these fish to acute confinement stress, but interestingly the robustness of the response was greater in the LR compared to the HR fish. The differences in the metabolic response of LR and HR fish to stress is not explicable on the basis of differences in plasma cortisol levels or cortisol receptor numbers between these two groups. The underlying basis for the divergent metabolic stress response between HR and LR fish is not clear but the implication is that breeding of these two strains for high and low cortisol responses to stress has also coincidentally selected these two strains for (as yet) undefined additional phenotypes that are involved in the stress response. These observations underscore the complexity of the stress response and also imply that other phenotypes may be selectively linked to the high stress responder phenotype.

Feeding, Adiposity and Metabolic Homeostasis

Investigating the inter-relationships between feeding, adiposity and metabolic homeostasis has become an extensive and expanding field of research. However, a framework defining these inter-relationships is beginning to take shape. As background to this discussion, it is important to remember that in humans, appetite, feeding and metabolic homeostasis all evolved under the pressure of an environment of food scarcity not one of food abundance, the situation that currently exists.

Although, much of the data on metabolic homeostasis comes from studies using mammals, many of the signaling networks and genes involved have been conserved across vertebrate groups and as reviewed by Schlegel and Stainer (2007) much can be learned from worms, flies and zebra fish about human energy metabolism.

In the section on Glucose sensing mechanisms b) brain; populations of hypothalamic neurons that express appetite promoting or appetite suppressing peptides were discussed. As reviewed by Schwartz (2001), insulin and the adipocyte- cytokine leptin regulate the actions of these neuron populations. Infusion of leptin or insulin into the cerebral ventricular system leads to a decrease in food intake. The hypothalamic arcuate nucleus is an area of the brain rich in leptin and insulin receptors and it is also the location of two populations of neurons; one expresses neuropeptide Y and agouti related peptide (NPY neurons) and one expresses melanocortin peptides (POMC neurons). NPY is a potent orexigen (appetite stimulant) while melanocortins inhibit appetite and food intake. The agouti related peptide blocks melanocortin receptors and hence acts as an appetite stimulant similar to NPY. Hence, these and other observations underlie the construct that information concerning changes in energy balance and fat mass are transmitted by insulin and leptin to these specialized populations of hypothalamic neurons. Peptides expressed by these neurons regulated appetite and food intake thereby restoring energy balance and fat mass to previous baseline values. Again, it is important to recall that this physiological mechanism evolved to defend metabolic balance and fat mass under conditions of food scarcity. This same physiological mechanism will result in different and most likely adverse effects in a setting of food excess, as are the present day circumstances.

In recent publications, more details concerning this "core" appetite and feeding mechanism have been reported. Wu et al., (2012) examined in mice the neuronal circuits related to hypothalamic NPY/agouti-related protein- expressing neurons. The NPY/agouti neurons express gamma-aminobutyric acid (GABA) and send inhibitory (GABA) signals to a sub population of glutamatergic neurons in the hypothalamic parabrachial nucleus (PBN). Unopposed activity of these PBN neurons, achieved by ablation of NPY/agouti neurons, resulted in cessation of appetite and food intake. The PBN glutamatergic neurons were excited directly by a population of glutamatergic neurons in the nucleus tractus solitaries (NTS) which neurons in turn were excited by serotonergic neurons located more caudally. These various neuron populations also receive information related to the metabolic status and energy balance of the animal, which information inputs into the balance of neuronal activity determining feeding behavior. For example NPY/agouti neurons carry receptors for insulin and leptin which indicates that these peptides can communicate "metabolic" information to these neurons. In summary, this circuitry defines a complex mechanism located in the hypothalamus which regulates feeding behavior. A subpopulation of glutamatergic neurons in the PBN inhibits feeding and these neurons are in term activated by glutamatergic neurons in the NTS and more caudally located serotonergic neurons. The NPY/agouti neurons in the arcuate nucleus restore feeding by inhibiting this population of glutamatergic neurons in the PBN. Hormonal peptide signals feed into the neurons in the NTS and arcuate nucleus (NPY/agouti neurons) so that feeding behavior can be adjusted appropriately for the metabolic state and energy balance of the animal.

This core appetite and feeding mechanism is part of a larger more elaborate system which regulates feeding behavior. This more elaborate system includes feeding behaviors that are not driven by metabolic need and endogenous signals of nutrient depletion but rather by other factors that include environmental cues (Berthoud et al., (2011). The non-metabolic aspects of feeding are based upon a variety of sensory stimuli, emotional states and reward-seeking behaviors. Dopaminergic neurons play a significant role in the reward –seeking behaviors involved in food ingestion. The non-metabolic aspects of feeding behaviors share a number of the features described for salt appetite and salt ingestion behaviors (discussed in the section; Hypertension, Social environment b) salt intake). In fact, the same neural mechanisms most likely underlie non- metabolic feeding behaviors and non-physiologic salt appetite and salt ingestion behaviors. As stressed by Berthoud et al., (2011), the evolved inherent bias of the homeostatic regulatory system is to defend against energy depletion more strongly than energy surplus. This same observation would apply to the salt homeostatic mechanism as well.

As discussed in the section on salt intake (section Hypertension), one of the determinants of an offspring's salt appetite is the salt intake of its mother during pregnancy and the early post-partum period. A similar observation has been described for feeding behaviors; offspring feeding behaviors can be determined by maternal nutritional intakes during pregnancy.

George et al., (2012) conducted an interesting series of experiments on ewes and their offspring. From days 28 to 78 of pregnancy, dams were fed either 50% (NR group) or 100% (C group) of the National Research Council (NRC) dietary nutrient recommendations. Beginning on gestation day 79 the NR group was realimented to 100% of the NRC recommendations. The 100% diet was maintained in both NR and C groups for the remainder of pregnancy (total gestational period about 150 days) and lactation. Offspring birth weights were similar in both groups. For the next six years, the offspring from both maternal groups (NR and C) were fed regulated amounts of NRC recommended diets. At six years of age, female offspring from both maternal dietary treatment groups were studied. The study period consisted of an eleven week period during which these female offspring were allowed ad libitum feeding. Study parameters included; feeding behaviors, body weight changes, intravenous glucose challenge with assays for insulin and glucose levels, leptin and cortisol plasma levels and body composition (lean tissue and fat) measured by X- ray absorptiometry. At the beginning of the eleven week period of unlimited food intake both NR and C offspring had similar body weights, fasting glucose and insulin levels as well as comparable body compositions. During the unlimited food intake period the feeding behaviors of the two groups differed. Average daily feed intake and feed efficiency (weight gained per unit feed consumed) were both higher in the NR offspring. As a result the NR offspring gained significantly more body weight than the C offspring during the eleven week period. Percent body fat gained was increased in both groups of offspring to the same extent. During the eleven week feeding period, fasting blood sugar levels were comparable in the NR and C groups, but fasting plasma insulin, cortisol, and leptin levels were higher in the NR offspring. An intravenous glucose challenge elicited different responses in the NR and C offspring. Insulin sensitivity was lower in the NR group and the NR group showed a much greater increase in insulin levels in the first 10 minutes following the glucose challenge. The hyperinsulinemia of NR offspring noted during the feeding period and the reduced insulin sensitivity of the NR offspring to a glucose load are indicative of a state of insulin resistance in these animals.

This study reports several very interesting observations. First, the data demonstrate that when NR offspring were fed only to metabolic requirements there were no differences in body weight or fasting levels of glucose or insulin compared to the C offspring. Only when both groups were allowed unlimited food intake did differences between the two groups become evident. During this period, the NR offspring gained more weight and displayed higher levels of insulin, cortisol and leptin than the C offspring. When challenged with a glucose load, the NR offspring displayed features of insulin resistance. A second important observation is that the metabolic phenotype of an animal can be determined during intrauterine development by the quality and quantity of nutrient ingestion by the mother during pregnancy. This observation is consistent with the "thrifty phenotype" hypothesis (George et al., 2012) and in addition echoes the observations that the stress response of offspring can be determined by the quality of maternal care during the early post-partum period and that the salt appetite of offspring can be set by the quantity of salt ingested by the mother during pregnancy. These examples clearly demonstrate that the nature of maternal behaviors can have a profound influence on the nature of their offsprings' behaviors and metabolic state.

Adipose tissue by virtue of its endocrine functions plays both a dynamic and central role in the area of metabolic homeostasis. Kershaw and Flier (2004) reviewed the endocrine functions of adipose tissue and their metabolic consequences. Adipose tissue secretes a number of peptide hormones and also contains enzymes involved in steroid hormone metabolism. Adipose tissue depots can be subcutaneous or visceral in location and the differences in the metabolic effects between these two fat depots are believed to be due to their different anatomic locations; visceral adipose tissue secretes peptide hormones into the portal system while subcutaneous fat secretes endocrine peptides into the systemic circulation.

One of the first adipocyte peptide hormones described was leptin. Secretion of this peptide is greater from subcutaneous relative to visceral adipose tissue, but the circulating level of leptin is directly proportional to the total amount of fat in the body. Leptin expression is increased by a number of factors including insulin, glucocorticoids estrogens and its expression is decreased by activated peroxisome proliferator-activated receptor (PPAR) gamma. Leptin acts as an appetite suppressant by inhibiting the activity of NPY/agouti neurons and increasing the activity of neurons expressing melanocortin peptides. As noted by Kershaw and Flier (2004), the leptin-appetite and food intake mechanism is more sensitive to starvation than overfeeding i.e. the primary role of leptin is to regulate energy sufficiency not excess. Leptin levels rapidly decline with caloric restriction and weight loss and the most sensitive portion of the leptin/energy sufficiency dose- response curve lies in the physiological range between energy deficiency due to food restriction and energy sufficiency achieved by refeeding and not in the supraphysiological range associated with obesity. Leptin can also be considered an insulin sensitizing peptide since leptin deficient mice are not only obese but also insulin resistant (Kubota et al., 2002). Leptin also has other biological actions not directly related to energy homeostasis; promotion of angiogenesis by increasing levels of vascular endothelial growth factor (VEGF) and regulation of reproductive function and immune function.

A second peptide hormone expressed in adipocytes is adiponectin (Kershaw and Flier, 2004). As with leptin, adiponectin expression is higher in subcutaneous than visceral adipose tissue. This peptide exists in multiple isoforms as a result of extensive post-translational modification and can exist as full length or as a smaller globular fragment. Adiponectin has been identified as having an insulin-sensitizing effect (Kodowaki and Yamauchi, 2005). In an insulin resistant lipo-atrophic mouse model, the insulin resistance was completely reversed by physiological doses of leptin and adiponectin but only partially by either alone. Adiponectin improves insulin sensitivity in liver and skeletal muscle by a number of mechanisms as described by Kershaw and Flier (2004) and Kodowaki and Yamauchi (2005).

The contrasting biological actions of leptin and adiponectin were demonstrated by Kubota et al., (2002). These investigators studied mice that had been made either heterozygous or homozygous for adiponectin deficiency. At 6 weeks of age both homozygous and heterozygous adiponectin deficient mice exhibited body weight gain similar to wild type mice. This is in contrast to homozygous leptin deficient mice which become quite obese. The adiponectin deficient mice were insulin resistant with the homozygous mice showing a greater degree of resistance than the heterozygotes. After ingestion of a high fat diet, heterozygotes and wild type mice showed comparable weight gains. The high fat diet appeared to increase the insulin resistance of the adiponectin deficient mice with the homozygous deficient mice having greater resistance than the heterozygous mice. As noted by Kubota et al., (2002), leptin plays a much greater role in the regulation of appetite, weight gain and energy balance than adiponectin. However, leptin and adiponectin also have overlapping functions since both peptides act to promote insulin sensitivity.

Adipose tissue also contains the enzyme 11 beta- hydroxysteroid dehydrogenase which converts inactive glucocorticoid metabolites to hormonally active forms; cortisol in humans and corticosterone in mice. Overexpression of this enzyme in adipocytes of a mouse model leads to visceral obesity and insulin resistance even though circulating glucocorticoid levels remain normal (Kershaw and Flier, 2004).

In addition to its capacity to secrete peptide endocrine hormones, adipose tissue also regulates metabolic and energy balance through a system of complex inter-related molecular events occurring within adipose tissue itself. There is an extensive body of experimental studies in this area so what follows is only a brief discussion of some of the mechanisms operative within adipose tissue itself that help to regulate metabolic homeostasis. However, even this limited number of studies underscores the complexity of the multiple interacting biological processes at work within adipose tissue.

Although increased activity of NPY and its receptors in the brain have been reported in a number of experimental models of obesity, Kuo et al., (2007) examined whether NPY had specific actions in adipose tissue. In an in vitro cell culture preparation of preadipocytes and endothelial cells, NPY (acting through its receptor NPY2R) stimulated proliferation of preadipocytes and endothelial cells as well as promoting adipogenesis (differentiation of preadipocytes). In another set of experiments, Kuo et al., (2007) fed mice a high fat and sugar diet (HFS) and subjected them to a standardized cold water exposure stress (immersion in cold water for one hour per day for between 14 and 90 days). These mice developed gross obesity with evidence of impaired glucose tolerance and increased plasma levels of insulin and leptin. These mice also showed up regulated expression of NPY and its receptor NPY2R in white adipose tissue. The source of the NPY in fat tissue is believed to come from sympathetic nerves as well as macrophages. Mice treated with an antagonist to NPY2R and fed a HFS diet plus being exposed to the cold-stress, developed less obesity and showed improved glucose tolerance compared to the HFS diet/cold stress mice that did not receive the NPY2R antagonist. The cold exposure stress up regulated the enzyme 11B-hydroxysteroid dehydrogenase in (white) adipose tissue. This enzyme converts inactive corticoid metabolites to the active form (cortisol in humans, corticosterone in mice) and as a result, the fat content of corticosterone was increased. Glucocorticoids up regulate the expression of the genes for NPY and its receptor NPY2R and hence this mechanism is probably responsible for the increased amounts of NPY and its receptor in adipose tissue. These observations of Kuo et al., (2007) indicate that within fat tissue, NPY plays a significant role in the genesis of diet plus stress induced obesity and the metabolic syndrome.

The nuclear receptor peroxisome proliferator-activated receptor gamma (PPAR-g) is a key factor in the differentiation and maintenance of adipocytes. To clarify the role of this nuclear receptor, Sugii et al., (2009) created transgenic (TG) mice with a gain of function form of PPAR-g; a significant level of transgene was expressed in adipose tissue. TG and wild mice fed a high fat diet for 12 weeks showed comparable increases in weight and fat mass, but the TG mice displayed enhanced insulin sensitivity on testing. TG mice (compared to wild mice) had lower fasting glucose and insulin levels. Leptin levels were also lower in the TG mice but adiponectin levels were comparable in TG and wild mice. Adipose tissue from TG mice fed a high fat diet had smaller but more numerous adipocytes than high fat diet-fed wild mice. Genes that were up regulated in the adipose tissue of TG mice (compared to wild mice) were ones involved in the insulin/IGF 1 signaling pathway; insulin receptor substrate proteins 1 and 2, PI3K, and GLUT 4. The experimental observations reported in this study indicate that transgenic activation of PPAR-g improves insulin sensitivity in adipose tissue by increasing the expression and post translational activation of key insulin signaling components.

In a related study, Jonker et al., (2012) defined additional mechanisms linking adipose tissue PPAR-g and metabolic homeostasis. These investigators reported that fibroblast growth factor 1 (FGF 1) is selectively induced in visceral white adipose tissue in mice fed a high fat diet (HFD). FGF 1 exists as two alternative splice variants (a and b) and it was the "a" variant (FGF 1a) that was selectively expressed in mice fed a HFD. When mice deficient in FGF 1 (FGF 1 -/-) were fed a HFD they showed equivalent changes in weight and serum levels of leptin and adiponectin as wild type mice fed a HFD. However, compared to wild type mice, the FGF 1-/- mice displayed increased fasting levels of glucose and insulin and an abnormal glucose tolerance curve; features of insulin resistance. In addition FGF 1 -/- mice fed a HFD had a fatty liver and structurally abnormal fatty tissue. Feeding FGF 1-/- mice a HFD was associated with up regulation of a number of genes (including those for VEGF and PPAR-g) in visceral adipose tissue. Further testing indicated that the increased HFD –induced expression of the nuclear receptor PPAR-g in adipose tissue was responsible for the up regulation of FGF 1a observed in the adipose tissue of mice fed a HFD. The promoter region of the FGF 1 gene contains a PPAR response element (PPRE) to which the nuclear receptor PPAR binds. This PPRE is functionally conserved across a number of mammals. In summary, feeding a HFD to mice leads to up regulation of PPAR-g in visceral adipose tissue. This nuclear receptor binds to the PPRE in the promoter region of the FGF1 gene and increases the expression of the splice variant FGF1a. Loss of the FGF 1 gene is associated with severe insulin resistance, a fatty liver and structurally abnormal adipose tissue.

The studies by Kuo et al., (2007), Sugii et al., (2009) and Jonker et al., (2012) indicate that PPAR-g- FGF 1 interactions in adipose tissue are important for maintaining insulin sensitivity while glucocorticoid-NPY (and its receptor NPY 2) interactions promote obesity and insulin resistance when the animal is fed a high fat/sugar diet and is under stress. These observations underscore the complex molecular events that occur within adipose tissue that regulate the size and function of this tissue and as well regulate the metabolic effectiveness of insulin. Add to this mix the endocrine functions of adipose tissue and it becomes clear that this tissue plays a pivotal and dynamic role in the maintenance of metabolic/energy balance.

Another Layer of Complexity

In recent years, a new layer of complexity has been added to our understanding of metabolic homeostasis; host-gut microbiota interactions. Gut microbiota represent a dynamic ecosystem of multiple populations of bacteria residing in the gastrointestinal tract (Nicholson et al., (2012). At birth the primary "seed" populations are handed over by the mother, but subsequent shaping of this microbial ecosystem is driven by a number of dynamic interactions throughout life including diet, life style and antibiotic use. The gut microbiota and the host immune system share two-way communication signals and as well the microbiota contribute a number of small metabolites to the host (Nicholson et al., 2012). In addition, as reviewed by Nicholson et al., (2012), gut microbial populations appear to be an important agent in the genesis of obesity and insulin resistance.

Although the reference in this section is limited to the role of gut microbes in host metabolic homeostasis, it is important to realize that host-gut microbiota interactions are part of a larger issue; the two way inter-relationships between microbes and animal behaviors (Ezenwa et al., 2012).

The inter-relationships between the gut microbiota, toll like receptors and disrupted metabolic homeostasis have been investigated by Vijay-Kumar et al., (2010). Toll-like receptors (TLRs) are membrane spanning receptors that recognize molecules unique to microbes and are these receptors are considered part of the innate immune system. When a toll-like receptor binds its specific microbial- associated molecule, a signal pathway is activated which leads to the up regulation or suppression of genes that co-ordinate an inflammatory response. This TLR-mediated inflammatory response is part of the innate immune system's defense against a pathogenic microbial infection. In the experiments reported by Vijay-Kumar et al., (2010) mice rendered deficient in the Toll like receptor 5 (T5KO mice) were used as the model animal. TLR 5 is highly expressed in the intestinal epithelium and specifically recognizes bacterial flagellin. In order to "standardize" the gut flora between wild type mice and T5KO mice, T5KO mice to be used were transplanted as embryos into wild type mice. Hence the T5KO mice and wild type mice used in these experiments had similar gut microbiota. At 20 weeks of age T5KO mice had a greater body mass and visceral fat mass than wild type mice and had on average higher systolic and diastolic arterial pressures. Fasting glucose and insulin levels were higher in T5KO mice and in addition T5KO mice displayed an abnormal glucose tolerance curve. These differences between T5KO and wild mice were exacerbated by feeding both groups a high fat diet.

To investigate the role of the gut microbiota in the induction of the phenotypic differences between T5KO and wild type mice, Vijay-Kumar et al., (2010) treated both T5KO and wild type mice after weaning with broad spectrum antibiotics. This treatment reduced gut microbial load by about 90% and the mice were monitored for 12 weeks while being treated. After the twelve weeks, fasting blood sugar was reduced (and equivalent in both groups) compared to values obtained prior to antibiotic administration. In addition, food intake, and fat pad mass over the 12 week period remained equivalent in both T5KO and wild type mice. In a second series of experiments, germ-free wild type mice received intragastrically, the cecal microbiota from either wild type mice or T5KO mice. The mice were then monitored for 7 weeks. Food intake, percent gain in body weight and fat pad mass were greater in the mice that had received the cecal contents from T5KO mice. In addition, insulin sensitivity was reduced in wild type mice that had received T5KO gut microbes. In essence, the investigators demonstrated that the gut microbiota of mice deficient in Toll like receptor 5 had been altered in some as yet to be defined manner such that "signaling" from this changed gut flora was able to induce hyperphagia, obesity and reduced insulin sensitivity in the host.

Finally, it is important to remember that the "diabetic" phenotype is plastic. In susceptible animal models, ingestion of a high fat/sugar diet (environmental cue) is generally necessary to induce this phenotype. In addition the "diabetic" phenotype can be triggered by other environmental cues such as a viral respiratory tract infection (Chen eta l., 2012). Chen et al., (2012) performed "omics" (genomic, transcriptomic, proteomic and metabolomic) profiling of blood components in a healthy 54 year old male over a 14 month period during which time the subject experienced two viral infections. Whole genomic sequencing of the subject's DNA detected many sequence variations including SNPs, small insertions and deletions as well as larger copy number variants. Some of these sequence variations occurred in genes with reported disease risk including three variants associated with diabetes. On day 301, the subject contracted a viral (RSV) infection and on day 369 the subject had blood glucose and glycated hemoglobin values consistent with a diagnosis of diabetes type 2. By day 450 the blood glucose and glycated hemoglobin levels had returned to a normal range. Through this "omics" analysis, the investigators followed the subject's response to the RSV infection and the response included enrichment of a number of pathways including the IGF 1 and insulin signaling pathways. Presumably the immune/inflammatory response to the RSV infection triggered aberrant glucose regulation i.e. diabetes.

Tissue Damage

One of the hallmarks of the diabetic state is tissue damage in specific organs such as the eye and the kidney. In this section I will focus the discussion on the eye. Two major retinal problems cause most of the diabetic related vision loss; macular edema and retinal neovascularization (Crawford et al., 2009).

It is interesting that in humans, if the occurrence of retinopathy is used as a marker, an upper threshold value for blood glucose concentrations appears to be present. As discussed in the beginning of this section on Diabetes Mellitus, in cross-sectional studies the prevalence of retinopathy increases significantly for HbA1C values above 6.5% (Nathan et al., 2009). Longitudinal studies (McCance et al., 1994; Diabetes Control and Complications Trial Research Group, 1993) indicate that the cumulative incidence of retinopathy increases with time in those with sustained blood glucose concentrations above this threshold value. However, the cumulative incidence does not achieve a value of 100%. Not all individuals with a "diabetic" state develop retinopathy. This observation is consistent with the evidence that the "diabetic" state is comprised of a heterogeneous collection of metabolic phenotypes; some of these phenotypes will include retinal damage and some will not.

A number of mechanisms have been implicated in the genesis of the retinal changes observed in the "diabetic" state and two major rodent models have been preferentially used to explore these mechanisms; streptozotocin-induced diabetes and oxygen-induced proliferative retinopathy. Recent studies have underscored the important role that the pericyte plays in maintaining the "health" of the retinal vasculature and hence understanding the biology of pericytes is important for understanding the development of retinal damage.

Pericytes are vascular mural cells embedded within the basement membrane of micro vessels where they make specific focal contacts with the endothelium (Armulik et al., 2005). These cells do not function simply as scaffolding but display dynamic and complex interactions with associated endothelial cells (Bergers and Song, 2005). In fact, these two vascular cell types (endothelial cells and pericytes) are interdependent; primary defects in one cell type have obligated consequences for the other cell type. Pericytes are related to vascular smooth muscle cells (VSMC) although it is not clear whether pericytes and VSMC represent phenotypic variants of the same lineage or whether they have distinct progenitor cells. Pericytes are morphologically distinct in different organs; ranging from flattened cells encircling the capillary endothelium in the central nervous system to the rounded compact mesangial cell found in the kidney glomerulus. Interestingly, the retina has the highest pericyte density in the body (Bergers and Song, 2005). Since the retinal pericyte and renal mesangial cell belong to the same family, the experimental observations relating pericyte biology to retinopathy probably also apply to mesangial cell biology and the genesis of hyperglycemia-induced renal damage. Pericytes have a number of diverse functions. Pericytes contain contractile elements which allow these cells to produce vasoconstriction and vasodilation within capillary beds and hence regulate blood flow within the micro circulation. Pericytes are involved in the formation of the blood-brain barrier and in the retina, the blood-retinal barrier. Hepatic stellate cells and renal mesangial cells (both cell types are part of the pericyte family) have specialized functions as described by Bergers and Song, 2005). One of the earliest changes in diabetic retinopathy is loss of pericytes and this loss of pericytes is associated with the development of micro aneurysms , breakdown of the blood-retinal barrier and leakage of fluid into retinal tissue (edema) (Campochiaro, 2004; Bergers and Song, 2005).

A number of factors regulate pericyte function. Platelet-derived growth factor B (PDGF B) secreted by endothelial cells is an important regulator of pericyte proliferation and recruitment to vessels as well as maintenance of pericyte coverage of vessels (Armulik et al., 2005; Bergers and Song, 2005). PDGF B binds to a specific receptor tyrosine kinase (PDGR B) bound to the pericyte membrane. Angiopoietin 1 expressed by the pericyte binds to the Tie2 receptor on the endothelial cell and this signaling loop is important for vessel maturation and the stability of pericyte-endothelial contacts. On the other hand, angiopoietin 2, also expressed by the pericyte, destabilizes pericyte-endothelial contacts when it binds to the Tie2 receptor.

An important observation relates the mechanism by which PDGF B regulates pericyte function (Choudhury, 2001). Activation of the PDGF receptor B by binding of its ligand (PDGF B) results in the induction of several kinase signaling cascades. The predominant cascade involves phosphatidylinositol 3 kinase (PI3K) and its downstream target AKT/PKB. Choudhury (2001) clearly showed that the biological effects of PDGF B in pericytes (glomerular mesangial cells in these experiments) are mediated by the serine/threonine kinase AKT/PKB. This kinase has emerged as a critical and versatile signaling node and as already discussed a significant downstream component of the insulin/IGF 1 signaling pathway.

Three isoforms of AKT/PKB kinases have been identified and AKTPKB signaling mediates diverse and widespread biological functions through phosphorylation of multiple downstream targets (Manning and Cantley, 2007). AKT/PKB enhances the survival of cells by blocking the function of proapoptotic proteins and processes. AKT/PKB signaling promotes cell growth (i.e. an increase in cell mass) through activation of the mTOR complex 1 and regulates cell proliferation through a number of downstream targets effecting cell cycle dynamics. AKT/PKB signaling plays a role in angiogenesis. In endothelial cells, the PI3K-ATK/PKB pathway is activated by vascular endothelial growth factor (VEGF) and in pericytes by PDGF B (Choudhury, 2001). AKT/PKB kinase also plays a role in endothelial cell migration. Finally, the PI3K-AKT/PKB pathway, as already discussed, is an important downstream component of the insulin/IGF 1 signaling cascade and hence a critical mediator of the metabolic effects of insulin.

Geraldes et al., (2009) explored the interactions between PDGF, AKT/PKB signaling and pericyte biology in the genesis of diabetic retinopathy. They used a mouse model of streptozotocin- induced diabetes and were able to tease apart the biochemical steps leading to pericyte apoptosis, one of the earliest changes in diabetic retinopathy. Chronic hyperglycemia activated protein kinase C delta (PKC D) in pericytes, probably by increasing transcription of the encoding gene. A possible mechanism underlying this hyperglycemia- induced increased gene transcription could be an (epigenetic) change in the methylation state of histones associated with the PKC gene promoter (El-Osta et al., 2008). This increased PKC D activity was sustained and resulted in pericyte apoptosis and development of acellular capillaries. A downstream target of activated PKC D activation is a phosphatase (SHP 1). This phosphatase can dephosphorylate several receptor tyrosine kinases (PDGF R B, insulin receptor and VEGF R 2) and hence decrease their activity. In summary, chronic hyperglycemia activates pericyte PKC D which increases the expression of a downstream target phosphatase, SHP 1. SPH 1 dephosphorylates the pericyte PDGF receptor, thus blocking PDGF signaling from the endothelial cell. The reduction in endothelial PDGF signaling to the pericyte PI3K-AKT/PKB pathway leads to pericyte apoptosis. The loss of pericytes induces a "repair" process which includes increased expression of VEGF and its receptor (Bergers and Song, 2005). VEGF is a survival factor for endothelial cells, preventing apoptosis by activating the PI3K-AKT/PKB pathway in these cells (Ferrara et al., 2003; Manning and Cantley, 2007). However, the increased expression of VEGF will further enhance vascular permeability and promote neovascularization (Campochiaro, 2004; Antonetti, 2009). The actions of VEGF are very complex and include mitogenic, angiogenic and permeability enhancing functions as well as the inducing the expression of anti-apoptotic proteins.

Although the evidence appears strong that pericyte loss is the predominant event leading to retinal damage, other mechanisms have been described.

Brucklacher et al., (2008) using a rat model of streptozotocin induced diabetes measured retinal permeability and retinal gene expression in control and diabetic rats after 1 and 3 months. Retinal vascular permeability was significantly increased in rats after 3 months but not 1 month of diabetes. The expression (mRNA) patterns of thirty two genes were assessed. Genes were classified into three categories; micro vascular, inflammatory and neuronal functions. Among the micro vascular genes, some showed increased expression while others, in particular, VEGF, showed a decrease in expression. The observation that retinal VEGF mRNA expression decreases in diabetic animal models together with a previous observation that the level of retinal VEGF protein increases in diabetic animals suggests that VEGF protein levels are regulated by a post translational mechanism. Brucklacher et al., (2008) acknowledged that their data are hypothesis generating in nature rather than being confirmatory of any specific mechanism. However, it is interesting that genes encoding for factors such as PDGF, PKC, PI3K, and AKT/PKB were not been included in their assessment.

A specific post translational mechanism for regulating retinal VEGF protein levels has been described by Schrufer et al., (2010). Using a mouse model of diabetes, these investigators examined VEGF expression in the retina as well as in retinal Muller cells. They observed that VEGF protein abundance but not VEGF mRNA expression was increased at early time points in three different models of diabetes. The eukaryotic initiation factor 4E binding protein (4E-BP) also increased in abundance in the retina of diabetic animals in the absence of an increase in its mRNA expression and this increased 4E-BP was relatively less phosphorylated compared to retinal 4E-BP from control animals. The diabetes induced increase in VEGF protein abundance did not occur in mice made deficient in 4E-BP. In summary, diabetes induced an increase in unphosphorylated retinal 4E-BP which bound to a translational initiating complex which allowed for increased translation of VEGF mRNA. However, since mTORC1 signaling phosphorylates the 4E-BP binding protein which releases it from the translational initiating complex, dysregulation of mTORC1 signaling could also explain the observations of Schrufer et al., (2010).

Kondo et al., (2003) used a mouse model of oxygen-induced proliferative retinopathy to examine the role of endothelial insulin receptor (INSR) and endothelial insulin- like growth hormone 1 receptor (IGF1R) in this vascular process. Oxygen-induced retinopathy was induced in mice with either INSR or IGF1R gene knockouts and the extent of retinal neovascularization was compared in these mice to control mice. The degree of vascular changes was greatest in control mice, least in INSR knockout mice and intermediate in IGF1R knockout mice. Retinal protein staining for three vascular mediators; VEGF, endothelial nitric oxide synthase (eNOS) and endothelin 1 (ET1) showed a large increase in protein abundance for all three mediators in control mice with retinopathy. Endothelial receptor knockout mice had reduced protein levels for all three mediators but the levels were still significantly higher than baseline values in mice without retinopathy. The interpretation of these experimental observations is not straightforward. The increased expression of VEGF in humans with diabetic proliferative retinopathy has been well documented (Antonetti, 2009). However, the inter-relationships between insulin/IGF1 signaling and VEGF actions is quite complex. Insulin stimulates the expression of VEGF mRNA via activation of the PI3K-AKT/PKB pathway (Jiang et al., 2000; Mick et al., 2002). VEGF also activates the PI3K-AKT/PKB pathway in endothelial cells which accounts for its endothelial cell survival and angiogenic properties (Ferrara et al., 2003; Manning and Cantley, 2007). In the experiments of Kondo et al., (2003) there are several complementary processes occurring. Receptor deficient mice will have less signaling down the PI3K-AKT/PKB pathway which in itself will reduce angiogenesis (Jiang et al., 2000; Manning and Cantley, 2007). In addition the reduced signaling down the PI3K-AKT/PKB pathway will reduce expression of VEGF (Jiang et al., 2000). Both of these mechanisms could account for their experimental observations.

The adipose tissue peptide hormone adiponectin has also been implicated in the retinal microvasular changes of the diabetic state. Higuchi et al., (2009) created mice with an adiponectin gene knockout (APN KO) and subjected these mice to oxygen-induced proliferative retinopathy. APN KO mice displayed much more neovascular retinal changes than wild type mice. Retinal expression levels (mRNA) of VEGF, angiopoeitin 1 and 2, endothelial nitric oxide synthase and VEGF receptor 2 did not differ between APN KO and wild type mice. However, retinal mRNA levels of tumor necrosis factor alpha (TNF A) were much higher in APN KO mice than wild type mice. The source of TNF A in the retina is probably macrophages and microglia cells and the observations of Higuchi et al., (2009) implicate this cytokine in the neovascularization of oxygen induced retinopathy and by analogy in the genesis of proliferative diabetic retinopathy. In addition, it has been demonstrated that TNF A through binding to its receptor (TNF R) can interfere with insulin signaling through "cross talk" at the level of insulin receptor substrates (Taniguchi et al., (2006). However, adiponectin has other vascular effects as well. Kubota et al., (2002) showed that adiponectin deficient mice formed twice as much neo-intima in response to a femoral artery cuff injury (which did not directly damage the intima) than wild type mice. The signaling pathways responsible for the development of new intima in these adiponectin deficient mice were not elucidated.

Even this brief survey underscores the complex interactions involved in the genesis of diabetic retinopathy. It appears that retinal pericyte loss due to impaired endothelial signaling may be the initiating factor. Impaired endothelial signaling appears to be a consequence of defective insulin signaling within the context of an insulin "resistance" state. Pericyte apoptosis results in a weakened vessel wall, micro aneurysm formation and increased fluid leakage from the vessel. Repair processes initiated in response to the loss of pericytes actually compound the problem. VEGF is recruited, but this endothelial cell survival factor also promotes increased endothelial proliferation and new vessel formation. Vessel permeability is further enhanced with the development of macular edema. A vicious cycle is put in place between injury and repair processes. However, this somewhat simplistic synthesis is but a framework defining the problem. Other factors known to be involved include various signaling proteins; PDGF, PKC, PI3K, AKT/PKB, adiponectin, insulin, IGF 1, TNF A, angiopoietin 1 and 2, Tie 2 receptor to name just a few. However, I think it is fair to say that the inciting event in the development of the retinal changes is an "injury" that occurs as a byproduct of the metabolic phenotype responsible for the insulin resistance. Once the injury has occurred, the subsequent repair process appears unfortunately to compound the physiological and structural abnormalities.

Summary and Perspectives

Across vertebrate groups there is a diversity of glucose homeostatic mechanisms. The insulin/IGF1 pathway is central to glucose regulation and the ancestral pathway was characterized by a single receptor that bound insulin- like peptides. This pathway became more complex with the evolution of additional specific receptors. Fish possess the peptides glucagon, GLP 1 and GIP, but since the fish has only one receptor, a glucagon-type, all three of these peptides have similar effects in this vertebrate. Birds have distinct glucagon and GLP 1 receptors but as yet an incretin role for GLP1 in the bird has not been demonstrated. Among mammals, there are species with unusual glucose regulating mechanisms that also possess insulins with unusual properties. This group includes the hystricognathi suborder of rodents. One member of this group, the naked mole rat, not only displays a "diabetic" type response to a glucose challenge but is also characterized by extreme longevity and negligible senescence. All of these diverse glucose regulating mechanisms evolved under the pressure of specific environmental conditions. For the human species, the environmental context in which our species evolved included a scarcity of food and a need for endurance activities.

Humans are built for long distance endurance running and most likely early humans hunted for food by chasing down and tiring their prey. The scarcity of food required that metabolic homeostatic mechanisms were set to defend against energy deficiency rather than energy excess. Temporary storage of metabolic energy in fat depots was also important for times that food was not available. Humans have a complex glucose regulating mechanism. The central component is the insulin/IGF1 signaling network which in addition, participates in extensive cross talk with other nutrient and mitogenic/growth networks such as the mTOR signaling network. In addition, the insulin/IGF network plays an important role in the ageing process and longevity as well as being implicated in the neoplastic transformation of cells.

Humans possess a complex system of glucose sensing mechanisms including glucose sensing neurons. These neurons are tied into the appetite and feeding behavioral system which is partly regulated by peptide hormones such as insulin and leptin. In addition, appetite and feeding have been integrated into a set of reward seeking behaviors in the human; feeding, salt-appetite and salt intake and the “runner’s high” are all reward-seeking behaviors. Glucose and metabolic homeostatic mechanisms are also shaped by both a dynamic input from adipose tissue which has been recognized as an endocrine organ and by the metabolic effects on the host of the gut microbial ecosystem. Other factors contribute significantly to the complexity of glucose regulating mechanisms such as the stress hormones which have wide spread effects on metabolic homeostasis and on vascular remodeling and repair and arterial blood pressure regulation as discussed in previous sections.

The genome and epigenome of the individual human is unique and this genetic variation across individuals will shape glucose regulating mechanisms within that individual. Environmental cues also modify glucose regulating mechanisms probably through epigenetic alteration of gene expression patterns. Important environmental cues include; nature of maternal care during and after pregnancy which modifies in the offspring food and salt feeding behaviors as well as the stress response, availability, at least in the developed world, of abundant high caloric foods, feeding behaviors which are tied into the reward- seeking system and have become uncoupled from metabolic need, an urban social structure that fosters inactivity.

Genome wide association studies (GWAS) have revealed only modest genetic influences. The Wellcome Trust Case Control Consortium (2007) performed a GWAS for seven common diseases including diabetes type 2. The Consortium examined for an association between SNPs and diabetes across all chromosomes. Three SNPs located respectively on chromosomes 6, 10 and 16 showed a statistical association with diabetes. This association was strongest for the SNP on chromosome 10. However, effects were modest with homozygous odds ratios varying from 1.5 to 2.10 for all three SNPs. The same Consortium (2010) examined (GWAS) for associations between CNVs and eight common diseases. In the case of diabetes, a weak statistical association was found for a CNV located on chromosome 12. These GWAS confirm that diabetes (type 2) is clearly a polygenic disorder with inputs from multiple genomic loci each having a small effect size.

The data are consistent with the conclusion that the “diabetic” state does not represent a single phenotype but rather a collection of metabolic phenotypes. For a given individual, glucose homeostasis will be determined by that individual’s unique genome and epigenome overlaid by the epigenetic effects of various environmental cues on gene expression patterns. As a result, some individuals will develop a metabolic phenotype characterized by dysregulation of the insulin/IGF 1 signaling network. This phenotype will manifest as reduced insulin sensitivity and elevation of blood glucose concentrations. However, the specific molecular mechanisms underlying the dysregulation of the insulin/IGF 1 signaling network will vary across individuals. Given the extensive cross talk between the insulin/IGF 1 signaling network and other signaling networks such as the mTOR kinase cascade, the metabolic phenotypic resulting in reduced insulin sensitivity might also include impairment in “cell- survival” signaling through the PI3K- AKT/PKB pathway. In the case of retinal pericytes, this impairment of cell- survival signaling would lead to pericyte apoptosis. Loss of retinal pericytes constitutes an “injury” and as such would invoke a repair process. A component of the repair process includes increased expression of VEGF protein which unfortunately enhances retinal vascular permeability and stimulates an angiogenic response (neovascularization). However, impaired "cell survival" signaling is not present in all individuals with reduced insulin sensitivity since about half of those with chronically elevated blood glucose concentrations above the "threshold" value do not show retinal edema or vascular changes. Hence, some of the metabolic phenotypes underlying the diabetic state will include altered cell-survival signaling and some will not.

Is the diabetic state a disease? I believe the data are most consistent with the "diabetic" state being a variant of the ageing process. As discussed in the section; Background; Ageing; at the individual level, senescence is partly the result of accumulation of incompletely repaired damage. DNA structural variants (mutations) can occur for a variety of reasons; ionizing radiation, meiotic recombination, as a consequence of repair of double strand breaks and errors during DNA replication. In addition, as noted in the section; Background; Genetics; certain regions of the genome are more susceptible to mutations (regions of low DNA methylation) than other regions. There are repair mechanisms to correct DNA damage but these mechanisms can be incomplete. As was discussed in the section; Background; Genetics; double strand DNA breaks are difficult to repair if they occur near telomere sites. Cellular and tissue damage can also occur for "natural" reasons. One example of "naturally" occurring cellular damage is the occurrence of focal intimal cushions in the arterial tree at sites of non-laminar blood flow such as bifurcations, branch points and regions of high curvature. These cushions are particularly prominent in the coronary circulation by virtue of the unusual hemodynamic forces occurring as a result of the intramyocardial location of these vessels. These cushions represent a repair process in response to altered shear stress. If the stimulus for vascular remodeling is extensive, the repair process can result in the progression of these cushions into atherosclerotic-type lesions.

Ageing represents in part the accumulation of DNA and cellular damage that has been incompletely repaired. The extent of accumulated damage will increase with advancing chronological age since repair processes become less robust with advancing age. Within this framework, diabetes represents a part of the ageing process. Blood glucose concentrations in various populations show a unimodal distribution with a distinct right sided skew (higher blood glucose concentrations). This right-sided skew is much more pronounced in older populations consistent with the observations that glycated hemoglobin levels increase with age in "non-diabetic" individuals and the diabetic state has a much higher prevalence in older individuals (Schulz et al., 2006). These two observations indicate that insulin sensitivity decreases with chronological age which is to be expected since "repair" processes are less robust in older individuals. In addition, the diabetic state represents a heterogeneous collection of metabolic phenotypes so if we did call diabetes type 2, a disease, we would have to consider it to be not one disease but a collection of many diseases. Also, sequencing of the human genome has revealed that a significant fraction of DNA is structurally polymorphic and that, in essence, no two human genomes are identical. This DNA structural polymorphism across individuals means there is no such entity as a wild-type human (Olson, 2011).

How do all of these considerations apply to the diabetic state? By virtue of the uniqueness of each human genome, the molecular details of glucose regulatory mechanisms will vary across individuals. Blood glucose concentrations will show a distribution within a population of individuals but will be right skewed because of the "left wall effect" discussed at the beginning of the section; Diabetes Mellitus (Type 2). The extent, nature and sites of an individual's genomic structural variants will determine where in the distribution of blood glucose concentrations a given individual resides. In addition, an individual's (unique) genome will influence how that individual responds to environmental cues such as the availability of a surfeit of high caloric foods and an urban social setting which creates a barrier to adequate levels of physical activity (Schulz et al., 2006). Environmental cues probably affect glucose homeostasis via epigenetic mechanisms; altering gene expression patterns, although the molecular details are largely unknown. As the individual ages, DNA damage accumulates and glucose homeostasis becomes less well regulated. In addition, those with extensive DNA structural polymorphisms, will likely have alterations in many signaling networks including those related to cell survival e.g. of pericytes. As discussed in the section; Tissue damage; apoptosis of retinal pericytes sets up a repair process which contributes to the retinal vascular changes observed in a significant fraction of individuals with chronically high blood glucose concentrations (extensive impairment of glucose regulating mechanisms).

Environmental influences, such as a highly complex urban societal structure and labor saving technologies which act to prevent adequate levels of activity, although working at the level of the individual actually represent societal issues as discussed in a recent report issued by the Institute of Medicine (Glickman et al., 2012). The committee responsible for the report proposed a number of recommendations to be implemented at the societal level such as; making physical activity an integral and routine part of life and creating a food and beverage environment that ensured that healthy food and beverage options are the routine, easy choice. In essence these recommendations are an attempt to re-direct the "social environment" back towards an environment more in keeping with our evolved metabolic design features.

A final note: Most of the experimental studies of glucose regulating mechanisms have used inbred rodent models (usually the mouse) with engineered specific gene deletions (loss of function) or specific gene gain of function mutations. These experiments do give valuable information as to the functions of the mutated (loss of function or gain of function) genes, but these animal models are quite displaced from the natural state. First, highly inbred animals have less genetic diversity than natural animals. Secondly, the assumption is made that deleting or inducing a gain of function mutation in a specific gene does not cause other genetic functional changes. It is now understood that signaling pathways are not simple linear cascades but complex signaling networks which engage in extensive cross talk with other signaling networks. Engineered mutations in single genes could lead to wide spread gene functional abnormalities on the basis of this network- type organization. Such wide spread effects are generally not considered in these experiments with traditional rodent models. With these considerations in mind, I am perplexed as to why a natural animal model such as the bird has not been embraced as a suitable model for studying the biological effects of chronically high blood glucose concentrations (Singer, 2007). For example, birds do not have a retinal vascular network like that of mammals, but instead have a special structure called the pectin oculi. However, this structure does contain endothelial cells (with abundant GLUT 1transporters) and pericytes (Raviola and Raviola, 1967; Micali et al., 2012). How are the pericytes, in this structure able to avoid the apoptotic effects of a high blood glucose concentration as occurs in mammals? Studying cell survival signaling networks in the bird could give an answer to this question?

Chapter V

Dementia

As discussed in the section Background; Evolution; the genetic underpinnings for the evolution of morphological diversity across species are becoming better defined. Different morphologies arise from the differential spatial and temporal expression of the genes contained in a highly conserved genetic toolkit. In contrast, the genetic underpinnings for the evolution of behavioral diversity across species are not as well understood. A genetic toolkit comparable to that for morphology has not been described. There are however, highly conserved genes such as FOXP2 which play a central role in the behaviors of vocal imitation and language development. However, even though a genetic toolkit for behaviors has not been defined, it is clear that humans have evolved, body and mind, from earlier primates. The ways in which humans think reflect this evolutionary origin just as surely as the ways in which their limbs are articulated, their immune systems defend against pathogens and the cones in their eyes process colored light (Editorial, Nature, 2007). One of the premises of this section is that the complex behaviors of humans, even those considered "unique" to our species, evolved from our ancestors and hence aspects of these so-called unique behaviors can be found in other vertebrates. As Jones (2007) noted, even the human moral faculty- the psychological systems that make judgments about right and wrong, what is permissible and what is not- has arisen from pre-existing brain systems over millions of years of biological and cultural evolution.

In a recent publication, Jonsson et al., (2012) reported that humans having a specific structural variant (SNP)in the gene coding for amyloid-B precursor protein (APP) are not only "protected" from developing Alzheimer's disease but also have less age- related cognitive decline. The investigators proposed that Alzheimer's disease may represent the extreme of the age-related decline in cognitive function. This proposal relates to the second and principal premise of this section which is that dementia is not a disease but a variant of the ageing process.

Evolution of the Mammalian Brain

Demystifying the complex functions of the brain has turned out to be a daunting scientific task that clearly will require a multipronged approach. One component of this approach involves understanding the selective pressures that shaped the evolution of the vertebrate brain and in particular that of the mammal. However, before examining the nature of these selective pressures, a few general observations are in order to highlight some of the unusual features of the vertebrate brain.

The vertebrate brain is organized into anatomical areas that sub serve relatively specific functions. This spatial and functional organization has been well documented in humans using both static and dynamic neuroimaging techniques. The mammalian brain also displays a considerable amount of plasticity both in terms of its circuitry and in terms of the production of new neurons in the adult brain (Doidge, 2007; Singer, 2011). At the cellular level, neurons and synapses are organized into networks which appear to be the regulated elements rather than the individual cells themselves (Prinz et al., 2004; Hooper, 2004). Prinz and colleagues (2004) used a rather "simple" system, the pyloric rhythm generated by the somatogastric ganglia of lobsters, to examine network organization. The circuitry and neurons involved in this system have been well characterized. Over 20 million neural networks were simulated using three different neurons existing in five or six different states interconnected by synapses of five or six different strengths. Using fairly stringent selection criteria, about 2% (over 400 thousand) of the model circuits produced correct "pyloric' outputs. Similar network outputs could be generated by a large variety of combinations of synaptic strengths and intrinsic neuronal properties which suggests that network performance rather than individual neuronal activity or synaptic strength, might be the regulated property. The overall proposal is that the different properties of the neurons and the different strengths of the synapses that make up the network can be fitted to many different combinations that nonetheless produce very similar network outputs. Such a mechanism could partially explain neuronal circuit plasticity. The investigators compared this neuronal network organization to the network arrangement of biochemical signaling cascades (e.g. insulin/IGF 1 network). As pointed out by Hooper (2004), this model is appealing since evolution selects out for correct network output (the phenotype) and not for the intrinsic properties of individual neurons or synapses comprising the network. This model is supported by the observation that within a single class of neuron, there is considerable variation across individual cells in their physiological properties. Variation in individual cell physiology appears to occur when there is variation in input activity (Urban and Tripathy, 2012).These few observations highlight the very complex functional organization of the brain both at the macro level and at the cell/synapse circuit level.

One model, the "social brain hypothesis" has been used as a basis for understanding the evolution of the mammalian brain and in particular the primate brain. This hypothesis has recently been reviewed by Dunbar and Shultz (2007). The hypothesis is rooted in the proposal that one or more ecological problems (survival, foraging, rearing offspring) are more effectively solved socially than by an individual's unaided efforts. Brain size and functional capacity had to increase to allow the animal to cope with the demands of a social living arrangement. The data reviewed by Dunbar and Shultz (2007) indicate that in primates, brain volume (or more specifically neocortex volume) correlates with sociality (defined in terms of the complexity of social interactions). However, the relationship between sociality and brain size is also shaped by a number of constraints, as noted by Dunbar and Shultz (2007), which set boundary conditions for this relationship. Only long lived animals that experience low mortality rates can sustain the growth and learning period necessary to develop large brains. In addition, an animal must have an adequate diet to supply the energy required to support a large brain. Within the boundaries set by these and other constraints, the survival advantage of extensive social interactions and cooperation as a means of solving ecological problems serves to drive the expansion of brain (neocortex) capacity thus enabling the animal to engage in such interactions and cooperation.

Eusociality refers to the highest level of organismal social organization and is defined as a form of social organization in which groups display cooperative care of young, overlapping generations and reproductive division of labor where one or a few individuals monopolize reproduction within the colony. Animals fulfilling these criteria include; ants, bees, wasps, termites, naked mole rats and Damaraland mole rats. Primates are clearly social but not eusocial, since there is not a reproductive division of labor within primates. Sociality arose through the interplay between ecological pressures and natural selection; a social living arrangement provided species such as humans with a powerful tool for solving ecological problems and such a living arrangement required a large brain characterized by a sophisticated set of behavioral traits. But what do we know about the genetic changes that accompanied the development of sociality? Investigators have begun to examine the molecular evolution of eusociality in insects and given the conservative nature of evolutionary processes, the general genetic mechanisms underlying the evolution of insect eusociality probably also apply to the mechanisms underpinning social living arrangements in general.

As discussed in the section Background; Evolution; the morphological diversity across species is now understood in terms of modifications in highly conserved suites of toolkit genes such as the HOX genes which regulate anterior-posterior morphology in developing animal embryos. Phylogenetic diversity of form arises primarily through changes in the regulation of the temporal and spatial function of these toolkit genes. Adaptive divergence in morphology and behaviors across species correlates to a greater extent with changes in gene regulatory elements (non protein coding DNA) than with changes in protein coding genes. Within the context of this evolutionary development (evo-devo) approach, Toth and Robinson (2007) and Bloch and Grozinger (2011) have examined the molecular evolution of eusociality in bee colonies.

Toth and Robinson (2007) point out that complex animal behaviors can be viewed as being built upon simpler behavioral modules and that changes in the temporal and spatial expression of genes are more important than changes in DNA coding sequences in the evolution of novel behaviors. In addition, there is evidence for the existence of genetic toolkits for phylogenetic behavioral diversity as there is for phylogenetic morphological diversity. The solitary life style is the ancestral state and hence social animals have evolved from solitary ancestors (Bloch and Grozinger, 2011). Building upon the evo-devo approach, it is likely that genetic toolkits and pathways that regulate specific behaviors in solitary species have been co-opted to regulate complex social behaviors in social species. Toth and Robinson (2007) consider behavioral modules in the honeybee concerning foraging, reproduction and division of labor and how these interacting modules have evolved from solitary to social insects.

For example, in the fruit fly (a solitary insect); alleles of the foraging gene (For) which encodes an isoform of cyclic GMP- dependent protein kinase (PKG) are associated with different foraging behavioral phenotypes. Fruit flies carrying the “rover” allele move large distances while feeding while flies carrying the “sitter” allele are relatively inactive in the presence of food (Schafer, 2002; Engel et al., 2000). The For locus has no effect on locomotion rate in the absence of food. The foraging gene has been conserved across fruit flies, bees and nematodes. The honeybee ortholog (amfor) of this gene is associated with age related changes in worker bee foraging behaviors. Expression of amfor (mRNA levels) is higher in the brain of workers which forage out of hive compared to bees performing in hive nursing activities. This observation indicates that genetic pathways orchestrated by the For gene which regulate foraging behaviors in solitary insects (such as the fly) can be modified to regulate division of labor and task functions (foraging versus nursing activities) in the eusocial honeybee. The For locus could be considered a behavioral toolkit gene, although it encodes a signaling kinase rather than a transcription factor. As summarized by Bloch and Grozinger (2011), modifications in conserved core physiological and metabolic pathways such as the insulin/IGF 1 signaling network, the circadian system of molecular clocks, reproductive and endocrine signaling networks all play key roles in the molecular evolution of solitary behaviors into social behaviors.

Evolutionary processes generally involve trade- offs and sociality is no exception. The observation that many vertebrates form social groupings indicates that group solutions to ecological problems have advantages over an individual- based approach. Humans are probably the most socialized species in many ways and our sociality has allowed us to control many of our ecological pressures through a number of strategies; development of a reliable and adequate food supply, transfer of goods and services between social groups, urbanization with creation of clean water supplies and safe sewage systems. However, the trade-off is that our complex and extensive social interactions can alter biological processes at the individual level as discussed in the sections; Atherosclerotic Vascular Disease, Hypertension and Diabetes Mellitus (Type 2). For a given individual, our complex social environment and social interactions can modify the nature of the vascular remodeling and repair process in response to injury, change the setting of arterial blood pressure levels and alter appetite and feeding behaviors such that food intake is no longer driven by metabolic need. However, on balance the trade-offs associated with our sociality are clearly net positive.

The social brain hypothesis (sometimes also referred to as the social intelligence hypothesis) has been used to explain the evolution of large brains (chiefly neocortex) in primates, elephants and cetaceans (dolphins and toothed whales) (Connor, 2007). Dolphins and toothed whales have large and spatially highly organized brains (Marino et al., 2007). The cognitive sophistication of cetaceans has been well documented (Marino et al., 2007) and the evidence favors sociality as the main driving force for the evolution of their large brains. As summarized by Connor (2007), primates, dolphins, toothed whales and elephants rely on the mutual dependence of group living to reduce predatory mortality risk, to better access resources and to provide protection for their offspring who are extremely vulnerable during a prolonged period of their early life. Group living involves complex social interactions (mutual dependence, social competition) and primates, elephants, dolphins and toothed whales have evolved an expansive and highly organized neocortex which has the capacity for sophisticated cognitive functioning which makes group living feasible. Other advantages of cohesive social groups are that this type of structure facilitates information transfer in the form of social learning and is the basis of culture and inter-generational cultural knowledge transmission in humans.

Birds are also social animals but bird sociality differs from that of mammals. Most birds are monogamous and only form large flocks outside of the breeding season (Emery et al., 2007a). As reviewed by Emery et al., (2007a), birds display a high level of cognitive functioning and these investigators discuss the empirical evidence that the pair-bonding between birds involves sufficiently complex interactions to serve as a driver for the evolution of avian social intelligence. An additional aspect of avian brain physiology is its extreme neuronal plasticity. New neurons originate in the ventricular zone and migrate to various regions of the forebrain. There is experimental evidence that the survival of these new neurons is determined by the complexity of the bird's social environment (Singer, 2011; Emery et al., 2007a). Hence, the sizes of parts of the avian brain vary as a function of the complexity of its social groupings. These groupings vary from pair bonds during the breeding season to large social groups (flocks) at other times.

In summary, the social intelligence (or social brain) hypothesis proposes that the major influence in the evolution of a large mammalian brain (i.e. neocortex) is the requirement for a cognitive capacity to meet the challenges of life in a social group. Humans are the most social species and given the existence of (Darwinian) evolution, cognitive functions such as consciousness and the "mind" have not arisen in humans de novo but as extensions of similar but more rudimentary functional forms in our ancestors (Emery et al., 2007 b).

Recent experimental studies have begun to explore the genetic underpinnings of mammalian brain evolution. Pollard et al., (2006) looked at regions of the human genome that showed significant evolutionary acceleration and identified 49 "human accelerated regions (HARs)" which displayed a significantly accelerated nucleotide substitution rate in humans. The highest ranking HAR (HAR1) was well conserved across vertebrates showing only two base substitutions between chicken and chimpanzee but eighteen substitutions in the human since humans and chimpanzees diverged from their common ancestor. This region (HAR1) is transcribed as part of two overlapping genes, HAR1F and HAR1R. These two genes are not protein coding genes but transcribe novel noncoding RNA. HAR1F is strongly and specifically expressed in the developing human neocortex early in embryonic development and may play a critical regulatory role in cortical neuron migration and cell specification (Amadio and Walsh, 2006). At later stages of embryonic brain development, expression of HAR1F was no longer detectable. On the other hand, HRA1R was not detected in embryonic neural tissue but only in adult brain tissue where it was coexpressed with HRA1F. One speculation is that HRA1R is expressed later in neural development and is responsible for down regulating HRA1F (Amadio and Walsh, 2006).

Haygood et al., (2007) examined the promoter regions (defined as the region immediately upstream from a transcription start site) in about 17,000 genes from humans and non-human primates. A significant number of genes in humans which displayed within their promoter regions a high nucleotide substitution rate (high positive selection) were involved in neural development and function (axon guidance, synapse formation, neurotransmission).

In a recent paper, Konopka et al., (2012) compared gene expression (transcriptome) in three brain regions in the human, chimpanzee and rhesus macaque. The greatest differences in gene expression between the human, chimpanzee and rhesus macaque were found in the frontal pole region of the brain. This observation is consistent with the construct that this brain area is involved in higher cognitive functions. In addition, the results define a number of gene coexpression (connectivity) patterns that have rapidly evolved in the human frontal cortex. Compared to the two other primates, the human brain is characterized by a greater degree of transcriptional regulation and complexity and transcriptional connectivity particularly in the frontal pole region. Morphologically human neurons contain a greater number and density of dendritic spines compared to other primates. Konopka et al., (2012) also described gene coexpression networks that were centered on certain core genes. One such module had as its hub gene CLOCK, a component of molecular clocks and this module contained genes linked to neurobehavioral disorders. A second coexpression network had FOXP2 as its hub gene. FOXP2 encodes a transcription factor important in cognitive and language capacities. These gene coexpression networks or modules were specific to the human lineage.

The experimental observations of Pollard et al., (2006), Haygood et al., (2007) and Konopka et al., (2012) indicate that the genetic basis for the evolution of large brains in humans appears to be primarily due to changes in gene regulatory mechanisms rather than in the development of "novel" protein coding genes. This observation is consistent with the concepts discussed in the section; Background; Evolution; in which the degree of animal biological complexity correlates with the extent of non-protein coding DNA. In addition, these observations support the notion that the so called higher cognitive functions of humans are derived from similar functions in our ancestors; humans have essentially co-opted existing ancestral protein coding genes but have re-fashioned their tissue specific temporal and spatial expression.

One final observation concerning the genetics of mammalian brain evolution; As noted in the section; Background; Genetics; genomic regions of hypomethylation (methylation deserts) appear to be hotspots of DNA structural polymorphisms and show a tenfold enrichment for structural rearrangements that have occurred in the human genome since humans and chimpanzees diverged from their common ancestors (Li et al., 2012). Li et al., (2012) noted that methylation deserts were also enriched for DNA regions involved in the regulation of tissue specific gene expression. These investigators examined for enrichment of two specific classes of regulatory DNA sequences; genomic regulatory blocks (GRBs) and DNA sequences coding for transcription factors (TFs). A gene regulatory block (GRB) is a chromosomal region containing a highly conserved non coding sequence which acts as a regulator for a target gene also within that region (Akalin et al., 2009). The target genes of GRBs are generally genes that code for transcription factors which are involved in embryonic development and differentiation. As described by Akalin et al., 2009), GRB target genes have unique properties that allow them to respond to regulatory inputs from very long distances. Li et al., (2012) found that GRB target genes showed a twelve- fold enrichment in methylation deserts whereas GRBs themselves displayed about a three-fold enrichment. Transcription factors (TFs) are a class of proteins that binds to DNA in a sequence specific manner and regulate the transcription of genetic information from DNA to mRNA by controlling the recruitment of RNA polymerase. Vaquerizas et al., (2009) looked at the array of transcription factors in humans. They were able to identify about 1400 genomic loci that coded for TFs and for the majority of identified TFs, their regulatory functions were poorly understood. Li et al., (2012) measured the genomic locations of these 1400 TF encoding genes and found that there was almost a four-fold enrichment in regions of hypomethylation (methylation deserts). In addition, two clusters of TFs identified by Vaquerizas et al., (2009) to be fast evolving in primates had an even higher enrichment (fifteen-fold) in methylation deserts.

Since hypomethylated DNA regions are enriched for both fast evolving loci and loci involved in regulation of gene expression patterns, it is likely that the novel non-coding RNA genes (HAR1F and HAR1R) described by Pollard et al., (2006) are to be found in such hypomethylated genomic regions. The genes, HAR1F and HAR1R, are part of a fast evolving region in the human genome that has a gene regulatory role in brain cortical development.

Cognition

Although cognition is a commonly used term, there does not appear to be an agreed upon definition. One definition describes cognition as comprising a group of mental functions which include attention, memory, communication, decision making and problem solving. Measuring such cognitive functions across various animal groups is problematic. Making such measurements in the wild involves a number of technical challenges. Designing what to actually measure and how to make the measurement have not been standardized. In humans, assessing cognitive functions generally involves verbal communication with the subject which is not possible in other species. In all other animal groups, assessing cognitive functions can only be done by observing specific behavioral responses to various experimental test situations; direct communication with the animal is not possible. In addition, we humans tend to judge the utility and sophistication of animal "cognitive" behaviors through a human lens. Should we not be viewing these behaviors from the perspective of the animal? However, such an animal- oriented perspective is not possible. We can objectively compare physiological functions of organs such as muscle, heart and bone across various animal groups including humans. However, we cannot make similar objective comparisons with respect to cognitive functions between humans and non- humans. Given the reality of evolution, our inability to compare directly human and non- human cognitive functions, does not mean that human cognitive capacities are somehow mysterious, ethereal and unrelated to the cognitive capacities of non- humans.

Before describing examples of cognitive behaviors in different animal species, it is useful to review what is known about the genetic underpinnings of such behaviors. Although the heritability of various cognitive traits has been well known, it is only with the development of newer genetic techniques that investigators have been able to explore the genomic mechanisms underlying cognitive behaviors.

Songbirds engage in complex social interactions that are mediated by their songs, which are learned vocal signals. For example, when the male zebra finch hears the singing of another male bird, the expression of the gene EGR1, an immediate early gene, is induced in a specific sub region of the auditory forebrain devoted to hearing (Robinson et al., 2008). EGR 1 codes for a transcription factor and its target genes are believed to be involved in the neural process of storage of song memories. In songbird societies, individual birds recognize and differentiate conspecifics from members of other species according to their vocalizations. It is speculated that the genomic response involving EGR1 allows the songbird to update its representations of stored vocalizations, hence aiding in the recognition of "friends" and "foes" (Robinson et al., 2008). In this example an environmental cue (singing) induces a genomic response responsible for memory storage.

Donaldson and Young (2008) reviewed the role of neuropeptides such as vasopressin and oxytocin in social cognition and behaviors. Oxytocin and vasopressin homologs have been highly conserved across vertebrates as has their roles in facilitating species specific social and reproductive behaviors. Oxytocin has a single identified brain receptor while vasopressin has two brain receptor subtypes, V1a and V1b (Donaldson and Young, 2008). The anatomical localization of V1a receptors within the brain has a marked effect on mammalian social behavior. Male monogamous prairie voles unlike male polygamous meadow and montane voles, show selective mating-induced partner preferences, care for offspring and selective aggression against conspecifics. This difference in social behaviors between prairie and meadow and montane moles correlates with differences in the brain regional distribution patterns for V1a receptor expression between these different species. When a viral vector is used in the polygamous meadow vole to artificially increase the expression of V1a receptors in those brain areas characteristic of the monogamous prairie vole, the meadow vole begins to display a selective preference for a particular mate. Oxytocin also modulates social behavior. In female rats, central infusion of oxytocin stimulates maternal behavior and maternal-infant bonding, but not selection preference for a particular partner; rats do not form pair bonds. In female prairie voles, central administration of oxytocin facilitates preference selection for a particular partner as well as maternal- infant bonding. Blockade of the oxytocin receptor in female prairie voles inhibits selection preference for a particular partner. Donaldson and Young (2008) also note that structural variants in the gene for V1a in humans have been associated with differences in human social behavior, personality traits relevant to social interactions and the onset of reproduction.

These observations on the selective effects of oxytocin and vasopressin on patterns of social (cognitive) behaviors teach several lessons. A single neuropeptide (oxytocin) which normally promotes one type of social behavior, maternal bonding, can be co-opted to promote a different type of social behavior, male-directed bonding, as well and that altering the anatomical distribution of receptor gene expression in the brain can have significant effects on the nature of social behaviors. As an aside, the importance of receptor type in determining the effects of ligand binding, in this case vasopressin, is illustrated by the observation that binding of vasopressin to a different receptor type in the kidney induces biological processes that regulate water reabsorption by the renal tubule. Hence the same ligand, vasopressin, can regulate a wide range of biological processes ranging from diverse social behaviors to water handling by the kidney as determined by receptor type and receptor tissue localization and distribution.

As discussed in the section; Background; Evolution; the gene FOXP2 is an important regulator of vocal learning, an experience-based form of learning, and language acquisition. FOXP2 is a highly conserved gene which codes for a transcription factor which can function as a transcriptional repressor or activator. In mammals the gene is expressed in multiple sites other than the brain; lung, heart and gut. It is clear that the gene FOXP2 is quite relevant to (cognitive) linguistic abilities in humans and the effects of mutations in this gene are well described by Fisher (2006). However, it is important to realize as pointed out by Fisher (2006), that the grammatical difficulties in humans with mutations of the FOXP2 gene are just one aspect of a more extensive multifaceted disorder of speech, language and the impaired ability to coordinate the mouth movements underlying speech. The observation that FOXP2 is expressed in multiple tissues indicates that this gene plays a role in the development and function of organs other than the brain. A guiding principal in complex biological systems is to use the same regulatory factors to control multiple pathways in different tissue and functional contexts. It is rare to find a transcription factor that has an exclusive role specific to only one context (Fisher, 2006).

In humans, the genetic basis of cognitive behaviors has been probed by looking for associations between gene variants or genomic loci and either known cognitive disorders or the test scores of standardized psychological tests (Goldberg and Weinberger, 2004). For example, executive cognition and cognitive control processing are centered in the prefrontal cortex and dopamine is an important neurotransmitter in these neurobiological processes.

SNPs in the gene catechol-O-methyltransferase (COMT; located on chromosome 22) which codes for an enzyme involved in the degradation of dopamine, are associated with differences in prefrontal cortex cognitive function. One of the SNPs is located in exon 4 and the nucleotide substitution results in a valine substitution for a methionine in the resulting protein. The two different amino acids cause differences in enzymatic activity. The valine allele displays more enzymatic activity and hence is associated with greater catabolism of dopamine. Using scores attained on a standardized test for prefrontal cognitive function, individuals with two methionine alleles achieved on average the highest scores and individuals with two valine alleles had on average the worst scores. Individuals with a combination, one valine and one methionine allele, have on average intermediate scores. This study indicates that the gene COMT is involved in prefrontal cortical cognitive functions; the enzymatically weaker methionine allele allows more dopamine to become available at the synapse which could explain its association with better cognitive functioning.

These examples illustrate that the genetic underpinnings of cognitive functions are becoming better understood. The observation that evolutionarily conserved genes such as FOXP2 and neuropetides such as vasopressin sub serve comparable functions in diverse species underscores the inter-connectedness between humans and non-humans with respect to cognitive functions. In the next sections, other examples of complex cognitive functions in different animals are reviewed. In most of these examples, corresponding genomic studies have not been done.

In the section; Background, Evolution; several examples of complex cognitive behavioral traits in non- humans were discussed. Vocal learning, which is considered an important step in language acquisition, has been documented in songbirds, some species of parrots, hummingbirds, certain bats, elephants, whales and dolphins (cetaceans). Australian magpies use the gesture of pointing in a definitely intentional manner as do primates. The scientific literature is replete with other examples of complex cognitive behaviors in non- humans.

Honeybees can learn spatial relational concepts of “above” and “below” (Chittka and Jensen, 2011) and pigeons appear to be on a par with rhesus monkeys in acquiring an abstract numerical ordinal rule (Scarf et al., 2011). Marino et al., (2007) have reviewed the complex cognitive capacities characteristic of cetaceans (toothed whales and dolphins). Lunau (2011) reported on the Dominica Sperm Whale Project which is a longitudinal study of families of whales. The investigators involved in this project have observed that these mammals appear to have a nuanced communication system based upon a system of clicks which differ from echolocation clicks.

Migratory birds rely on experiential learning and memory to aid in their migrations. Mettke-Hofmann and Gwinner (2003) examined long term memory in garden warblers, a long distance nocturnal migrant, compared to Sardinian warblers, a non-migrant. The experimental design consisted of an exploratory phase and then a memory test. During the exploratory phase, birds were allowed to access two rooms only one of which contained food. The memory test was applied at different time intervals following the exploratory phase. Food was removed from the one room but otherwise the experimental setup was unchanged. The percent of time birds spent in the “correct” room (i.e. the room that had contained food) constituted the memory test. The long distance migrant warbler was able to remember the correct feeding site for up to a year whereas the non-migrant warbler could only remember such a site for only about two weeks. Hence, migratory behavior requires that the bird be able to learn and remember the features of quality (i.e. food resources) habitat sites. In a related study, Pravosudov et al., (2006) observed that migratory white-crowned sparrows had better spatial memory and more neurons in the right hippocampus than non-migratory white-crowned sparrows. A comparison of adult and juvenile members of both subspecies suggested that the differences in hippocampal neuron numbers between the migratory and non-migratory subspecies were probably experience- dependent.

Henderson et al., (2006) studied free-living Rufous hummingbirds and noted that these birds were able to remember both the location of nectar containing flowers and also when they had visited (emptied the nectar) these various flower locations. Hence, these hummingbirds appear to possess episodic-like-memory processes previously thought to be restricted to mammals.

This survey, although limited, illustrates that non-humans possess cognitive abilities which have evolved to allow groups of animals to solve their ecological problems. Cognitive functions are part of the adaptive "toolbox "by which animals cope with environmental demands. Foraging honeybees can recognize spatial relationships, which is one of the cognitive tools that this invertebrate uses to search out suitable food sources. Migratory birds have the capacity to remember the features of topographical maps which allow them to select and return to resource rich habitats. Hummingbirds can remember not only the location of nectar containing flowers but also when they fed from the various flower locations; this capacity maximizes feeding efficiency for this bird. These observations in migratory birds and hummingbirds indicate that these vertebrates are capable of experience based learning and memory. Whales have a cognitive skill set which appears to include a communication system such that these mammals can survive in an ocean environment. Humans have evolved a sophisticated set of cognitive skills as an adaptation to or perhaps better stated as a pre-requisite for our highly social living arrangement. The repertoire of cognitive capacities characteristic of a species is adaptive for its ecological niche and hence, the distribution of cognitive abilities across species can only be understood within the specific ecological contexts that apply to those species (Bald et al., 1996). In addition, within a species there will also be individual variation in cognitive abilities.

What about environmental influences as determinants of cognitive functions? Ramus (2006) has pointed out that there is really no distinction between genetic and environmental influences at the mechanistic level. In order to affect brain functions, environmental influences (experiences) must first "enter" the organism through genetically designed sensory pathways which provide a first filter on the environmental cue. The environmental cue or experience would in general be composed of multiple sensory inputs; sight, sound and touch. As soon as the environmental cue is encoded by our sensory receptors, all external signals become in fact internal neural signals, subject to all the constraints imposed by our neural architecture. Any changes that these now internalized neural signals induce on brain functions are the product of molecular processes that are under strict genetic control. The effects of experience (environmental cues) selectively alter the expression pattern of our genes thereby modulating the execution of our genetic program. As summarized by Ramus (2006), there are no pure environmental influences; experiences can only influence an organism through the filter of its own genome. Within this context what mechanisms are known to link environmental cues (sensory and motor experiences) with cognitive functions?

Perhaps the best studied mechanism involves the induction of immediate early genes (IEGs). IEGs are a class of genes which are activated transiently and rapidly in response to a wide variety of cellular stimuli including growth factors and neural activity. There are approximately 30-40 neuronal IEGs which can be classified into two groups (Davis et al., 2003; Tzingounis and Nicoll, 2006).One group known as regulatory genes e.g. C-FOS, C-JUN and ERG1, encode transcription factors while the second group, known as effector genes, code for growth factors, signal transduction molecules, metabolic enzymes and cell surface proteins. The link between neuronal activity and induction of IEG expression is clearly demonstrated by a novel experiment by Schoenenberger et al., (2009). These investigators "inserted" a light- gated cation channel into pyramidal cells in hippocampal slice culture. Pyramidal cell activity was induced by brief light pulses and this neuronal activity triggered the expression of the IEG C-FOS in the neuronal cell. The expression of C-FOS was detected within 30 minutes of light stimulation.

Immediate early genes play a role in synaptic plasticity, learning and memory storage. Expression of an IEG occurs as a result of the stimulation of various cell membrane receptors (including NMDA glutamatergic receptors and voltage gated calcium channels) which activate signaling cascades and downstream transcription factors that bind to the promoter region of a given IEG activating transcription (Davis et al., 2003; the induction of ERG1 is the example they discuss). This process results in increased expression of the immediate early gene. Induction of IEG expression is involved in a variety of brain cognitive functions such as; song learning in birds, visual paired associations in the monkey, fear associated learning tasks in rats and spatial learning in rats (Davis et al., 2003). Combinations of IEGs appear to be necessary for the long term storage of information and consolidation of memories (Davis et al., 2003). Guzowski et al., (2000) showed that the IEG, ARG.3.1 (ARC), functions in rats to regulate activity-dependent synaptic strength plasticity (capacity of chemical synapses to change their strength) and to promote long term memory consolidation.

A very interesting system for looking at the effects of IEGs is that of the whiskers-barrel cortex of rats and mice (Filipkowski, 2000). Mice and rats use their whiskers (a mechanosensory organ) for a variety of functions; balance, orientation, spatial learning, distinguishing objects, depth perception as well as aggressive, predatory and copulatory behaviors. The sensory signal from the whiskers travels from the brainstem through the thalamus to the somatosensory cortex (barrel cortex). In the unstimulated barrel cortex there is a very low expression of the IEGs, C-FOS and ERG1. Treating rats with a dopamine agonist resulted in increased expression of C-FOS and ERG1 mRNA in various brain regions, including the barrel cortex. Stimulating learning and exploration by introducing animals to a new cage environment also increased C-FOS expression. The whisker-barrel cortex system of mice and rats allows investigators to examine relationships between various sensory inputs, different cognitive behaviors and the expression patterns and effects of IEGs. (Experiments describing the effects of new sensory experiences on structural synaptic plasticity in the barrel cortex and the role of the dopaminergic system in determining plasticity are discussed in a subsequent section; Mechanisms underlying cognitive ageing; c) Synaptic plasticity).

Another mechanism linking environmental cues with brain function is epigenetic modulation of gene expression patterns. Several examples of environmental cues influencing behavioral and morphological phenotypes through induction of epigenetic mechanisms are reviewed in the section; Background; genetics. Epigenetic mechanisms operate over a much longer time frame than the induction of IEGs which is very rapid process. In addition, considering the two main epigenetic mechanisms, DNA methylation is a much more permanent gene silencing mechanism than post translational histone modifications.

No doubt the effects of environmental cues (experiences) on brain cognitive functions involve multiple mechanisms. The rapid induction of IEGs and the effects of their protein products on multiple downstream target genes would represent a rapid immediate linkage between an experience and a cognitive behavior. This rapid IEG- mediated link is also involved in memory storage of the experience. Epigenetic mechanisms might induce longer term changes in gene expression patterns in response to an experience and hence could potentially lead to a more long lasting alteration in cognitive functions as a result. The IEG and epigenetic mechanisms are themselves inter-linked (Borrelli et al., (2008) as discussed in the section; Mechanisms underlying cognitive ageing, c) Synaptic plasticity.

In summary, although our understanding of the genetic underpinnings of cognitive behaviors is still incomplete, based upon current data as well as the data related to evolution of the mammalian brain, certain general principles appear to apply. First, the genes and neuropeptides involved in cognitive behaviors appear to play comparable roles across many vertebrate groups. In addition, these genes and neuropeptides have functional roles in many tissues other than the brain. This principle underscores the economical nature of evolution; the same or similar genes have comparable functions in different species and also have multiple functional roles within the same species. Secondly, modification of gene regulatory elements rather than "creation" of new protein coding genes appears to be the principal mechanism underlying the diversity of cognitive functions across species.

Cognition and Ageing

What happens to an animal's cognitive skills over its life history? Although this is clearly an important question, it has not been addressed for animals other than primates. An exception is the honeybee (Singer, 2011) and possibly some bird species.

The honeybee is a social insect that lives in colonies consisting of a single egg-laying queen, about 10,000-30,000 sterile female workers and from zero to a few thousand males (drones). The female workers nurse the queen's offspring and perform a number of exterior hive tasks such as foraging and guarding. Activities within the hive such as nursing are generally done by young workers while riskier outside the hive functions such as foraging are performed by older workers. The switch from in-hive nursing tasks to outside-hive foraging activities usually occurs at about three weeks of age. Forager bees have a higher extrinsic mortality rate, a shorter life span and a more rapid senescence pattern than nurse bees. Ageing in honeybees is a plastic process tied to role function. As reviewed by Singer (2011), cognitive senescence in worker bees is principally determined by social role (foraging rather than nursing tasks) and correlates with the duration of foraging activities. However, the senescence does not affect global cognitive capacities but one of selected cognitive impairments. In addition, cognitive ageing in the forager bee is at least partially reversible in that cognitive skills in foragers are improved if they revert back to nursing activities.

Cognitive functioning in birds has not been specifically examined over the life history of a particular species. Perhaps, the closest study was one done by LeComte et al., (2010). These investigators measured ageing in the long-lived wandering albatross and one of the variables included was foraging behavior.

This seabird has a lifespan in excess of fifty years and both males and females show evidence of declining reproductive success after the age of about thirty years. The foraging area for this bird is extensive (thousands of kilometers) and is only patchily distributed with prey. Finding restricted numbers of prey in such a vast area represents an impressive cognitive task. Older birds displayed a different foraging pattern than younger birds with the age-dependent changes in foraging behavior essentially restricted to males. Most striking was the observation that young and old males tended to segregate into different foraging areas. Other significant changes in foraging behavior with age included; distance travelled and foraging range increased with age and foraging activity declined with age (old males spent more time flying between foraging locations and when at a location spent more time sitting on the water). In summary, older males show a decline in foraging efficiency with age. The investigators did not have a ready explanation for their observations but several explanations are possible. Foraging behavior is both an energetically and cognitively demanding task. Given that these investigators found no age related changes in humeral immunity, or anti-oxidant enzyme levels (in erythrocytes), I would tend to favor the possibility that the decline in foraging efficiency in older males represents at least partially a decline in the specific spatial cognitive skills required for foraging across wide areas containing limited amounts of prey.

In mammals, age related declines in cognitive skills have been well documented in non-human primates and in humans. Herdon et al., (1997) measured age related cognitive functioning in rhesus monkeys. The subjects were 22 female and 31 male rhesus monkeys studied at the Yerkes Regional Primate research Centre. Males ranged in age from 4.5 to 27.6 years and females from 4.1 to 30.9 years. A number of individual cognitive tests were applied and as well an overall cognitive performance index was devised. The time course for age related declines in the various cognitive tasks measured varied across these different tasks. Tasks involving spatial components appeared to be particularly sensitive to age related impairment. However, nearly all monkeys surviving to ages of 29 years or more showed significant impairments in all of the cognitive tasks tested. Jonsson et al., (2012) measured cognitive functioning in older humans using a cognitive performance scale. The subjects for this study were residents in Icelandic nursing homes in the age range 80-100 years (without a diagnosis of Alzheimer's disease) and the data consisted of 23,831 measurements made in 3,673 individuals. Most of the individuals had multiple measurements made over a number of years. The data showed a slow but definite progressive decline in cognitive functioning over the age range 80 to 100 years.

The limited available data suggest that a decline in cognitive capacities with ageing is probably a general feature of animals although this suggestion is based upon studies restricted to the honeybee, one species of seabird, non-human primates and humans. If this is the case, what might be the mechanisms underlying such an age related decline in cognitive functioning?

Mechanisms Underlying Cognitive Ageing

A number of mechanisms have been implicated as underlying cognitive ageing and these mechanisms should not be considered mutually exclusive.

a) Molecular Clocks

Ageing in the honeybee appears to be primarily determined by behavioral traits and in particular task functions. Forager honeybees age more rapidly than nurse bees and this senescence includes cognitive ageing. Toma et al., (2000) and Bloch et al., (2001) studied the role of molecular clocks in regulating honeybee role function. Foragers must have a highly functional circadian system in order to integrate various navigational inputs with the purpose of timing visits to flowers for maximum nectar and pollen availability, The topic of circadian rhythms and molecular clocks was discussed in the section on Atherosclerotic Vascular Disease. Toma et al., (2000) looked at circadian rhythms for loco motor activity as well as the expression pattern for the molecular clock gene period (Per). They observed that circadian loco motor rhythmicity was age- related appeared in worker bees at about 8 days after birth and the proportion of rhythmic bees increased significantly with age. Whole brain levels of Per mRNA increased with age and were greater in foragers than young bees. Bloch et al., (2001) expanded on these observations and found that a number of factors in addition to role function influenced brain per mRNA levels. The importance of task function was confirmed; foragers had higher (whole) brain levels of Per mRNA than young bees and foragers displayed significant circadian rhythms in brain Per mRNA whereas nurse bees did not. However, although foragers always had high levels of brain Per mRNA, levels in nurse bees could be manipulated. For example, foragers that had reverted to nursing activities had brain Per mRNA levels similar to those of bees which continued to forage. Chronological age itself did not seem to be an important factor since there was no consistent association between Per mRNA brain levels and honeybee chronological age. An interesting observation was that social housing environment appeared to influence brain Per mRNA levels. Young bees in single cohort colonies in the field had brain levels of Per mRNA similar to foragers but young bees housed individually in the laboratory had lower brain levels of Per mRNA than foragers. Bloch et al., (2001) concluded that the expression of brain clock genes in the worker honeybee was a complex function of social environment (housed individually or in a colony), developmental programming and task behavior. At a minimum, brain molecular clocks in the honeybee are intimately involved in regulating honeybee task behavior (nursing versus foraging) which in turn is a strong determinant of cognitive ageing in the worker bee. The honeybee represents a wonderful natural animal model for studying the molecular links between molecular clocks, circadian rhythms, and cognitive ageing.

Ageing of the circadian system has been studied in the zebra fish and in this animal ageing is associated with a decline in circadian loco motor activity, a reduction in nighttime "sleep" duration and a decrease in cognitive functioning (Singer, 2011). With ageing, nighttime levels of melatonin levels decline and a decrease in mRNA expression of several clock genes also occurs (Singer, 2011). These observations in the zebra fish point to a relationship between age related changes in the functioning of molecular clocks and age related changes in circadian rhythms and cognitive capacities.

Molecular clocks by regulating daily rhythms in brain activity establish awake-sleep cycles and such cycles are important modulators of synaptic strength (Herzog, 2007).The importance of molecular clocks with respect to cognitive behaviors is underscored by observations that disruptions in the functioning of molecular clocks have significant neurobehavioral consequences (Barnard and Nolan, 2008). Modifications in the clock genes of mice are associated with effects varying from sleep disorders to cognitive disturbances.

SNPs in human clock genes have been linked to sleep disorders and features of bipolar behavior (Barnard and Nolan, 2008). Dysregulation of circadian rhythms such as sleep cycle, activity pattern and temperature are observed in neurodegenerative disorders and most likely reflect disruptions in the functioning of molecular clocks. However, whether age related alterations in molecular clock functioning contributes to cognitive ageing has not been definitely established although this topic is discussed in a following section; Alzheimer's disease; d) Sleep impairments.

b) Amyloid Deposition

Although the deposition of B-amyloid in the brain is thought to play a role in the genesis of Alzheimer's disease, the accumulation of this peptide in the central nervous system has been well documented in a number of vertebrate groups.

Spawning kokanee salmon, a landlocked subspecies of sockeye Pacific salmon, displayed extensive deposits of amyloid precursor protein (APP) and B-amyloid in the brain (Maldonado et al., 2000). These deposits were found in regions of the spawning salmon important for visual, olfactory, coordination and rhythmic functions, but did not appear to interfere with function. Since spawning salmon use their olfactory system to return to their natal stream, this system must be functionally preserved despite the deposits of APP and B-amyloid. Maldonado et al., (2002) also examined the time courses of neuronal degeneration and B-amyloid deposition in fish varying in reproductive stages from sexually immature to spawning. These reproductive stages correlate with increasing somatic ageing of kokanee salmon which die after spawning. In general, low levels of neuronal degeneration first became evident in sexually immature fish, were more extensive in maturing fish, and greatest in spawning fish. Neuronal degeneration and deposition of B-amyloid occurred in the same brain regions and in fourteen out of sixteen brain areas neuronal degeneration either preceded or appeared more or less simultaneously with B-amyloid deposition. The data of Maldonado et al., (2002) are consistent with the notion that B-amyloid deposition is part of the ageing phenotype not the cause of neuronal degeneration in fish, but perhaps part of a repair process.

Amyloid deposits have also been documented in aged birds. Nakayama et al., (1999) reported the autopsy findings for a great spotted wood pecker of 16 years of age. Grossly, the major organs showed signs of atrophy although the brain appeared normal. Histology of the cerebral cortex showed deposition of B- amyloid in vessel walls. The cortex also contained a few senile plaques which also stained positive for B- amyloid. The investigators reported that autopsies on young birds of two other species did not show brain amyloid deposits consistent with the notion that the amyloid angiopathy in the sixteen year old wood pecker was a senescence- specific lesion.

With ageing, B-amyloid is also deposited in the brains of primates (Fukumoto et al., 2004; Hof et al., 2002). Hof et al., (2002) reviewed the neuropathology of brain ageing in non-human primates and noted the frequent occurrence of B-amyloid protein deposits in the cortical brain areas of monkeys, gorillas, orangutans and chimpanzees. In non-human primates, there is no decrease in cortical neurons with ageing, but alterations have been observed in subcortical nuclei. A substantial loss of dopaminergic neurons in the substantia nigra has been reported in old macaque monkeys and in aged monkeys the development of cognitive and memory impairments have been correlated with morphological alterations of catecholaminergic circuits. Fukumoto et al., (2004) measured formic acid extractable B-amyloid protein and B-secretase activity (one of two enzymes that cleave amyloid precursor protein to yield B-amyloid protein) in brain samples from rhesus monkeys and humans of various ages. There was an age related increase in the amount of extractable B-amyloid and in B-secretase activity in both monkey and human brains. The investigators raised the possibility that the increased activity of brain B-secretase with ageing could be, at least partially, responsible for the increased production and accumulation of B-amyloid protein in the brain of older monkeys and humans.

In summary, deposition of B-amyloid protein in the brain with ageing appears to be a common occurrence in diverse vertebrate groups; fish, birds and mammals. The functional consequences of this process are unclear. In fish, neuronal degeneration precedes B-amyloid accumulation and in non-human primates, age related cognitive impairments correlate with alterations in subcortical neuronal systems whereas B-amyloid accumulates in cortical areas. These observations in non- humans suggest that the production and deposition of B-amyloid in the brain with ageing is not responsible for the age related decline in cognitive functioning. Perhaps, the deposition of B-amyloid represents part of a repair process in response to some other form of "damage".

c) Synaptic Plasticity

The earliest manifestation of Alzheimer's disease involves the inability of individuals to encode new memories (Selkoe, 2002). As reviewed by Selkoe (2002), the initial stages of cognitive decline correlate with both synaptic functional alterations and synaptic loss. Cholinergic and glutamatergic synapses are particularly involved. Quantitative morphometric studies in temporal and frontal cortical brain biopsies of individuals with early stages of Alzheimer's disease revealed a significant decrease in both the numerical density of synapses and the number of synapses per cortical neuron. Studies in genetically engineered animals showed a correlation between loss of presynaptic terminals and the extent of the soluble pool of cortical B-amyloid protein.

Synapses can show plasticity in terms of strength (measured as inducible changes in the magnitude of post synaptic membrane potentials) and structure. Although both synaptic structural and strength plasticity are involved in memory acquisition and consolidation, this discussion will principally focus on structural plasticity.

In the adult human brain, structural plasticity in terms of synapse formation and elimination are thought to underlie aspects of long term memory formation (Holtmaat and Svoboda, 2009). Bailey and Kandel (1993) point out that a wide variety of memory processes of differing complexity across vertebrates and invertebrates are accompanied by alterations in the structure of synaptic connections. Although long term memory storage is associated with changes in preexisting synapses, alterations in the number and pattern of synaptic connections appear to be the most important structural substrate for this behavior. Another important observation is that neuronal activity is a critical substrate for synaptic structural plasticity. Monocular visual deprivation during early development (lack of visual experience) results in permanent changes in perceptual capacities and in alterations in the number and pattern of synaptic connections (Bailey and Kandel, 1993). Enriching the visual sensory environment of animals by including many objects within their housing space resulted in a thickening of the occipital cortex due to a significant increase in the extent and branching of dendrites and a parallel increase in the number of synapses per neuron. Changes in the number and pattern of synaptic connections have also been shown to accompany various motor learning paradigms. In rodents, motor learning resulted in an increase in the number of synapses per cerebellar Purkinje cell. Bailey and Kandel (1993) concluded that new synapse formation was a highly conserved feature of long lasting behavioral memory.

Newer imaging technologies which allow investigators to directly visualize brain dendritic spines have allowed a more detailed understanding of synaptic structural plasticity in the mammalian brain. Holtmaat and Svoboda (2009) reviewed the general features of synaptic structural plasticity. Dendritic spines are the post synaptic sites of excitatory cortical synapses in the brain and hence changes in spine morphology and formation/elimination are a good proxy of synaptic plasticity. Typically, one spine and one axonal bouton correspond to one synapse. Compared to synaptic strength changes alone, structural synaptic plasticity would greatly increase the memory storage capacity because of the large number of neuronal circuit patterns attainable (Holtmaat and Svoboda, 2009). Spines have widely different lifetimes. Under baseline laboratory conditions, most dendritic spines are stable over one month of imaging and some may persist for the lifetime of the animal, but a substantial fraction appear and disappear over days (transient spines). In rodents, as the brain ages, the density of transient spines (lifetime less than 4 days) significantly decreases up to 6 month of age, the last time point measured (Holtmaat et al., 2005). In addition, the density of transient spines in 6 month old mice was lower in the visual cortex than in the somatosensory cortex perhaps reflecting differences in the capacity for experienced-based synaptic plasticity in these brain regions. In summary, as a baseline characteristic, the brain shows a very active level of synaptic structural plasticity with a significant formation and elimination of dendritic spines and by inference a significant creation and loss of synapses. An important modulator of synaptic structural plasticity is the learning of new motor tasks or the acquiring of new sensory experiences. These experiential learning situations are associated with the formation of new sets of synaptic connections in motor and sensory regions of the brain respectively.

Xu et al., (2009) used an imaging technique to follow synaptic remodeling in the motor cortex of mice taught a motor skill; single- seed reaching task. Even a single motor learning session was sufficient to induce the rapid formation of new dendritic spines in the motor cortex on the contralateral side to the reaching forelimb. A 10% addition of new spines, detected by direct brain imaging, was observed within one hour of the training session. More prolonged training sessions resulted not only in an increase in spine formation but also in spine elimination compared to control mice; the result was that total spine density approached baseline levels observed prior to training. This coupled increased formation and elimination of spines most likely reflected a rewiring of neuronal circuitry in response to the learning experience. The new spines formed in trained mice were more stable (persisted longer) than new spines formed in control mice whereas pre-existing spines in trained mice were less stable than pre-existing spines in control mice over the same time period ; hence motor learning selectively stabilizes learning-induced new spines and destabilizes pre-existing spines. The prolonged persistence of the stabilized learning-induced new spines provides a cellular mechanism for the consolidation of long lasting motor memories. In addition, subjecting the trained mice to a new motor task- learning experience did not affect the stabilized synapses formed during the previous learning experience. This observation that new learning experiences continue to induce synaptic reorganization without affecting the stability of synapses formed during previous learning suggests that different motor behavior memories are stored in different sets of synapses in the brain.

Yang et al., (2009) did comparable experiments using a direct brain imaging technique in mice to look at the effects of both a motor learning and a sensory experience on synaptic structural plasticity. The motor task was learning to use a rotarod. Motor training resulted in a significant increase in new spine formation compared to control mice in the forelimb area of the motor cortex. The novel sensory experience consisted of transferring animals from a standard housing environment to an enriched environment. When animals were switched from the standard to the enriched environment there was an increased formation of spines in the barrel cortex (brain area for whisker sensation). Sensory deprivation by whisker trimming prevented the increase in enriched environment- induced spine formation indicating that the creation of experience-dependent new spines required continued neural input activity. Novel experiences (sensory or motor) also increased the elimination (pruning) of existing spines. The investigators concluded that the structures responsible for long lasting memory storage following novel (new) sensory or motor experiences were new neuronal circuits formed from a combination of a small number of stabilized learning-induced new spines together with a stabilized fraction of pre-existing spines that had survived the experience-dependent pruning (elimination) process.

There are also observations that memory and "emotional" behaviors (mood) are dependent upon the generation of new neurons (neurogenesis) in discrete regions of the adult mammalian brain (Eisch and Petrik, 2012). The connections and cross-interactions between the processes of neurogenesis and new synapse formation in the acquisition and consolidation of memories have as yet been elucidated.

An interesting observation of Xu et al., (2009) was that the brains of mice given a motor task similar to the "learning" task but under conditions in which learning could not occur or mice that failed to learn the motor task, did not show any increase in new spine formation greater than that observed in the control mice. However, all of these groups (those exposed to the motor skill learning paradigm, those given a "non-learnable" motor task and those that failed to learn the motor task) experienced similar amounts of forelimb activity. Ziv and Ahissar (2009) suggested that this observation indicated that there was a behaviorally driven component to the learning-induced process of new spine formation. They proposed that this behavioral component was a reward related one; new experience –dependent spine formation and stabilization occurred only if the resulting new circuit was functionally related to a rewarded action. Furthermore, since the dopaminergic system is involved in various forms of reinforcement or reward-driven learning, Ziv and Ahissar (2009), suggested that this system was the probable modulator of experience- dependent learning and memory acquisition.

The complexity of the dopaminergic system has recently been underscored by the observation that dopamine releasing neurons can actually co-release two neurotransmitters; dopamine and gamma amino butyric acid (GABA) through a common vesicular mechanism (Williams, 2012). This co-release mechanism allows these neurons to induce a variety of responses in post synaptic receiver neurons.

These observations on synaptic plasticity particularly structural plasticity, underscore the strong association between learned tasks and specific groupings of novel synapses whose strength might remain relatively constant once formed. These synaptic groupings might be viewed as the fundamental cellular structures underlying learned sensory and motor experiences (Ziv and Ahissar, 2009). This notion is consistent with the proposal of Prinz et al., (2004; see section; Evolution of the mammalian brain) that similar neural network outputs can be generated by a large variety of combinations of synaptic strengths and intrinsic neuronal properties; neural network output and performance, not individual neuronal activity or synaptic strength, becomes the regulated parameter. In both constructs, the emphasis is on a variety of specific groupings of neural connections as the units of regulation, rather than the properties of individual neurons and synapses.

In the section on Cognition, the question of how environmental cues influence cognition was considered. Two mechanisms were considered; activation of immediate early genes (IEGs) and epigenetic modulation of gene expression patterns.

The role of IEGs in learning, memory acquisition and synaptic strength plasticity is well documented (Davis et al., 2003; Tzingounis and Nicoll, 2006). For example ARG3.1 knockout mice are unable to form long term spatial, fear or taste memories. However there is also evidence that IEGs are important in the control of structural synaptic plasticity. Sanyal et al., (2002) using as a test system the neuromuscular junction of fruit fly larvae, examined the cellular effects of AP1. Activator 1 (AP1) is a generic term used to describe dimeric transcription factors composed of FOS and JUN proteins that bind to a DNA enhancer sequence (Frigo et al., 2004; Karin et al., 1997). FOS and JUN proteins are products of the IEGs C-FOS and C-JUN. Sanyal et al., (2002) observed that neuronal AP1 regulated both synaptic strength and synaptic number and that both FOS and JUN were required for these effects. Increased neural expression of the FOS/JUN heterodimer resulted in a 30% increase in evoked junctional currents (a measure of synaptic strength plasticity) and a comparable increase in synaptic number (assayed as the number of axonal boutons; a measure of synaptic structural plasticity).

Epigenetic processes represent another mechanism by which environmental cues can influence cognitive functions. The activation of IEGs and epigenetic processes are not separate, but intertwined. This interaction between activation of IEGs and epigenetic processes was examined by Crosio et al., (2003). These investigators looked at histone protein modifications and activation of IEGs in mouse hippocampal neurons. The mammalian hippocampus has been strongly implicated in learning and memory acquisition and retention with dopaminergic, cholinergic and glutamatergic neural pathways being the major systems involved. Crosio et al., (2003) used agonists of dopamine, acetylcholine and (ionotropic) glutamate receptors to induce neuronal activity. Stimulation of neuronal activity by these agonists was associated with a rapid phosphorylation of histone protein H3 N-terminal tail. In addition agonist induced neural activity also increased expression of the C-FOS IEG in the same hippocampal areas. However, induction of H3 phosphorylation always preceded induction of C-FOS expression. A significant enrichment of phosphorylated H3 occurred in chromatin associated with the C-FOS gene. The investigators proposed that neural activity induced by neurotransmitters (dopamine, acetylcholine or glutamate) resulted in rapid phosphorylation of unmodified H3 with subsequent acetylation of a proportion of the phosphorylated H3. This chromatin remodeling is at least partially responsible for the change in gene expression pattern that follows neurotransmitter induced neural activity and this change includes the rapid induction of IEG (e.g. C-FOS) expression. This neural activity-induced change in gene expression pattern (including activation of IEGs) provides a genetic basis for the learning and memory functions of the hippocampus. Two observations emanating from this study by Crosio et al., (2003) need to be underscored; epigenetic modulation of chromatin structure can occur quite rapidly and epigenetic chromatin remodeling can activate IEGs.

Miller and Sweatt (2007) examined the role of DNA methylation in the memory functions of the brain. Rats were the test subject and were exposed to a contextual fear conditioning training paradigm. Animals trained in contextual fear conditioning showed increased levels of DNA methyltransferase (DNMT) 3Aand 3B mRNA as well as increased levels of C-FOS mRNA in the hippocampus compared to control animals within 30 minutes after the training. When a DNMT inhibitor was infused into the hippocampus after the training period, the animals showed less memory for the fear conditioning paradigm when tested 24 hours later. Interestingly, the ability of these animals that had been treated with a DNMT inhibitor, to learn the fear conditioning task 24 hours later suggested that changes in DNA methylation in the adult nervous system are not necessarily permanent; i.e. DNA methylation maybe a more plastic process that previously envisaged. Fear conditioning trained animals displayed increased methylation of the gene, protein phosphatase 1 (PP1) and reduced expression of this gene (reduced mRNA levels) compared to control animals within one hour after the training. The gene PP1 is involved in suppressing memory consolidation and in reducing synaptic strength plasticity. These changes in the methylation state and expression of PP1 could be blocked with a DNMT inhibitor. The investigators also looked at the methylation state and activity of the gene reelin in fear conditioning trained animals and controls. This gene promotes synaptic strength plasticity as well as memory retention. Trained animals (one hour after training) showed reduced methylation of the gene reelin as well as increased mRNA levels compared to control animals. The investigators proposed the following scheme. Within the hippocampus, activation of neuronal receptors triggers a signaling network which increases expression of DNMTs and demethylases in the nucleus. Genes such as reelin that promote learning and memory are demethylated and the associated histones acetylated; the result is a more open chromatin structure and increased expression of these genes. Genes which suppress memory and learning such as PP1 are methylated and methyCpG binding proteins are recruited to these loci. These proteins orchestrate chromatin remodeling (deacetylation). The result is transcriptional silencing of these genes. In summary, learning experiences lead to dynamic alterations in DNA methylation patterns in the hippocampus which promotes the learning and memory retention of the experience.

A study by Graff et al., (2012) also looked at epigenetic regulation of memory function. The test subject was a genetically modified mouse with a neurodegenerative phenotype considered analogous to Alzheimer's disease; various types of memory impairments, neuronal loss, B-amyloid accumulation, reduced synaptic density, all most prominent in the hippocampus and cortex. Compared to controls, these mice showed an increase in neuronal nuclear histone deacetylase (HDAC 2) protein. HDAC2 was significantly enriched at genes involved in learning, memory and synaptic plasticity and was bound to both promoter and coding regions. These genes included IEGs, glutamate receptor subunits, neurofilament light chain, synaptophysin and synaptotagmin. The binding of HDAC2 to these genes was associated with hypoacetylation of histone residues in the promoter regions. Histone deacetylation leads to chromatin remodeling and a more compact chromatin structure which is associated with DNA transcriptional repression. The investigators observed reduced expression of all these genes which were enriched with HDAC2. Next, the investigators used a viral vector to insert a modified RNA targeted against HDAC2 into the hippocampal area of these mice. Such treated mice showed a significant improvement in various memory tasks such that their performance was comparable to control animals. The treated mice also demonstrated reduced levels of hippocampal HDAC2, increased histone acetylation at promoter regions and increased expression of the various genes under study. The treated mice did not have any increase in the number of surviving neurons as compared to untreated mice but did have an increase in synaptic density and dendritic abundance comparable to control mice. Also treated mice showed improved synaptic strength plasticity. Hence, treatment of the mice (i.e. reduction of HDAC 2 activity) re- instated synaptic structural and strength plasticity but did not improve neuronal survival. The investigators found a glucocorticoid response element (GRE) in the promoter region of the HDAC2 gene and observed increased binding of glucocorticoid receptor to this GRE in the subject mice compared to controls. The investigators cloned the HDAC2 promoter with and without the GRE and used a luciferase construct to monitor activity. Binding of glucocorticoid receptor to the GRE markedly increased luciferase activity. In summary, the neurodegenerative phenotype of this genetically modified mouse was due to increased HDAC 2 gene transcription with histone deacetylation in the promoter region of various genes involved in learning, memory and synaptic plasticity. The histone deacetylation led to a more compact chromatin structure around these genes resulting in repression of DNA transcription. The increased expression of HDAC 2 appeared to be mediated through increased binding of glucocorticoid receptor to a GRE in the HDAC2 promotor region.

Other observations supporting epigenetic mechanisms (DNA methylation, histone methylation and acetylation patterns) as underlying environmentally mediated changes in gene expression have been reviewed by Miller (2012) and Nestler (2012).

In summary, a principal mechanism underlying learning and memory storage of sensory and motor experiences is the formation of new dendritic spines and new synapses. Exposure of the animal to new motor and sensory experiences induces neural activity which in turn triggers several events; the rapid up regulation of IEGs and rapid changes in DNA methylation and histone modifications (phosphorylation/ acetylation/deacetylation). These two processes are interconnected since post translational modifications of histones can up regulate IEG expression. DNA methylation and post translational histone modifications alter chromatin packing and DNA transcriptional activity (enhancement or repression). These epigenetic processes occur at the promoter regions of various genes involved in learning and memory retention. These changes in the pattern of gene expression (up regulated IEGs and epigenetic induced alteration in DNA transcription) result in new dendrite formation. A subtraction of these new dendrites becomes stabilized and pruning of pre-existing dendrites takes place. Together these two processes result in the establishment of new synaptic connections and neural circuits in response to the animal's exposure to novel sensory and motor experiences. In addition, to these morphological changes (synaptic structural plasticity), alterations in synaptic strength (synaptic strength plasticity) also occur in response to the new experiences. I suspect that the efficiency of synaptic plasticity in response to new experiences declines with age although I am not aware of any direct studies addressing this question. However, as already noted, the density of transient spines (defined as spines that have a lifetime of only a few days) in mice decreases with age and this age related decrease in dendritic spine density varies between brain regions (Holtmaat et al., 2005). Probably, transient spines are the pool of spines that respond to novel experiences. If so then an age related decrease in density of transient spines would translate into an age related decrease in memory acquisition and storage.

Although formation of new neural connections and changes in synaptic strength are crucial for the learning process and acquisition of memory, the quality of the social environment experienced by an individual as a child can set limits on these cognitive capacities. It has been well documented that childhood isolation and neglect can produce lasting cognitive damage ranging from emotional instability to intellectual impairment (Underwood, 2012). The effects of social isolation on cognitive functioning were recently studied by Makinodan et al., (2012) using mice as the test subject. Male mice at the time of weaning were housed in one of three social settings; isolation (IS), regular environment (four mice per standard cage, RE) and enriched environment (large cage with eight mice and novel toys, EE). Four weeks later the mice were tested for sociability (interaction with other mice) and learning and remembering a swimming task. General motor activity was not altered by isolation, but the IS mice did much worse in the sociability and swimming task test than the RE and EE mice. Two weeks later the histology of the medial prefrontal cortex was examined in the mouse groups. In the IS group, oligodendrocytes showed a much simpler morphology with shorter processes, less branching and fewer internodes compared to the RE and EE groups. Axonal myelin thickness and the mRNA levels of two myelin genes were reduced in IS mice compared to RE and EE mice. The influence of social isolation on myelination and cognitive and social functions was limited to a short critical two week time period after weaning. These effects persist even when the socially isolated mice are re-exposed to social interactions.

The effects of social isolation on oligodendroycte morphology and myelination were mediated by the neuregulin 1(NRG1)-ErbB3 (receptor) signaling pathway. Mice that were socially isolated during the critical post weaning period showed reduced medial prefrontal cortex expression of the type III protein isoform of the neuregulin I gene. In addition, mice that had oligodendrocyte ErbB3 receptor expression reduced during the critical post weaning time window (i.e. lost ErbB signaling) displayed the "social isolation" phenotype (reduced myelin gene expression, reduced myelin thickness, and alterations in sociability and task learning and memory) even though these mice had not been socially isolated. Hence, social isolation during a critical post weaning time window resulted in reduced type III NRG 1 expression, reduced oligodendrocyte ErbB3 signaling and incomplete oligodendrocyte maturation and myelination. In summary, juvenile social experiences can regulate prefrontal cortex myelination, through neuregulin 1-ErbB3 signaling, which can result in long lasting alterations in cognitive functioning.

d) Regulation of Protein Folding

The correct folding of proteins is an essential biological function. Proteins are ultimately responsible for almost all cellular processes and their requisite functioning depends upon their primary structure and their three dimensional folded structure. The three dimensional structure of a globular protein was first determined about 50 years ago yet as summarized by Dill and MacCallum (2012) the biophysics of protein folding is still poorly understood. Unfolded or misfolded proteins tend to aggregate and this aggregated state has been linked to many "disease" processes; so called conformational diseases (Yoshida, 2007; Guerriero and Brodsky, 2012). Although proteins can fold spontaneously in vitro, within the cell productive folding can only occur after a complete protein or at least a domain has emerged from the ribosome (Vabulas et al., 2010). Molecular chaperones (a class of proteins that aid non-native proteins acquire their native three dimensional folded structures) interact with nascent polypeptides to inhibit premature misfolding and aggregation by shielding the hydrophobic surfaces of the folding chain and to effect the correct folding of the polypeptide. There are several groups of chaperones in the cytosol; the 90kDa heat shock protein (HSP90), the 70kDa heat shock protein (HSP 70) and small HSP proteins (10-40kDa). Chaperones facilitate folding through ATP regulated binding and release cycles; blocking hydrophobic sites prevents aggregation but transient release of binding is necessary for folding to proceed.

For proteins that undergo the major part of their folding in the cytoplasm, the ribosome remains within the cytosol. Chaperones stabilize the nascent polypeptides while on the ribosome and initiate their folding. About 20% of polypeptides achieve their native state during this step. For other polypeptide chains, chaperones (HSP 90) acting downstream to the ribosome complete the folding process (Vabulas et al., 2010). For a small subset of polypeptides that cannot be folded by the binding-release cycles of the chaperones, a second group of molecules called chaperonins are involved in the folding process. Chaperonins are large double ring protein complexes which promote folding through ATP regulated cycles of global protein encapsulation. These complexes enclose unfolded proteins one molecule at a time (Vabulas et al., 2010).

This description refers to the chaperone system responsible for the regulation of folding of cytoplasmic proteins. An analogous system regulates folding of proteins synthesized in the endoplasmic reticulum (ER).

The ER is a cellular organelle where secretory proteins (proteins excreted into the extracellular space) or membrane proteins are synthesized. Transcription of secretory proteins is similar to that of other proteins. The mRNA is transported to the cytosol where it interacts with the ribosome. The first part of the polypeptide chain produced contains a signal sequence with hydrophobic side chains and this signal sequence binds to a ribonucleoprotein complex (signal recognition particle, SRP). The binding of the signal sequence to the SRP results in translational arrest and movement of the ribosome-nascent polypeptide chain complex to the ER membrane. At the ER membrane, the SRP docks to a receptor, translation resumes and the nascent polypeptide chain is trans located into the ER lumen. During the translocation of the chain into the ER lumen the signal sequence is removed (Guerriero and Brodsky, 2012). After signal sequence cleavage, nascent proteins undergo post translational modifications in the ER. Within the ER, molecular chaperones and folding enzymes (foldases) facilitate the proper folding of the nascent polypeptide chains.

Accumulation of misfolded proteins within the cytosol or in the ER triggers processes to correct or eliminate these misfolded proteins.

In the cytosol, transcriptional up regulation of molecular chaperones occurs via the action of heat shock transcription factors (HSFs) such as HSF1 (Vabulas et al., 2010; Kubota, 2009). Under normal physiological conditions HSF 1 is present as an inert monomer bound to molecular chaperones. An increase in the amount of unfolded or misfolded proteins leads to displacement of HSF 1 from chaperones by these misfolded proteins. HSF 1 trimerizes, trans locates to the nucleus, and there undergoes post translational modifications. The activated HSF 1 trimer induces the transcription of a number of HSP genes which help to promote folding of the unfolded or misfolded proteins and also induces the expression of ubiquitin (Vabulas et al., 2010; Kubota, 2009). The increased concentration of chaperones also acts as a negative regulator of HSF 1 by binding the monomeric and trimeric forms thus attenuating the activity of HSF 1. In addition, terminally misfolded proteins can be degraded through the ubiquitin-proteasome and autophagy-lysosome systems (Kubota 2009). Misfolded proteins are "recognized" by chaperones and ubiquitin molecules are added to the chaperone identified misfolded protein through a cascade of enzymatic steps. The ubiquitin molecules tag the misfolded protein for transfer to the proteasome for degradation (Guerriero and Brodsky, 2012). The tagged protein enters the proteasome where it undergoes proteolysis. The ubiquitin-proteasome system mostly functions to degrade monomers of misfolded proteins while the autophagy-lysozyme system degrades soluble protein aggregates (Kubota, 2009). Soluble misfolded protein aggregates (identified by chaperones) are ubiquinated and sequestered in membrane vesicles. The vesicles fuse with lysozymes and the sequestered protein aggregates are degraded by lysozymal enzymes (Kubota, 2009).

The accumulation of misfolded proteins in the ER leads to a series of corrective processes analogous to those described for handling cytosolic misfolded proteins. These collective processes are referred to as the unfolded protein response (UPR). The UPR is a conserved response that results in translational repression and expansion of the folding and degradative capacity of the ER (Guerriero and Brodsky, 2012). Misfolded proteins in the ER activate a resident ER protein kinase (IRE 1) which through a series of steps induces the transcription of genes encoding chaperones, folding enzymes and genes involved in degradative pathways. Although chaperones and foldases can help promote folding of misfolded chains, ER associated degradative pathways (ERAD) represent the fastest mechanism for eliminating misfolded proteins from the ER. ER associated chaperones identify misfolded proteins which are then polyubiquinated. These ubiquitin tagged molecules are retrotranslocated to the cytosol where they are degraded by proteasomes. An additional component of the UPR is the induction of pathways resulting in cellular apoptosis (Yoshida, 2007).

The regulation of protein folding has become an extremely active area of research and the accumulation of misfolded proteins is thought to play a role in many "disease" states including neurodegenerative diseases such as Huntington's and Alzheimer's (Guerriero and Brodsky, 2012; Yoshida, 2007). The references; Vabulas et al., 2010, Kubota, 2009, Yoshida, 2007, Guerriero and Brodsky, 2012, Ron and Walter, 2007; describe in detail the molecular events underlying the biological response to protein misfolding in the cytosol and endoplasmic reticulum. Quality control against misfolded proteins shows an age related decline (Balch et al., 2008; Vabulas et al., 2010; Chiang et al., 2012). The link between ageing and the effectiveness of quality control against misfolded proteins maybe partly explained by the link between the insulin/IGF 1 signaling network and the cytosolic heat shock transcription factor HSF 1 which up regulates the transcription of cytosolic molecular chaperones. Signaling down this network negatively regulates the expression of the gene encoding HSF 1 in worms (Chiang et al., 2012; Cohen et al., 2006; Balch et al., 2008). Reduced signaling down the insulin/IGF 1 network in worms increases life span and the expression of HSF 1.Overexpression of HSF 1 or inhibiting the activity of HSF 1 leads to increased and reduced longevity respectively (Chiang et al., 2012).These observations suggest that the insulin/IGF 1 signaling network might, at least in part, influence life span by regulating the heat shock response. Since this signaling network is highly conserved a similar relationship might exist in mammals.

In summary, the learning process involves acquisition of sensory and motor experiences and development of memory for the learned task. Experiences are acquired through sensory receptors and the associated neural activity leads to the rapid induction of immediate early gene (IEG) expression as well as the epigenetic modification of gene expression patterns. The morphological correlate of the learning process is a burst of new dendritic spines and the formation of new neuronal synaptic connections. This morphological process is dynamic but does establish stable new patterns of neural circuitry associated with the newly learned task. There are numerous mechanisms and processes underlying this overall scheme. Since brain functions are organized anatomically, newly stabilized neural circuits, depending upon the nature of the learned task, will be brain region- specific. Molecular clocks are essential to the learning process by supplying temporal cues but also in other ways not yet defined. Maintenance of protein quality and in particular correct folding of newly synthesized proteins within neural cells is also essential to the learning and memory of experienced tasks. Molecular clocks show age related changes and the efficiency of protein folding mechanisms declines with age. Older animals show a reduced density of transient dendritic spines and hence the efficiency of forming new neural connections will decline with age. In addition, adult cognitive functioning can be altered by social experiences during critical childhood periods; the quality of such social experiences can modify prefrontal cortex myelination patterns which in turn alter the learning process and acquisition of memory.

However, there is still so much that is unknown about learning and memory. It is one thing to study the properties of contractile proteins or solute specific trans membrane channels and relate these properties to an understanding of the functioning of the heart as a pump or the capacity of the kidney to regulate salt and water balance. But understanding learning and memory represents a whole different level of complexity. What is a memory? How is memory encoded by neural circuits? Memories have attached sensations (sounds, sights, smells) and emotions (fear, joy, sadness). What neurochemical processes and neural circuit patterns underlie the genesis and storage of memories and their sensory and emotional attachments? How do experiences and other environmental cues shape learning and the genesis and storage of memories? There is also the distinct possibility that we may never fully understand the cognitive functions of the brain; can the brain study itself?

With this background information on mammalian brain evolution, cognitive functions and age related changes in cognition, we return to the primary premise of this book; dementia is not a disease state but a variant of the ageing process. Two well defined neurodegenerative states, Alzheimer's and Huntington's diseases, will be used to examine this premise.

Alzheimer's Disease

I have divided this discussion somewhat arbitrarily into separate sections although clearly these sections show considerable overlap.

a) Amyloid Cascade Hypothesis

Perhaps the most important and influential hypothesis proposed to explain the behavioral and brain structural changes in Alzheimer's Disease (AD) is the amyloid cascade hypothesis (Karran et al., 2011). The term amyloid refers to the highly ordered B-pleated sheet structure that can be formed by certain proteins. The central feature of this hypothesis is the deposition of amyloid B-protein in the brain parenchyma which is ultimately responsible for the morphological and behavioral features of AD. The amyloid plaques and neurofibrillar tangles that have been considered the pathognomonic histological features of AD are composed of amyloid B-protein and hyperphosphorylated tau protein respectively. Tau is a protein that stabilizes cellular microtubules and is abundant within neurons. Amyloid aggregation and deposition is viewed as an early event that can trigger tau pathology; the accumulation of amyloid B-protein precedes and drives the deposition of tau protein in neurons and their processes. Tau protein appears to mediate the downstream effects of amyloid B-protein on neurons (Selkoe et al., 2012 b). However, most data show a disconnection among a number of variables; levels of amyloid B-protein in the brain, location of amyloid B-protein in the brain, neuronal loss and cognitive impairments. Many apparently healthy older humans have substantial amounts of amyloid in their limbic and association cortices upon post mortem examination (Haass and Selkoe, 2007). Amyloid deposits have been almost universally observed in the brains of the elderly and have even been detected in the brains of about 20% of cognitively normal people who had died in their fifties (Schnabel, 2011). These observations have cast doubt on the role of amyloid plaques as the culprit responsible for the early cognitive impairments found in Alzheimer's disease.

Amyloid B protein is formed by the sequential cleavage of amyloid precursor protein (APP), a ubiquitous type 1 trans membrane glycoprotein, by B-secretase and g-secretase. Amyloid B-proteins, isoforms of 38-43 amino acid residues, are generated normally throughout life in virtually all mammalian cells by the proteolysis of APP (Haass and Selkoe, 2007; Selkoe, 2004). The longer protein isoforms containing 42 or 43 amino acids (AB 1-42; AB 1-43) are considered to be the "toxic" forms.

Autosomal dominant mutations in three genes involved in the generation of amyloid B-protein have been associated with early onset AD; APP gene and the genes presenilin 1 (PSEN 1) and presenilin 2 (PSEN 2) (Karran et al., 2011). The genes, PSEN 1 and PSEN 2 code for proteins that form the catalytic active site of g-secretase. An allele of the apolipoprotein E gene (APOE 4) has also been linked to early onset AD. Over 30 coding mutations in the APP gene have been described; 25 of these lead to autosomal dominant AD with an early onset (Jonsson et al., 2012).These mutations fall into three categories; those inducing changes at the B and g-secretase cleavage sites of APP and those in the mid-domain amyloid B region of APP. Mutations at the first two sites result in overproduction of either total B-amyloid protein or a shift in the ratio of AB 1-42/AB 1-40 towards formation of the more "toxic" AB 1-42 protein. Mutations within the APP gene sequence coding for amyloid B- protein are believed to result in formation of a protein with an increased tendency to aggregate (Jonsson et al., 2012).

Jonsson et al., (2012) reported a rare SNP in the APP gene of an Icelandic population that appears to protect against the development of the more common late onset AD. This SNP resulted in an alanine to threonine substitution in APP close to the B-secretase cleavage site. This SNP was much more common in an elderly control group than in an AD group. In addition, the investigators compared cognitive functioning in two groups of subjects aged 80-100 years; one group consisted of 41 individuals heterozygous for this SNP and the second group comprised 3673 subjects without AD who were non carriers of this SNP. Both groups showed an age related decline in cognitive functioning but the cohort who were heterozygous for the SNP did significantly better on cognitive testing than the group that did not carry the SNP. Using an in vitro cell assay, these investigators showed that the mutated APP underwent less enzymatic cleavage than wild type APP with the result that the production of amyloid B-protein (1-40) and amyloid B-protein (1-42) were reduced by about 40% compared to wild type APP. This SNP seems to "protect" carriers (heterozygotes) from developing late onset AD and also appears to reduce the extent of cognitive decline in the elderly. Although the in vitro experiments of Jonsson et al., (2012) raise the possibility that the protective effect of this SNP is due to reduced formation of "toxic" amyloid proteins, it is also possible that this mutation in the APP gene leads to the formation of amyloid peptides with altered aggregation properties (De Strooper and Voet, 2012).

The g-secretase complex is formed from four proteins and one of those proteins is either PSEN 1 or PSEN 2. However, PSEN 2 containing g-secretase complexes are not as important in the production of amyloid peptides as PSEN 1 g-secretase complexes (Karran et al., 2011). There are currently more than 180 mutations in the PSEN 1 gene linked to autosomal dominant AD (Karran et al., 2011).All of these PSEN1 mutations are missense or in-frame deletions or insertions (Wang et al., 2010).Most of these mutations lead to a reduction in the total amount of amyloid B-protein produced but an increase in the ratio of the "toxic" (1-42) amino acid isoform to the "less toxic" (1-40) amino acid isoform.

The g-secretase complex cleaves various other type 1 trans membrane proteins in addition to APP. Wang et al (2010) described a family suffering from acne inversa in which all of the affected members carried a mutation in one of the copies of the PSEN 1 gene; the mutation resulted in a frame shift and delayed termination codon. Interestingly, none of the affected members of this family showed evidence of AD even though fifteen of the fifty affected members were 50 years or older. This observation suggests that simple inactivation of a single PSEN 1 allele may not be sufficient to cause autosomal dominant AD and raises some interesting possibilities. As discussed in the section; Background; Genetics; loss of function variants in human protein coding genes are not uncommon. MacArthur et al., (2012) reported that individuals harbor on average about 97 such variants with about 18 being present in a homozygous state. In addition, Chakravarti and Kapoor (2012) point out that in autosomal dominant Mendelian disorders the phenotypic expression of the mutant allele will depend upon the presence or absence of associated variants in the regulatory elements for that gene. These regulatory elements can be close to, within or at some distance from the target gene and the effects of the regulatory variants will depend upon whether the variant occurs in an enhancer, silencer or insulator. For example, if the regulatory variant decreases the transcriptional activity of the mutant allele then wild-type expression will be greater than mutant expression. The observations of Wang et al., (2010) raise the possibility that a loss of function mutation in one allele of the PSEN 1 gene is not sufficient to result in AD unless there is an appropriate associated variant in the regulatory elements for the PSEN 1 gene. Could this possibility also hold for mutations in the APP and PSEN 2 genes that have been linked to early onset AD?

The APOE 4 allele is also considered a significant risk factor for the development of AD and in individuals carrying this allele, the age of onset of AD is earlier than in the more common sporadic cases of AD in the elderly. The proteins encoded by the APOE gene are involved in the clearance of amyloid B-proteins with APOE 2, APOE 3 and APOE 4 being increasingly less effective in mediating amyloid protein clearance.

APP is an integral trans membrane protein and the product of an evolutionary conserved gene family (Muller and Zheng, 2012). APP is the vertebrate member of this gene family and it possesses a unique amyloid beta protein sequence. The amyloid B-protein has been detected in mammals (Fukumoto et al., 2004), birds (Nakayama et al., 1999) and fish (Maldonado et al., 2000).The APP gene is expressed in many tissues but has a particularly high expression in neurons. Normal processing of the APP protein by secretases leads to the generation of various cleavage products including amyloid B proteins (Muller and Zheng, 2011). The details of the cleavage steps have now been defined. The extracellular domain of APP is removed by the action of B-secretase. The membrane associated stub then undergoes an intramembranous cleavage by the g-secretase complex, a special type of protease with a unique active site and cleavage mechanism (Haass and Selkoe, 2007). The amyloid B-protein sequence is located just outside and within the trans membrane domain of APP (Selkoe, 2004). It should be noted that the generation of amyloid B-protein is a minority processing pathway. The majority of APP is cleaved by A-secretase to release a large soluble ectodomain and retention of a smaller membrane fragment (Lahiri and Maloney, 2010).

The extracellular domain of the APP protein interacts with various extracellular matrix components and hence APP proteins are considered to function as synaptic adhesion molecules. This synaptic adhesion function requires the activity of both the intracellular and extracellular domains of the APP protein. Ashley et al., (2005), using the fruit fly neuromuscular junction as a test system, showed that the fly homolog of APP (APPL) interacted with Fasciclin II (a trans membrane cell adhesion molecule) to form a complex that regulated new synapse formation. This APPL- Fasciclin II complex also modulated synaptic strength plasticity. APP proteins appear to also serve a trophic function since hippocampal neurons deficient for APP protein show initially reduced neurite outgrowth. APP knock- out mice display impaired learning and spatial memory and impaired synaptic strength plasticity. However, these impairments are not associated with any gross structural changes such as a loss of neurons or synapses. However, as noted by Muller and Zheng (2011), the full functional repertoire of the APP protein is currently unknown and hence the role this protein might play in age related cognitive decline or in the development of AD has yet to be defined.

b) Protein Misfolding and Prions

Protein folding, Alzheimer's Disease and prions share common features (Schnabel, 2011).The folding of a nascent protein can be understood in terms of the shape of the energy surface or energy "landscape" for that particular protein. The energy landscape, which is unique for a specific protein is defined by the amino acid sequence of that protein (Dobson, 2003). Although details are not known, the elements of the folding process appear to be largely determined by the pattern of hydrophobic and polar residues in the protein. As already reviewed (section; Mechanisms underlying cognitive ageing; d) Regulation of protein folding), proteins undergo the major part of the folding process either in the cytosol or in specific cell vesicular compartments such as the ER. Given the enormous complexity and the stochastic nature of the folding process, it would be remarkable if misfolding did not occur. Protective mechanisms are in place to deal with this situation; up regulation of molecular chaperones and mechanisms to degrade misfolded proteins. Alzheimer's disease represents a situation in which proteins with a high propensity to misfold escape these protective processes. There are a number of proteins that can form amyloid which is defined by the characteristic cross-B fiber structure of its aggregates. The formation of amyloid involves the association of unfolded or partially folded proteins to form oligomers which undergo further assembly into protofibrils and then mature insoluble amyloid fibrils (Dobson, 2003). Fibrils can aggregate into large spherical plaques (Schnabel, 2011; Selkoe, 2004). This is the sequence of events that occurs in the case of amyloid B-proteins, particularly the longer isoforms e.g. amyloid B-protein (1-42). Monomers, which are produced normally, can oligomerize within intracellular vesicles and a portion of these oligomers is released into the extracellular fluid of the brain. In experimental studies, intracellular and secreted soluble dimeric and trimeric oligomers have been described in cultured cells containing a mutated form of the human APP gene (Haass and Selkoe, 2007; Selkoe, 2004). The prion analogy relates to the "seeding" mechanism by which amyloid B-protein oligomers form aggregates. The oligomer serves as a nucleation seed to promote an aggregation process (Schnabel, 2011). Prion replication and the formation of amyloid plaques are thought to involve a similar seed-nucleation type of process (Soto et al., 2006).

c) Neurotoxic Species

There seems to be a consensus that one of the neurotoxic species involved in the cognitive impairments of Alzheimer's disease is the oligomeric form of amyloid B-protein. Soluble extracellular oligomers can diffuse into synaptic clefts and bind to synaptic plasma membranes (Schnabel, 2011). Oligomers have been shown to reduce excitatory postsynaptic potentials in the rat hippocampus (Haass and Selkoe, 2007). Although, the cellular and molecular mechanisms underlying the neurotoxicity of soluble oligomers are at present not well defined (Haass and Selkoe, 2007), excitotoxicity due to over excitation and hyperexcitability of NMDA receptors (glutamatergic synapses) has been implicated as one of the principal mechanisms involved (Ittner and Gotz, 2011).

Since the generation of amyloid B-protein appears to be a normal cellular function, what then is the physiological role of this protein? This question has been almost ignored since the research effort fostered by the amyloid cascade hypothesis (and its newer versions) has been almost exclusively focused on the toxicities of amyloid B-protein isoforms.

Koudinov and Berezov (2004) have summarized data concerning physiological roles for amyloid B-protein. These investigators have shown that amyloid B-protein can restore synaptic strength plasticity in rat hippocampus under certain experimental settings (prolonged maintenance ex vivo) and that inhibition of cholesterol biosynthesis by a statin (HMG-CoA reductase inhibitor) abolished this effect of amyloid B-protein. According to these investigators, amyloid B-protein is essential for the regulation of synaptic structural and strength plasticity and that this function is mediated by its regulation of cholesterol trafficking.

Morley et al., (2010) presented experimental data that amyloid B-protein is an important mediator for learning and memory. Young mice were cognitively tested with a T-maze training task and with object recognition experiments. Intracerebroventricular (ICV) injections of amyloid B-protein isoforms (1-42) and (12-28) immediately after a T-maze training session improved the training performance and memory retention of the treated mice compared to control mice. In these experiments, enhancement of learning and memory were associated with low concentrations of the amyloid proteins while higher concentrations inhibited learning and memory. Conversely, blocking amyloid B-protein with specific antibodies or reducing brain levels of amyloid B-protein with an antisense oligonucleotide directed against APP resulted in impaired T-maze task learning and memory compared to control mice. IVC administration of amyloid B-protein (1-42) improved object recognition memory in treated mice compared to control mice. In hippocampal slices, amyloid B-protein (1-42) facilitated long term potentiation, a measure of synaptic strength plasticity. These experimental observations indicate that in normal healthy young mice, amyloid B-proteins are important mediators of task learning and acquisition of memory. These physiological effects of amyloid B-proteins show an inverted U-shaped dose response curve; low concentrations enhance learning and memory whereas higher concentrations inhibit these cognitive functions. This data implies that the generation of amyloid B-proteins by sequential cleavage of APP must be closely regulated so that only the production of small physiological amounts occurs while the production of greater amounts, which are neurotoxic are avoided. With respect to such a regulator mechanism, Lahiri and Maloney (2010) present experimental evidence that amyloid B-protein (1-42) can bind to the promoter region of the gene encoding B-secretase and up regulate its transcription. However, a mechanism (as yet unknown) must be available to down regulate B-secretase transcription when the amounts of amyloid B-protein produced are "too much"and approach a neurotoxic range.

Amyloid B-protein also appears to have a physiological role in modulating the immune and inflammatory response (Hohlfeld and Wekerle, 2012). Mice with experimental autoimmune encephalomyelitis (EAE) showed substantial improvement in the extent of paralysis and inflammation when treated with intraperitoneal amyloid B-proteins (the 1-40 and 1-42 amino acid isoforms were both beneficial). The amyloid B-proteins appear to work by modulating the effects of CD4+ T cells, reducing the proliferation of other subsets of T cells and decreasing the production of pro-inflammatory cytokines (Jones, 2012). As noted by Hohlfeld and Wekerle (2012) amyloid B-protein appears to be a possible "remedy' for immune mediated disorders but can be an "enemy" to the nervous system.

Another molecule involved in the cognitive impairments of Alzheimer's disease is tau protein. The neurofibrillary tangles which are one of the signature histological features of Alzheimer's disease are composed of hyperphosphorylated forms of tau. This protein contains three major domains one of which is a microtubule binding domain (Ittner and Gotz, 2011). Tau is found predominantly in axons and to a lesser extent in dendrites. This protein functions to stabilize microtubules and regulate axonal transport. Tau has multiple phosphorylation sites and the extent of phosphorylation negatively regulates the binding of tau to microtubules. Interestingly, mice with a tau gene knock out show almost normal development but when old manifest behavioral changes such as aggression and memory deficits (Ittner and Gotz, 2011); indicating that tau protein is an important physiological mediator of cognitive behaviors. Ittner and Gotz (2011) review mechanisms by which tau and amyloid B-protein interact to induce neurotoxicity. These investigators proposed that tau mediates downstream amyloid B-protein neurotoxicity according to the following scheme. In dendrites (post synaptic compartment) tau activates a tyrosine protein kinase which phosphorylates NMDA receptors. The strength of the kinase activation is a function of the extent to which tau is phosphorylated. This step leads to the formation of a complex between NMDA receptors and the post synaptic density protein 95. This interaction is believed to be a requisite step for amyloid B-protein to induce over excitation of NMDA receptors (excitotoxicity), memory deficits and in animal models premature mortality.

In summary, the cognitive impairments of Alzheimer's disease are considered to be mediated by both tau protein and oligomers of amyloid B-protein. However, this model is definitely too simplistic given that the full range of normal physiological roles for APP, amyloid B-protein and tau protein in the processes of learning and memory acquisition have not been clarified (Bissette, 2009).

d) Sleep Impairments

In the section; Mechanisms underlying cognitive ageing; a) Molecular clocks; it was noted that disruptions in the functioning of molecular clocks were associated with a spectrum of neuropsychiatric behaviors. Gerstner et al., (2012) and Roh et al., (2012) have presented recent experimental studies looking at the relationships between sleep pattern, ageing and Alzheimer's disease (AD). The amount and quality of sleep decline with ageing and more so in those with AD. Young transgenic AD-model mice and wild-type mice displayed a diurnal cycle for concentrations of amyloid B-protein in brain interstitial fluids. Concentrations were highest during wakefulness and fell during sleep. A similar diurnal cycle for CSF concentrations of amyloid B-protein was also found in young healthy humans. In aged transgenic AD-model mice, in which amyloid plaques had been deposited in the brain, the diurnal cycle for amyloid B-protein concentrations in brain interstitial fluid was lost and the mice showed increased wakefulness. In humans with mutations in the PSEN 1 gene (but no brain amyloid plaques) and in non-carriers of the mutation, a diurnal concentration cycle for amyloid B-protein was found in the CSF. However, like the transgenic AD-model mouse, in humans with the PSEN 1 mutation and amyloid deposits in the brain detected by positron emission tomography, the CSF diurnal concentration cycle was lost. Young transgenic AD-model mice also displayed a similar interstitial fluid concentration cycle for the metabolite lactate and when these mice developed amyloid brain aggregates, the lactate concentration cycle was lost similar to that observed with amyloid B-protein. These studies suggested a complex inter-relationship between glial and neuronal metabolic coupling, amyloid deposition and wakefulness and sleep cycles. Molecular clocks no doubt play a role in these inter-relationships but this possibility has not yet been examined.

The relationship between sleep patterns and various behaviors is complicated by the observation that despite the fact that sleep is universal among birds and mammals no specific physiological function of sleep has been identified that can explain the huge variation in sleep times within and between species (Siegel, 2012). Sleep duration varies enormously in mammals ranging from 20 hours per day in the big brown bat to 2 hours per day in the horse. No physiological hypothesis is currently available to explain the underlying basis of such variation. In addition, sleep deprivation studies in birds and mammals have yielded conflicting results with respect to survival and other "health" outcomes (Siegel, 2012).

e) Positron Emission Tomography (PET); Diagnostic Biomarkers

Substrates have been developed to detect amyloid brain deposits in vivo using the technique of PET. The chemical currently being used is called Pittsburgh Compound B (PIB); this compound binds to fibrillar amyloid B-protein deposits, crosses the blood-brain barrier very well and is rapidly cleared from normal brain tissue. Klunk et al., (2004) used PIB-PET to examine for brain amyloid deposits in nine cognitively healthy controls (three aged 21 and six ranging in age from 59-77 years) and sixteen individuals with AD, ranging in age from 51-81 years. Six of the individuals with AD were homozygous for the APOE 4 allele. As expected, on average, amyloid deposits detected by PIB uptake were much more prominent in those with AD compared to the healthy controls. However, even the healthy controls did show a low level of PIB uptake. Among the healthy controls and those individuals with AD, there were some definite outliers. Three of the individuals with mild AD showed minimal PIB uptake similar to that of the healthy controls. Conversely, the oldest healthy control showed a level of PIB uptake similar to that of individuals with AD. The investigators questioned whether the amyloid deposits in this particular cognitively healthy individual represented a manifestation of the normal ageing process.

This study, although very limited in the number of subjects examined, shows that individuals with AD and cognitively healthy controls do not form two discrete populations; rather there appears to be a continuum between these two groups suggesting that the deposition of brain amyloid protein is part of "normal" senescence.

Biomarkers have been investigated with the purpose of detecting cases of AD prior to the development of impairments in cognitive functions. The biomarkers that have been used include the CSF concentrations of amyloid B-protein (1-42), total concentration of tau protein and concentration of phosphorylated tau protein 181. A number of studies have reported that a low CSF amyloid B-protein (1-42) level and a high CSF total tau and phosphorytated tau protein 181 levels are predictive of AD with sensitivities between 75-100% and specificities between 65-90% (Herskovits and Growdon, 2010). These CSF biomarkers reflect the biochemical composition of developing amyloid plaques (amyloid B-protein) and neurofibrillar tangles (phosphorylated tau protein) in the brain. Post mortem studies have shown an inverse correlation between CSF amyloid B-protein (1-42) levels and brain amyloid B-protein amounts and a direct correlation between tau protein levels and the amount of brain phosphorylated tau. De Meyer et al., (2010) measured CSF levels of amyloid B-protein (1-42) and total tau and phosphorylated tau protein 181 in 114 healthy individuals, 200 individuals with mild cognitive impairment (MCI) and 102 individuals with AD. The investigators used the CSF levels of amyloid B-protein and phosphorylated tau to develop distinct signatures for two states; AD and healthy. They found that forty-one (36%) of the 114 cognitively healthy subjects had the AD biomarker signature. Twenty-two of these 41 individuals did not carry an APOE 4 allele while 19 were either heterozygous or homozygous for APOE 4. Hence, about 20% of cognitively normal individuals have an abnormal (AD) CSF biomarker signature but do not carry the AD associated APOE 4 allele.

This study by De Meyer et al., (2010) and the one by Klunk et al., (2004) show that the boundary between cognitively healthy individuals and those with AD as defined by in vivo measurements (PIB-PET scan and CSF biomarker levels) is quite blurred.

f) Genetics

As discussed in the section; a) Amyloid cascade hypothesis; autosomal dominant AD, which accounts for less than 1% of cases, is due to mutations in one of three genes, APP, PSEN 1 or PSEN 2. Affected individuals show a much earlier onset of signs and symptoms of cognitive impairment. AD causing mutations in the APP gene are either within or immediately flanking the small amyloid-B region. The two genes, PSEN 1 and PSEN 2, code for proteins that are involved in forming the g-secretase complex. Mutations in these three genes directly affect biochemical reactions that generate amyloid B-protein and result in changes in the amount and types of isoforms throughout life (Selkoe, 2012 a).

In 1993, an association between early onset AD and the e4 allele of the apolipoprotein E (APOE) gene was reported (van Es and van den Berg, 2009). The APOE gene has three different alleles called APOE 2, APOE 3 and APOE 4. It is the APOE 4 allele that is associated with an increase in risk of developing AD; two to three fold with one copy of the allele and about twelve fold in those with two copies (Kim et al., 2009).The APOE 4 allele may account for up to 50% of the genetic risk for AD (van Es and van den Berg, 2009). APOE is expressed in several organs with the highest expression in the liver followed by the brain. Non- neuronal glial cells are the major cell types that express APOE in the brain (Kim et al., 2009). In the brain, APOE and two other apolipoproteins are contained in distinct high density like lipoprotein particles. The role of APOE in cholesterol transport is thought to be the key to its importance in AD (Eisenstein, 2011) since cholesterol is important in the process of synaptogenesis and maintenance of synaptic connections. In addition to its function as a cholesterol transporter, APOE also helps to clear amyloid B-protein from the brain. Of the APOE isoforms, APOE4 is the least stable and least effective isoform in terms of cholesterol transport and clearance of amyloid B-protein (Eisenstein, 2011).

Genome wide association studies have identified two other gene variants statistically associated with sporadic AD (Harold et al., 2009; Eisenstein, 2011); SNPs associated with the genes CLU and PICALM. The CLU gene encodes a protein clusterin which is thought to be involved in both amyloid B-protein aggregation and amyloid B-protein clearance. Clusterin aids APOE in the transport of cholesterol in the brain. The gene PICALM is expressed in many tissues but has prominent expression in neurons. The protein encoded by PICALM is involved in clathrin-mediated endocytosis of proteins and lipids, an essential step in the intracellular transport of these molecules. One of the proteins whose intracellular transport is directed by PICALM is involved in the process of synaptic vesicle fusion to the presynaptic membrane during neurotransmitter release (Harold et al., 2009).

The genetic risk factors for AD were summarized in a figure by Eisenstein (2011). Mutations in the genes APP, PSEN 1 and PSEN2 increase the total production of amyloid B-protein or lead to the formation of the longer (1-42 amino acid) isoforms. Proteins encoded by the genes APOE, CLU and PICALM are involved in cholesterol trafficking; cholesterol is a key molecule in synapse formation and maintenance. APOE and CLU encoded proteins are also involved in the aggregation state of amyloid B-protein and its clearance from the brain. Mutations in the genes CLU and PICALM will lead to the generation of faulty less functional protein products and the e 4 allele of APOE expresses a protein that is “less” functional than the proteins encoded by the other two APOE alleles. However, this picture is complicated by several observations which are not consistent with this amyloid cascade hypothesis framework. Wang et al., (2010) identified a mutation in the PSEN 1 gene, which impaired its functioning, but has not been associated with the AD phenotype (Wang et al., 2010) and amyloid B-protein may actually be an essential molecule for regulating synaptic plasticity rather than being primarily a neurotoxin (Koudinov and Berezov, 2004).

In summary, the amyloid cascade hypothesis has dominated thinking about the mechanisms underlying the cognitive impairments observed in Alzheimer’s disease. To date, drugs designed to target these mechanisms (e.g. bapineuzumab, a monoclonal antibody to amyloid B-protein plaques) have proven to be unsuccessful in alleviating the cognitive impairments of AD (Miller, 2012). However, some investigators believe these therapies failed because they were given too late in the course of the disease. As a result three new clinical trials are planned to test drugs administered at a much earlier stage of the disease (Miller, 2012). The study populations in two of the trials will be carriers of autosomal dominant gene mutations (APP, PSEN 1 and PSEN 2 gene mutations) while the third trial will look at the more common sporadic form of AD. This trial population will include older individuals who have positive PET scans for brain amyloid deposits. In one of the trials the drug treatment will consist of an anti-amyloid antibody (crenezumab) developed by Genentech (Miller, 2012) while in the other two trials the drugs to be used have not yet been determined. As noted by Miller (2012), the results of these trials will have significant implications. If these trials fail, the prospects for a "disease altering "treatment for AD at least in the short term will be dealt a major blow. In addition, a failure in these trials will probably make the current amyloid cascade hypothesis untenable.

For most individuals, Alzheimer's disease is accepted as a disease. Yet, some in the biomedical research community appear to believe AD might actually be a variant of the ageing process. Jonsson et al., (2012) have proposed that AD may represent the extreme of the age –related decline in cognitive function. Whitehouse (2003) has remarked that the statement that AD is not normal ageing is more a political than a scientific statement. As noted by Abbott (2012), there is still many unknowns concerning the mechanisms underlying age-related cognitive decline and there is still uncertainty within the research community whether Alzheimer's disease is an abnormal pathological condition or simply an acceleration of normal ageing. Even within the disease construct, Selkoe (2012 a) has noted how AD represents an extremely complex problem. To quote; "The array of observations, some seemingly contradictory, is daunting; it has become an enormous challenge to synthesize available findings into an accurate schema of how the disease starts, unfolds, and gradually devastates cognition , leading to the patient's premature death." The premise of this monograph is that neurodegenerative "diseases" such as Alzheimer's disease and Huntington's disease are extreme variants of the ageing process. This premise will be discussed more fully in the section that follows the discussion of Huntington's disease.

Huntington's Disease (HD)

a) Genetics; Huntingtin Protein Structure

The gene (HTT) responsible for HD was discovered in 1993 and encodes a large ubiquitously expressed protein called huntingtin (Imarisio et al., 2008). The huntingtin protein is found mostly in the cytosol but a small proportion is intranuclear. HTT contains a tract of uninterrupted CAG trinucleotide repeats downstream of the initiator codon in exon 1. In normal individuals the number of CAG repeats is 35 or fewer with 17-20 repeats being most commonly found. The causative mutation responsible for HD is an expansion of the number of CAG trinucleotide repeats. Between approximately 27 to 35 CAG repeats tend to be meiotically unstable and can expand into the disease range of 36 and above when transmitted particularly through the paternal line (Imarisio et al., 2008). Most adult onset cases have 40-50 CAG repeats while 50 or more CAG repeats are associated with juvenile onset disease.

The CAG trinucleotide is a codon for glutamine so the encoded huntingtin protein contains a stretch of polyglutamines (polyQ) at the amino terminus of the protein. In higher vertebrate groups and specifically in mammals the polyQ stretch is followed by a polyproline (polyP) stretch (Zuccato et al., 2010). Downstream from the polyQ and polyP tracts are the HEAT repeats; multiple forty or so amino acid sequences that are involved in protein-protein interactions. Huntingtin protein also contains cleavage sites for proteolytic enzymes that cleave the protein and generate a wide range of fragments. In addition the protein contains a nuclear export signal and nuclear localization signal sequences near the carboxyl end (Zuccato et al., 2010).

The HTT gene shows anticipation (a phenomenon whereby a disease develops an earlier onset or more severe symptoms as it is transmitted through the generations), but predominantly with paternal inheritance (Bates, 2005). The CAG repeat in the HTT gene is unstable and changes size from one generation to the next (Bates, 2005). Large expansions in number of CAG repeats are more likely to occur during paternal transmission since meiotic instability (which leads to an increase in the number of CAG repeats) is greater in spermatogenesis than oogenesis (Imarisio et al., 2008).

Contrary to expectations, HD shows a high new mutation rate (Falush et al., 2001). Falush et al., (2001) used an HD database containing 1,830 genotyped individuals who possessed 36 or more CAG repeats in their HTT gene. The database also contained 451 parent- to -offspring transmissions. The investigators measured mutational flow which is calculated by relating the genotype of the parents to that of offspring. Mutational flow reflects the progression of the genotype within the population in each generation which in turn determines the rate at which new families with HD arise. The calculated mutational flow rate led to an estimated overall new mutation rate of 10% per disease chromosome per generation; i.e. about 10% of individuals who develop HD have parents who would not appear to be carriers of HD. Although the overall de novo mutation rate was 10%, the values for maternal and paternal transmission were 5% and 20% respectively.

There were a number of interesting observations reported by Falush et al., (2001). The severity of the phenotype was a function of the number of CAG repeats. The mutational point flow peaks at a CAG repeat number of 44 and the data indicate that about 100% of these individuals will be ascertained as having HD. For individuals with CAG repeat numbers of 40 and 42, the ascertainments are 40% and 80% respectively. The low ascertainment rates for individuals with CAG repeats in the range 36-39 (less than 5%) is probably because these individuals have on average a less severe phenotype than individuals with 42 or more CAG repeats. Within the database, eight paternal transmissions in which the parent was not a carrier resulted in an affected (HD) offspring. In no case did a maternal transmission from an unaffected (not a carrier) parent lead to an affected (HD) offspring. In six of the paternal transmissions involving an unaffected parent the increase in number of CAG repeats in the offspring varied from 9 to 19. In one case a father with 27 CAG repeats had an offspring with 38 CAG repeats and in another case a father with 30 CAG repeats had an offspring with 40 CAG repeats. In both cases a phenotypically normal father had a phenotypically abnormal child.

Expansion of the CAG repeat number in the huntingtin gene is the primary genetic change underlying HD, but it was clear that the CAG repeat size was not the only determinant of the age of onset. There is a wide variation in the age of onset with a given CAG repeat number and CAG repeat number explained only 50-77% of this variance in different populations (Bates, 2005). The residual variance in age of onset is due to other modifying genes and environmental factors (Imarisio et al., 2008) and this issue has been examined by Wexler et al., (2004).

Wexler et al., (2004) studied the role of genetic and environmental factors on the age of onset of HD in the well described and documented Venezuelan HD kindreds. In these kindreds alleles with 34 CAG repeats or fewer do not produce symptoms. Alleles containing 35-39 repeats produce incomplete penetrance while a repeat of 40 or more CAG repeats is fully penetrant. Age of onset of HD in these kindreds showed great variability even across individuals with the same number of CAG repeats in their longer allele. Depending upon which subpopulation of the kindreds was studied, CAG repeat number only accounted for 44% to 72% of the variance in age of onset of HD. The residual variance, not due to CAG repeat number, was due to other genetic influences (37%), shared sibling environmental factors (22%) and non-shared environmental factors (41%). Hence environmental influences account for about 63% of variation in age of onset of HD not explained by CAG repeat number.

In summary, HD is associated with an expansion of the number of CAG repeats in the HTT gene. Repeat numbers greater than 36 are associated with HD although the phenotype tends to be relatively "mild" until the repeat number reaches into the forties. Higher CAG repeat numbers are associated with an earlier age of onset and more severe "disease." However, as discussed in the previous paragraph, only 44% to 72% of the variation in age of onset is accounted for by the CAG repeat number of the huntingtin gene. The pool of mutated genes is maintained by a relatively high rate of de novo mutations in the parental germ line and de novo mutations are transmitted primarily by the father. The paternal transmission of de novo mutations is not unique to the HTT gene. As discussed in the section Background; Ageing; Kong et al., (2012), using entire genome sequencing of 78 parent-offspring trios, observed that de novo SNPs in the offspring were transmitted primarily by the father and that the number of de novo SNPs mutations transmitted by the father increased with the age of the father. It would be interesting to know if an age-related effect also applied to the father- to-offspring transmission of de novo mutations in the HTT gene.

b) Function of "Normal" Huntingtin Protein

It is interesting to compare in a global sense the research thrusts in the fields of AD and HD. In the case of AD, the presence of a dominant hypothesis (amyloid cascade hypothesis) to explain the cognitive impairments has focused research primarily on the neurotoxic properties of amyloid B-proteins. Research directed toward understanding the physiological roles of amyloid B-proteins and even the physiological roles of APP has taken a back seat. In the case of HD, the situation is somewhat different. The mutated gene associated with HD was identified in 1993, but the relationship between this mutation and the genesis of the cognitive impairments and other features of HD was unknown. Research was directed towards understanding the physiological functions of the protein, huntingtin, encoded by this gene. Hence, research in the field of HD has in general been more broad based than in the field of AD given the lack of a dominant hypothesis to account for the HD phenotype.

The global importance of the huntingtin protein was established early on using mutant mice studies. Duyao et al., (1995) created a mutant mouse with a targeted inactivating mutation of the murine homolog of the HTT gene. Heterozygous mice were indistinguishable from wild-type littermates and had a normal post natal course. Homozygous mutant mice (huntingtin protein expression was abolished in these mice) died as embryos. These mutant mice implanted normally but degenerated rapidly with death occurring at about embryonic day eight. These observations indicate that the huntingtin protein was a critical protein for early embryonic development before the emergence of the nervous system. In contrast, mice homozygous for a null mutation of the APP gene show limited abnormalities (Zheng et al., 1995). These mice were 15-20% underweight compared to wild type littermates and showed reduced forelimb grip strength and loco motor activity compared to control animals. In addition, APP null mice displayed learning and memory impairments (Muller and Zheng, 2012). Histologically the brains of homozygous null mice showed a reactive gliosis (Zheng et al., 1995).

The poly Q stretch in the human huntingtin protein is an ancient acquisition. Fish, amphibians and birds have a series of four glutamines (QQQQ), whereas the polyQ stretch has become greatly expanded in mammals with humans showing the longest and most polymorphic poly Q arrangement (Zuccato et al., 2010). As already noted, in mammals the poly Q stretch is followed by a polyproline (PolyP) series. Clearly, the presence of a polyQ stretch is a key functional element of the huntingtin protein and this stretch appears to be an important regulator of huntingtin binding to multiple other proteins. The polyQ stretch can adopt multiple flexible conformations and together with the polyP stretch and the multiple HEAT repeats, the huntingtin protein can engage in many protein-protein interactions (Zuccato et al., 2010). The polyQ tract is clearly a structural requisite underlying the complex interactions of the huntingtin protein. This tract has become expanded in mammals, particularly humans, to accommodate the multiple interactions characteristic of this protein. The tradeoff is genomic instability. In the germ line, particularly that of the male, de novo mutations arise which can result in a further increase in the polyQ repeat numbers which unfortunately changes the aggregation properties of the huntingtin protein.

The huntingtin protein is expressed ubiquitiously in humans with highest levels in neurons of the central nervous system. Within the cell, the protein is associated with various organelles and is also found at synapses. A phylogenetic analysis suggested that the neural expression of huntingtin was associated with the appearance of chordates (Zuccato et al., 2010). Nearly fifty proteins can interact directly with huntingtin or its fragments and the interaction occurs primarily at the amino terminal polyQ end of the protein. As noted by Zuccato et al., (2010) huntingtin- interacting proteins are involved in diverse cellular functions including clathrin mediated endocytosis, apoptosis, vesicle transport, cell signaling, morphogenesis and transcriptional regulation. Many of the proteins that bind to huntingtin are transcription factors. As already noted, studies using huntingtin knock-out mice have demonstrated that this protein is critical at different stages of embryonic development. Huntingtin has prosurvival properties and stimulates the production of brain- derived neurotrophic factor (BDNF) which is important for the survival of striatal neurons and the activity of cortico-striatal synapses (Zuccato et al., 2010). Huntingtin protein plays an important role in axonal and vesicular transport facilitating the movement of vesicles and mitochondria along neuronal projections (Imarisio et al., 2008). Huntingtin is highly expressed presynaptically and interacts with proteins involved in synaptic vesicle exocytosis and recycling. Currently, these diverse functions appear to be relatively independent of each other although in the future with a better understanding of this protein a unifying functional framework will probably be uncovered (Imarisio et al., 2008).

c) Toxicity of Mutated Huntingtin Protein

As already noted, HD develops when the number of poly Q repeats exceeds thirty six. There still appears to be controversy as to whether the underlying disease promoting mechanism is the result of the mutated protein having a gain of function (Imarisio et al., 2010) or loss of function (Zuccato et al., 2010).

Huntingtin has well characterized sites where proteolytic enzymes can cleave the protein into a range of fragments. There appears to be evidence that the amino terminal fragment of the mutant protein containing the poly Q expanded tract may be the "toxic" molecule (Imarisio et al., 2008). Some of the evidence in favor of this suggestion has come from various animal studies (Imarisio et al., 2008; Marx, 2005). In addition the capacity of mutant huntingtin protein to aggregate has also been considered a component of the mechanism(s) resulting in neurotoxicity. Mutant huntingtin can aggregate into amyloid fibrils in vitro (Bates, 2005) and abnormal deposits of mutant huntingtin fragments have been described in the neurons of rodent HD models and in the neurons and axons of patients who had died of HD (Marx, 2005).

A number of cellular mechanisms altered by mutant huntingtin or its amino terminal fragment have been proposed as responsible for the neurotoxicity of HD (Zuccato et al., 2010; Imarisio et al., 2008; Marx, 2005; Munoz-Sanjuan and Bates, 2011). Briefly, these cellular mechanisms can be summarized as follows.

1) Accumulation of misfolded or partially folded mutant huntingtin protein or its fragments. This accumulation occurs because the ubiquitination-proteasome system for protein degradation and removal becomes overloaded.
2) Impairment of cellular calcium homeostasis by amino terminal mutant huntingtin fragments.
3) Induction of mitochondrial dysfunction by binding of mutant huntingtin to the transcription factor p53.This binding increases p53 activity resulting in an abnormal flow of calcium across the mitochondrial membrane.
4) Amino terminal fragments translocate to the nucleus where they impair gene transcription and aggregate to form intranuclear inclusions.
5) Reduced transcription and production of BDNF and reduced transport of BDNF vesicles along axons.
6) Mutant huntingtin alters vesicular transport and recycling.
7) Mutant huntingtin can bind and inhibit a histone acetylase thus changing histone epigenetic marks.
8) Altered neurotransmitter release and receptor activity resulting in excitotoxicity. Medium spiny neurons which are innervated by glutamatergic axons and release gamma amino butyric acid (GABA) appear to be a particularly susceptible neuronal population.

This diverse list of cellular mechanisms altered in HD may have an underlying unifying mechanism. A number of neurodegenerative diseases including AD and HD are linked to genetic mutations that result in the expression of a single specific protein which is prone to aggregate; amyloid B-protein in the case of AD and mutated huntingtin protein in the case of HD (Bates, 2006). Gidalevitz et al., (2006) using a nematode model explored the effects of a known aggregating protein on overall cellular protein homeostasis. Transgenic nematodes were created expressing poly Q peptides of repeat number 24 or 40 in muscle or neuronal cells. In addition the nematodes co expressed temperature sensitive (ts) mutations that produced a specific phenotype at a restrictive temperature but not at a permissive temperature. For example, one such ts mutation called UNC 15 (a nematode homolog of a muscle paramyosin) leads to early larval lethality or slow movement in adults at a restrictive temperature of 25oC but not at the permissive temperature of 15oC. Another ts mutation in the neuronal protein dynamin 1 causes paralysis at the restrictive temperature of 28oC but mice have normal motility at the permissive temperature of 20oC. Gidalevitz et al., (2006) observed that mice expressing a ts mutation displayed the (restrictive temperature) phenotype at the permissive temperature if they also co-expressed a poly Q peptide of 40 repeats but not if they co-expressed a poly Q peptide of 24 repeats. They found that the interaction between poly Q peptides and ts mutants was cell specific i.e. the ts mutation and the poly Q peptide must reside within the same cell type (muscle or neuron). Hence, poly Q 40 (and not poly Q 24) destabilized ts mutant proteins such that their pathogenic phenotypes occurred under physiological conditions (i.e. at the permissive temperature) when such a phenotype should not normally occur. Conversely, the aggregation of poly Q 40 was greatly enhanced by the co- presence of a misfolded ts mutant protein compared to its aggregation state in the absence of the ts mutant protein.

The model proposed to explain these observations is as follows (Gidalevitz et al., 2006; Bates, 2006). Under normal physiological conditions, gene polymorphisms can give rise to the expression of proteins with mild folding variants. Such mild misfolding is corrected by the mechanisms discussed in the section; Mechanisms underlying cognitive ageing; d) Regulation of protein folding. On the other hand , in the presence of an aggregation- prone protein such as mutant huntingtin (poly Q >36) or amyloid B-protein (1-42), the protein folding and clearance mechanisms become overwhelmed and proteins that are normally innocuous are no longer correctly folded leading to impairments in a diverse set of cellular pathways. In addition, these structurally and functionally unrelated proteins which are misfolded exaggerate the misfolding and aggregation of the inciting protein e.g. mutant huntingtin or amyloid B-protein. This model, based upon an imbalance in protein folding homeostasis, would account for the variety of cellular mechanisms disrupted in neurodegenerative protein conformational diseases. Such a model could also explain the 40% variance in age of onset of HD not attributed to poly Q repeat length and to the wide variation in HD severity between individuals with the same poly Q mutation (Bates, 2006).

A recent study by Luk et al., (2012) presents observations consistent with this model proposed by Gidalevitz et al., (2006) and Bates (2006). Luk et al., (2012) demonstrated cell-to-cell transmission of an aggregated misfolded protein. Early onset Parkinson's disease is associated with a mutation in the gene encoding the neural protein, alpha-synuclein. The mutated alpha-synuclein protein is prone to misfolding and aggregation into amyloid fibrils. Luk and colleagues injected synthetic alpha-synuclein preformed fibrils intracerebrally into wild-type mice. Such fibrils can nucleate the aggregation and fibrillization of soluble endogenous alpha-synuclein protein in neuronal cell cultures. Following a single intracerebral injection of preformed fibrils, Luk et al., observed cell-to-cell transmission of "pathologic" alpha-synuclein aggregates in anatomically interconnected brain regions. The steps underlying anatomic propagation of alpha-synuclein aggregates following a single injection of preformed fibrils would involve seeding (nucleation) of cellular monomeric soluble alpha-synuclein protein leading to its misfolding and aggregation with concomitant overwhelming of the misfolded protein clearance mechanisms.

Are Alzheimer's (AD) and Huntington's (HD), diseases or part of the ageing process? Before addressing this question, the following contextual facts are important to consider. First genetic variation (mutations) and natural selection are the two critical ingredients of the evolutionary recipe. Mutations allow organisms to evolve and hence should not be viewed as "disease causative". Secondly, genomic sequencing data have clearly shown the wealth of DNA structural variants that make each human genome unique. In addition each human has a unique epigenome reflecting his/her individual specific experiences. These two facts alone make the disease construct untenable. Two individuals labeled as having HD or AD would clearly have different underlying molecular phenotypes.

In the case of AD, there are so called sporadic and autosomal dominant forms whereas HD is considered to be autosomal dominant only. Even though a single mutated gene has been identified in HD, this mutation does not completely account for variation in age of onset of neurological symptoms. In HD, between 30% and 60% of the variation in age of onset is due to other (non- huntingtin gene mutations) genetic factors and to environmental influences. Hence, both autosomal dominant HD and autosomal dominant AD are not actually the result of single gene-based mutations. Most likely the other genetic alterations required for these mutations to be phenotypically expressed will be in DNA regulatory elements. Although, research into AD has focused on the neurotoxicity of amyloid B-protein, this protein and its precursor protein (APP) clearly have important physiological functions which have yet to be documented. In the case of HD, huntingtin protein has been found to have a number of important functions which are mediated by its extensive interactions with numerous other proteins. The critical nature of huntingtin protein has been documented by the observation that animals missing this protein die as embryos.

A more important question is why the mutations underlying autosomal dominant AD and autosomal dominant HD have persisted.

In the case of HD a possible answer to this question may be available. The human HTT gene must contain a high number of CAG repeats so that the poly Q tract in the expressed huntingtin protein is long enough to allow for the multiple protein-protein interactions necessary for its diverse set of cellular functions. The tradeoff is that the high number of CAG repeats in the gene makes it "unstable" particularly during the multiple replications that occur during spermatogenesis. The result is that the huntingtin gene shows a high de novo mutation rate. If the mutation changes the CAG repeat number from 25 to 32 then the offspring will not show any neurological changes. If the CAG repeat number goes from 25 to 40 then the offspring will probably show the HD phenotype. But HD should not be labeled a disease. The trade- off between the necessity for a long poly Q tract in the huntingtin protein and the associated genomic instability is simply one of the costs of living.

With respect to AD, there are published data that the allele APOE 4 has been under positive selection even though this allele increases the risk of cognitive decline (Brown, 2012; Eisenberg et al., 2010). APOE is involved in cholesterol homeostasis and the allele APOE 4 is associated with increased levels of both total cholesterol and low density lipoprotein cholesterol. Of the three common alleles of APOE, the e4 allele is ancestral. Cholesterol is a very important molecular component of cellular membranes and also serves as a precursor in the synthesis of steroid hormones. Eisenberg et al., (2010) have postulated that environmental conditions which favor animals with an elevated metabolic rate will increase the demands for higher cholesterol levels in these animals and hence positively select for those individuals having the APOE 4 allele. To test this hypothesis, these investigators used geographical latitude as a proxy for temperature variation and indirectly a proxy for variation in metabolic rate. An equatorial latitude and a very high latitude will be associated with high and low environmental temperatures respectively and in both cases a higher metabolic rate will be adaptive (compared to an intermediate latitude). These investigators observed a curvilinear relationship between the population frequency of APOE 4 and absolute geographical latitude consistent with their hypothesis. These data are supportive of the notion that environments requiring a high metabolic rate as an adaptive phenotype positively select for the APOE 4 allele.

No comparable data are available to account for persistence of the mutations in the APP, PSEN 1 and PSEN 2 genes. Perhaps these mutations have persisted because they confer some advantages to the individual at an earlier life stage. This possibility can only be addressed when we know much more about the physiological roles played by APP and amyloid B-protein.

Finally the role of epigenetic mediated environmental influences on the development of the HD and AD phenotypes has not been studied even though in the case of HD about 60% of the residual variation in age of onset (not explained by CAG repeat number) is due to environmental factors (Wexler et al., 2004).

In summary, AD and HD do not represent "diseases." They are simply extreme variants of the ageing process shaped by the interplay between each human's unique genome and the epigenetic mediated effects of that individual's unique environmental influences (experiences) on genetic expression patterns.

Chapter VI

Conclusion

As discussed in the Introduction, the disease concept is a composite of a number of components (Duffin, 2005), the description of which is shaped by the cultural norms and the state of scientific knowledge existing at that point in time. The history of disease taxonomies or classifications (National Research Council, 2011) clearly reflects the influence of cultural and knowledge based factors.

Linnaeus attempted a classification of diseases in 1763, but the effort did not succeed because of a lack of understanding of the biological basis of disease. A better taxonomy was developed in 1911 and this classification was actually the forerunner of the present day International Statistical Classification of Diseases and Related Health problems (ICD). Today the ICD (currently version 10) is the most commonly used disease taxonomy. The ICD, even the current version, categorizes diseases based upon symptoms, histological analysis of "diseased" tissues, laboratory tests and various imaging studies. The ICD has a hierarchical organization in which individual diseases are successively subdivided into types and subtypes. The rigid structure of the ICD-10 inhibits the rapid inclusion of up to date molecular biological and genetic data at a time when new data regarding the molecular nature of disease are becoming available at an ever increasing rate.

In a recent publication (2011), a committee of the National Research Council (USA) proposed the development of a new more fluid type of disease taxonomy that would allow for continuous updating with emerging new biological and genetic data. This new taxonomy would dovetail with the concept of personalized medicine; the tailoring of medical treatment to the individual characteristics of each patient.

The evolution of disease taxonomies has been characterized by a progressively finer subdivision of diseases into types and subtypes as the biological knowledge base has expanded. The proposed new "molecular" taxonomy would extend this trend by framing diseases on an almost individual basis. The trend for ever increasing sub-categorizing of diseases as our understanding of cellular processes deepens will in the limit, force us to abandon the disease construct altogether. If eventually diseases are defined on an individual (personal) basis, then in reality, we are no longer describing diseases but rather phenotypic variation on an individual basis. As we develop a better understanding of the molecular basis of cellular and multicellular functions and an appreciation that these functions show variation across individuals, we will realize that phenotypic differences between individuals ("diseases") are just individual variants of the ageing process. Genomic data clearly demonstrate that each human has a unique genome and epigenome based on the mix of genes, structural DNA polymorphisms and epigenetic marks (DNA methylation pattern, histone acetylation/methylation marks) transmitted from mother and father. During an individual's life this unique genome and epigenome are further modified by tissue specific somatic mutations and individual specific environmentally induced epigenetic changes; i.e. experiences.

In essence, we all reside on one phenotypic landscape with each individual having his/her own unique location. On the other hand, the "disease" construct places a box for each "disease" state on this phenotypic landscape. Classifying individuals as having a specific disease puts all those individuals in the same box. Although disease boxes may have different sizes, a box still has vertical walls and the individuals in any given disease box will be separated by these vertical walls from "normal" individuals and individuals in other disease boxes. Our current understanding of genomic and epigenomic polymorphic differences across individuals makes this disease- box construct untenable. An individual's unique genome and epigenome determines that individual's unique location on the phenotypic landscape.

The living state is based upon a highly complex biological organization that is both wondrous and awe-inspiring. Our understanding of even the functioning and organization of single celled organisms is still rudimentary. In fact it is a "miracle" that organisms such as humans function as well as they do for as long as they do. The topics discussed in this book if nothing else, underscore the myriads of diverse biological processes that are associated with the living state and hence the possibilities for mistakes are also extensive. The living state has evolved various repair mechanisms to either prevent mistakes or if they occur to institute a corrective response. However, repair mechanisms are not perfect and if they were perfect evolutionary changes would not occur. Ageing is an inevitable part of the fabric of the living state since ageing at the individual level is the integrated consequences of accumulated genomic and cellular damage as well as the results of imperfect repair mechanisms. In fact as pointed out by Finkel et al., (2007), the ageing process and the development of malignant tumors, which on the surface appear to be unlikely "cousins," represent complex biological tapestries that are woven by similar molecular threads.

As noted in the section; Background; Ageing; ageing can be viewed conceptually at both the species and the individual levels. At the species level, the developmental programs which underlie morphological and behavioral traits set general boundaries for the ageing process and maximum lifespan of that species. Evolution has selected these boundaries as adaptive for that species within the particular ecological niche that it occupies. Within these boundaries, there will be considerable variation across individual members of that species with respect to both the ageing process and lifespan. Due to this variation, it is difficult to define a "normal" range for specific morphological and behavioral traits at the individual level. As a solution, we use a statistical approach to characterizing "normalcy." We measure a given trait in a number of individuals, calculate a mean and define "normal" as arbitrarily encompassing two standard deviations on each side of that mean. This methodology gives rise to the dichotomous nature of the normal/disease construct. For example, we recognize that cognitive functions show an age-related decline. As long as measured cognitive functions remain within two standard deviations of the age-standardized mean for whatever function is being measured, we label that individual as "normal". If that individual's measured cognitive functioning falls outside the two standard deviation limit then that individual is said to have a "disease" e.g. possible Alzheimer's disease.

Over thousands of years, we humans have developed a disease construct to explain both the ageing process and individual variations in this ageing process. In fact, for some scientists the ageing process itself has become a disease. This disease construct has had profound societal implications. We chase disease cures and we have unrealistic expectations as to our abilities to extend lifespan and to prevent ageing. In view of our present day understanding of the biology of the living state, our current disease construct is no longer tenable.

Excluding death by predation, trauma or infection, all animals will still die. Death represents the ultimate breakdown of the living system. However, there are extreme differences in maximum lifespan between species. The time period prior to death constitutes ageing. During this time frame physiologic and metabolic processes change as a result of epigenetic alterations in gene expression patterns induced by environmental cues such as the nature of an animal's social environment and the accumulation of genomic damage secondary to endogenous and exogenous agents. Another example of damage involves the arterial tree which by virtue of its design is subject to injury at sites of altered laminar flow such as bifurcations, branch points and regions of high curvature. The body has various repair processes and the best studied are those involved in the removal of genomic damage. However, repair processes are not perfect and are generally incomplete. For example genomic damage in the region of the telomere is difficult to repair by virtue of the functional features of the telomere itself. In addition, within the evolutionary framework, repair processes become less robust in the animal's post reproductive period. The sum of these physiologic and metabolic changes, structural injuries (e.g. arterial tree) and the associated incomplete repair processes comprise the ageing phenotype. The trajectory and features of the ageing phenotype vary across species and individual animals. However, we humans generally refer to these physiologic/metabolic/structural changes and the associated repair processes not as part of ageing but as specific diseases. We have developed a disease construct as if some external process has "high jacked" our "normal" physiology. This disease construct is deeply entrenched in Western medicine and has been supported by experimental observations gathered generally in a few highly select inbred animal species (usually rodents) which have been genetically, surgically or pharmacologically manipulated.

Another important influence on the ageing process has been a significant relaxation of evolutionary selection in developed societies. Within our societies there are no longer the ecological pressures that existed thousands of years ago. An easily accessible food supply and the availability of suitable housing arrangements, public health measures and advanced medical care have collectively reduced the selective pressures to eliminate deleterious mutations. The result has been a progressive decline in the mean fitness of humans in developed societies and a change in the ageing phenotype.

As discussed in the section Background; Genetics; the phenotypic variation across individual humans is due to extensive underlying genetic and epigenetic variation. As a result, studies in humans rely on statistical rather than biological end points. In contrast, studies with laboratory animals can have defined biological end points since these studies use highly inbred well characterized strains of animals. The most popular animal models are carefully maintained inbred strains of mice such as C57BL/6J. This particular strain has been inbred at the Jackson Laboratory for over 70 years (Watkins-Chow and Pavan, 2008). Such strains have become genetically homogeneous after so many years of inbreeding, although even strains such as C57BL/6J demonstrate detectable genetic variation in such features as copy number variants (Watkins-Chow and Pavan, 2008). Needless to say, strains of mice such as C57BL/6J do represent a legitimate control group. The experimental group is generally composed of wild-type mice (e.g. C57BL/6J) that have been genetically modified by creation of an engineered mutation that either silences or alters in some other way the expression of a particular gene. However, the dilemma with this experimental approach is that highly inbred laboratory animals are not natural models but rather genetically engineered (un-natural) models. The use of such genetically altered laboratory animals does give important information concerning the functioning of specific genes and their interactions with other genomic elements. However, the genome contains an extensive regulatory organization and gene function can be modulated by regulatory elements located a great distance away from its target gene. Metabolic signaling cascades are now known to be actually networks with significant cross-talk occurring between different networks. Teasing out all these nuanced details will require experiments in natural animal models. Studies using inbred animals involve a distinct trade-off between better defined more easily interpretable biological results and animal models that are significantly displaced from their natural state. However, despite this distinct and generally ignored trade-off, this experimental approach has become one of the pillars supporting the disease construct.

The ever expanding genomic and epigenomic data base has revealed that the genome contains highly complex gene regulatory networks and a very sophisticated transcriptional process and that the individual genome and epigenome are unique. Rather than clarify the nature of a "gene," the data have forced a rethinking of what constitutes the "unit of heredity." Gene regulatory networks appear to be both hotspots of genomic mutability as well as regions that are rich in the DNA sequence variants that have been found to be associated with "disease" states. The genomic and epigenomic data indicate that the molecular phenotypes underlying so called disease states are not the same across individuals. Two individuals may be diagnosed as suffering from diabetes or Alzheimer's disease but their underlying molecular phenotypes will not be the same. In essence their "clinical phenotypes" do not represent a "disease" state but just variants of the ageing process; the outward manifestations of the cumulative effects of genomic mutations, imperfect repair processes plus the superimposed influence of the epigenetic effects of environmental cues (e.g. social interactions, activity level, food habits etc.). In addition, the human ageing process has been modified by a relaxation of purifying evolutionary selection pressures engendered by our modern social organizational structure; these relaxed selection pressures allow deleterious mutations to persist.

Our fixation on the disease construct has created unrealistic public expectations; magic bullets and disease cures. In addition, labeling individuals as suffering from a "disease" has in some circumstances resulted in these persons being treated as outcasts; considered different in a negative sense from so-called "normal" individuals. Abandoning the disease construct does not mean abandoning the management of the "health issues" that constitute the ageing process.

The reality is that many to most humans today reside in huge urban societies with all the advantages this social structure provides. Humans have access to many labor saving technologies as well as access to a stable food supply and in many societies access to advance medical care systems. This highly organized societal structure has led to a relaxation of natural selection. As noted by Crow (2000), our high standard of living, improved sanitation and better medical care have resulted in the persistence of mutant genes that would have been selectively eliminated in the past. The prediction is that given the relatively high human mutation rate, a relaxation of natural selection will lead to a 0.1-1.5% decline in fitness (survival and reproductive success) per generation as witnessed in other animal species (Lynch, 2010; Shabalina et al., 1997). The study of relaxed selection and its consequences has become an important topic and one that has moved from the laboratory to the real world (Lahti et al., 2009). In the wild, there are a number of examples of relaxed selection resulting in a significant loss or change in a morphologic or behavioral trait (Lahti et al., 2009). An interesting and possible case of relaxed selection was presented by Post (1971). Post noted that the incidence of color blindness was much lower in societies of hunters and food gatherers than in more "civilized" countries i.e. Western European and the Scandinavian countries. Post made the assumption that color vision was much more important to hunters and gatherers and hence the relaxed selection in more developed societies failed to eliminate the genetic mutations underlying color blindness.

Is it important to make the distinction between what constitutes a "disease" and what constitutes a manifestation of the ageing process? Is this distinction simply a semantic issue? No, this is not simply a question of semantics. Within society at large the "disease" concept carries with it certain connotations as discussed in the section; Introduction. A disease is within an individual, bad and hopefully discontinuous (Duffin, 2005). Humans are quite willing to accept that skin becomes more wrinkled, hair loses its color and one becomes more forgetful as one ages. However, humans prefer to believe that cognitive decline, an elevated blood sugar, or cardiac issues such as an elevated arterial blood pressure are manifestations of a "disease". The disease concept, unfortunately, raises unrealistic expectations within society. One of these expectations is that perhaps with sufficient research, the "disease" can be cured. Accepting that so called "chronic degenerative diseases" are just variants of the ageing process does not mean that we do not manage these aspects of ageing. However, this management must be based upon a much more realistic conceptual basis. "Chronic degenerative diseases" and ageing itself cannot be cured. There are no magic bullets for these variants of the ageing process.

A possible exception to this statement might be phenotypic variants that have an essentially monogenic basis. One such example is that of hemophilia B which is due to a variety of mutations in the gene (located on the X chromosome) encoding factor IX, a serine protease (Ponder, 2011). Nathwani et al., (2011) treated six individuals with Hemophilia B by intravenous injection of an adenovirus-associated vector that contained a liver specific promoter and the factor IX coding sequence. The recipients maintained levels of factor IX between 2-12 % of normal levels for between 5-15 months at follow-up. There appeared to be minimal evidence of adverse effects with this treatment. How long this transgene will function is unknown. Whether this type of "reversal "of a monogenic based phenotype can be generalized to other situations is unclear, although like Hemophilia B the phenotype must be essentially monogenic in nature. It is interesting that it has taken about thirty years from discovery of the factor IX gene to this first successful somatic gene therapy of Hemophilia B.

The current era has been termed unofficially the anthropocene. This informal geologic and ecologic term refers to the present age (date of onset somewhat controversial) in which human activities have had and are continuing to have significant effects on the earth's ecosystems and atmosphere. I believe the term anthropocene age should also be used to represent the effects of human activities on human evolution. Modern urban societies have resulted in a relaxation of natural selection as already discussed. A relaxation of selection will clearly result in a change in the ageing phenotype. In addition, a byproduct of our large urban societal structure is that social interactions between individuals have become much more complex. As has been noted in several sections of this monograph, the complexity of the social environment can significantly affect the ageing phenotype through its effects on vascular biology, particularly vascular remodeling and the setting of arterial pressure levels. In addition, the complexity of interactions in large social groupings is considered the primary selection force that has driven the evolution of the large mammalian brain and in adult sexually mature male zebra finches, the complexity of the social environment sets the survival outcome of newly formed neurons (Singer, 2011). In summary, although the complex social structure of the modern human has made our current life style possible, the biological cost of this social structure has been an alteration in the ageing phenotype. The ageing process is characterized by features such as an extensive degree of reparative vascular remodeling, impairments in metabolic homeostasis and forms of cognitive decline; features which we humans have euphemistically labeled as diseases.

References

Abbott, A. The brain's decline. *Nature*, 2012 492, S4-S5.

Akalin. A; Friedman, D; Arner, E; Dong, X; Bryne, JC; Suzuki, H; Daub, CO; Hayashizaki, Y; Lenhard, B. Transcriptional features of genomic regulatory blocks. *Genome Biology*, 2009 10:R38.

Alderman, MH. Hypertension, silver bullets and faded dreams. *J. Hypertens.*, 2004 22, 2263-2264.

Allam, AH; Thompson, RC; Wann, LS; Miyamoto, MI; Thomas, GS. Computed tomographic assessment of atherosclerosis in ancient Egyptian mummies. *JAMA*, 2009 302, 2091-2094.

Aluru, N; Vijayan, MM. Stress transcriptomics in fish: a role for genomic cortisol signaling. *Gen. Comp. Endocrin.*, 2009 164-142-150.

Amadio, JP; Walsh, CA. Brain evolution and uniqueness in the human genome. *Cell*, 2006 126, 1033-1035.

Andolfatto, P. Adaptive evolution of non-coding DNA in Drosophila. *Nature*, 2005 437, 1149-1152.

Antonetti, D. Eye vessels saved by rescuing their pericyte partners. *Nature Medicine*, 2009 15, 1248-1249.

Araki, E; Lipes, MA; Patti, M-E; Bruning, JC; Haag III, B; Johnson, RS; Kahn, CR. Alternative pathway of insulin signaling in mice with targeted disruption of the IRS-1 gene. *Nature*, 1994, 372, 186-190.

Armulik, A; Abramsson, A; Betsholtz, C. Endothelial/pericyte interactions. *Circ. Res.*, 2005 97, 512-523.

Ashley, J; Packard, M; Ataman, B; Budnik, V. Fasciclin II signals new synapse formation through amyloid precursor protein and the scaffolding protein dXII/Mint. *J. Neurosci.*, 2005 25, 5943-5955.

Aubin-North, N; Renn, SC. Genomic reaction norms: using integrative biology to understand molecular mechanisms of phenotypic plasticity. *Molec. Ecology*, 2009 18, 3763-3780.

Austad, SN. Mixed results for dieting monkey. *Nature*, 2012 489, 210-211.

Austad, SN. Methusaleh's zoo: how nature provides us with clues for extending human health span. *J. Comp. Path.*, 2010 142, S10-S21.

Avivi, A; Albrecht, U; Oster, H; Joel, A; Beiles, A; Nevo, E. Biological clock in total darkness: the ClOCK/MOP3 circadian sysrem of the blind subterranean mole rat. *PNAS*, 2001 98, 13751-13756.

Avivi, A; Oster, H; Joel, A; Albrecht, U; Nevo, E. Circadian genes in a blind subterranean mammal II: conservation and uniqueness of the three Period homologs in the blind subterranean mole rat, Spalax ehren bergi superspecies. *PNAS*, 2002 99, 11718-11723.

Baggio, LL; Drucker, DJ. Biology of incretins: GLP-1 And GIP. *Gastroenterology*, 2007 132, 2131-2157.

Bailey, CH; Kandel, ER. Structural changes accompanying memory storage. *Annu. Rev. Physiol.*, 1993 55, 397-426.

Balch, WE: Morimoto, RI; Dillin, A; Kelly, JW. Adapting proteostasis for disease intervention. *Science*, 2008 319, 916-919.

Bardi, M; Bode, AE; Ramirez, SM; Brent. LY. Maternal care and development of stress responses in baboons. *Amer. J. Primatol.*, 2005 66-263-278.

Barnard, AR; Nolan, PM. When clocks go bad: neurobehavioural consequences of disrupted circadian timing. *PLoS Genetics*, 2008 4 issue # 5.

Bates, GP. One misfolded protein allows others to sneak by. *Science*, 2006 311, 1385-1386.

Bates, GP. The molecular genetics of Huntington disease- a history. *Nature Reviews Genetics*, 2005 6, 766-773.

Baudisch, A; Vaupel, JW. Getting to the root of aging. *Science*, 2012 338, 618-619.

Baylin, SB; Schuebel, KE. The epigenomic era opens. *Nature*, 2007 448, 548-549.

Balda, RP; Kamil, A; Bednekoff, PA. Predicting cognitive capacity from maternal history: examples from four species of corvids. In: Nolan Jr., V, Ketterson, ED. Editors. *Current Ornithology* volume 13, New York, Plenum Press, 1996; 33-66.

Beintema, JJ; Campagne, RN.Molecular evolution of rodent insulins. *Mol. Biol. Evol.*, 1987 4, 10-18.

Bell-Pedersen, D; Cassone, VM; Earnest, DJ; Golden SS; Hardin, PE; Thomas, TL; Zoran, MJ. Circadian rhythms from multiple oscillators: lessons from diverse organisms. *Nature Review Genetics*, 2005 6, 544-556.

Bergers, G; Song, S. The role of pericytes in blood vessel formation and maintenance. *Neuro-Oncology*, 2005 7, 452-464.

Berthoud, H-R; Lenard, NR; Shin, AC. Food reward, hyperphagia, and obesity. *Am. J. Physiol. Regul. Integr. Comp. Physiol.*, 2011 300, R1266-R1277.

Bickmore, WA. Expression control. *Nature*, 2012 489, 53-54.

Bissette, G. Mini-forum: roles of amyloid-B and tau phosphorylation in neuronal repair and protection. *J. Alzheimer's Dis.*, 2009 18, 369-370.

Blaustein, MP; Zhang, J; Chen, L; Hamilton, BP. How does salt retention raise blood pressure. *Am. J. Physiol. Regul. Integr. Comp. Physiol.*, 2006 290, R514-R523.

Bloch, G; Toma, DP; Robinson, GE. Behavioural rhythmicity, age, division of labor and Period expression in the honey bee brain. *J. Biol. Rhythmns*, 2001 16,444-456.

Bloch,G; Grozinger, CM. Social molecular pathways and the evolution of bee societies. *Phil. Trans. R. Soc. B*, 2011 366, 2155-2170.

Bodnar, AG. Marine invertebrates as models for aging research. *Exp. Geront.*, 2009 44, 477-484.

Bolhuis, JJ; Okanoya, K; Scharff, C. Twitter evolution: converging mechanisms in bird song and human speech. *Nature Reviews Neuroscience*, 2010 11, 747-759.

Bonier, F; Moore, IT; Roberston, RJ. The stress of parenthood? Increased glucocorticoids in birds with experimentally enlarger broods. *Biol. Lett.*, 2011 7, 944-946.

Bookout, AL; Jeong, Y; Downes, M; Yu, RT; Evans, RM; Mangelsdorf, DJ. Anatomic profiling of nuclear receptor expression reveals a hierarchical transcriptional network. *Cell*, 2006 126, 789-799.

Borghol, N; Sunderman, M; McArdle, W; Racine, A; Hallett, M; Pembrey, M; Hertzman, C; Power, C; Szyf, M. Associations with early-life socio-economic position in adult DNA methylation. *Int. J. Epidemiol.*, 2012 41, 62-74.

Borrelli, E; nestler, EJ; Allis, CD; Sassone-Corsi, P. Decoding the epigenetic language of neuronal plasticity. *Neuron*, 2008 60, 961-974.

Bosch, TCG. Hydra and the evolution of stem cells. *BioEssays*, 2009 31, 478-486.

Bossdorf, O; Richards, CL; Pigliucci, M. Epigenetics for ecologists. *Ecology Letts*, 2008 11, 106-115.

Brakefield, PM. Evo-devo and accounting for Darwin's endless forms. *Phil. Trans. R. Soc. B*, 2011 366, 2069-2075.

Bramble, DM; Lieberman, DE. Endurance running and the evolution of Homo. *Nature*, 2004 432, 345-352.

Braun, EJ; Sweazea, KL. Glucose regulation in birds. *Comp. Biochem. Physiol.*, 2008 part B 151, 1-9.

Breen, MS; Kemena, C; Vlasov, PK; Notredame, C; Kondrashov, FA. Epistasis as the primary factor in molecular evolution. *Nature*, 2012 490, 535-540.

Breno, MC; Prezoto, BC; Borgheresi, RAMB; Lazari, MFM; Yamanouye, N. Characteristics of neural and humoral systems involved in the regulation of blood pressure in snakes. *Comp. Biochem. Physiol.*, 2007 part A 147, 766-778.

Brondum E. et al., Jugular venous pooling during lowering of the head affects blood pressure of the anesthetized giraffe. *Am. J. Physiol. Regul. Integr. Comp. Physiol.*, 2009 297, R 1058-R1065.

Brown, EA. Genetic explorations of recent human metabolic adaptations: hypotheses and evidence. *Biol. Rev.*, 2012 87, 838-855.

Brucklacher, RM. et al., Whole genome assessment of the retinal response to diabetes reveals a progressive neurovascular inflammatory response. *BMC Medical Genomics*, 2008 1:26.

Buffenstein, R; Kang, J; Biney, A. Glucose intolerance and insulin sensitivity in an extremely long-lived rodent, the naked mole-rat. *The FASEB J.*, 2007 21, abstract 1423.

Buffenstein, R; Pinto, M. Endocrine function in naturally long-living small mammals. *Mol. Cell Endocrinol.*, 2009 299, 101-111.

Buffenstein, R; Negligible senescence in the longest living rodent, the naked mole-rat: insights from a successfully aging species. *J. Comp. Physiol.* B, 2008 178, 439-445.

Campochiaro, PA. Ocular neovascularization and excessive vascular permeability. *Expert Opin. Biol. Ther.*, 2004 4, 1395-1402.

Carlberg, O; Hayley, CS. Epistasis: too often neglected in complex trait studies? *Nature Reviews Genetics*, 2004 5, 618-625.

Carmeliet, P; Tessier-Lavigne, M. Common mechanisms of nerve and blood vessel wiring. *Nature Reviews*, 2005 436, 193-200.

Carnero, A; LLeonart, ME. Epigenetic mechanisms in senescence, immortalisation and cancer. *Biol. Rev.*, 2011 86, 443-455.

Carroll, SB. Evolution at two levels: on genes and form. *PLoS Biology*, 2005 3, (issue 7) 1159-1166.

Carroll, SB. Evo-devo and an expanding evolutionary synthesis: a genetic theory of morphological evolution, *Cell*, 2008 134, 25-36.

Carroll, RG; Opdyke, DF. Evolution of angiotensin II- induced catecholamine release. *Am. J. Physiol. Regul. Integr. Comp. Physiol.*, 1982, 243, R65-R69.

Carvalho, JJ; Baruzzi, RG; Howard, PF; Poulter, N; Alpers, MP; Franco, LJ; Marcopito, LF; Spooner, VJ; Dyer, AR; Elliott, P. Blood pressure in four remote populations in the INTERSALT study. *Hypertens*, 1989, 14, 238-246.

Carvunis, A-R et al., Proto-genes and de novo gene birth, Nature, 2012 467, 370-374.

Cedar, H; Bergman, Y. Linking DNA methylation and histone modification: patterns and paradigms. *Nature Reviews Genetics*, 2009 10, 295-304.

Cerra, MC; Imbrogno, S; Amelio, D; Garo-falo, F; Colvee, E; Tota, B; Icardo, JM. Cardiac morphodynamic remodeling in the growing eel (Anguilla Anguilla L). *J. Exp. Biol.*, 2004 207, 2867-2875.

Chakravarti, A; Kapoor, A. Mendelian puzzles. *Science*, 2012 335, 930-931.

Chan, SJ; Steiner, DF; Insulin through the ages: phylogeny of a growth promoting and metabolic regulatory hormone. *Am. Zool.*, 200 40, 213-222.

Chappell, MC. Emerging evidence for a functional angiotensin-converting enzyme-2-angiotensin-(1-7)-mas receptor axis: more than regulation of blood pressure? *Hypertens*, 2007 50, 596-599.

Chavin, W; Young, JE; Factors in the determination of normal serum glucose levels in goldfish. *Comp. Biochem. Physiol.*, 1970 33, 629-653.

Choudhury, GG. Akt serine threonine kinase regulates platelet-derived growth factor- induced DNA synthesis in glomerular mesangial cells. *J. Biol. Chem.*, 2001 276, 35636-35643.

Check, E. Genome project turns up evolutionary surprises. *Nature*, 2007 447, 760-761.

Chen, R et al., Personal omics profiling reveals dynamic molecular and medical phenotypes. *Cell*, 2012 148, 1293-1307.

Cheng, B; Anea, CB; Yao,L; Chen, F; Patel, V; Merloiu, A; pati, P; Caldwell, RW; Fulton, DJ; Rudic, RD. Tissue-intrinsic dysfunction of circadian clock confers transplant arteriosclerosis. *PNAS*, 2011 108, 17147-17152.

Chiang, W-C; Ching, T-T; Lee, HC; Mousigian, C; Hsu, A-L. HSF-1 regulators DDL-1/2 link insulin –like signaling to heat shock responses and modulation of longevity. *Cell*, 2012 148, 322-334.

Chittka, L; Jensen, K. Animal cognition: concepts from apes to bees, *Curr. Biol.*, 2011 21, R116-R119.

Cochrane, AL. The history of the measurement of ill health. *Int. J. Epidem.*, 1972 1, 89-92.

Coelho Jr, AM; Carey, KD; Shade, RE. Assessing the effects of social environment on blood pressure and heart rates of baboons. *Am. J. Primatol.*, 1991, 23, 257-267.

Coffman, TM; Crowley, SD. Kidney in hypertension: Guyton redux. *Hypertens.*, 2008 51, 811-816.

Coghlan, C; Hoffman, J. Leonardo da Vinci's flights of the mind must continue: cardiac architecture and the fundamental relation of form and function revisited. *Eur. J. Cardio-Thoracic. Surg.*, 2006 29 (suppl 1), S4-S17.

Cohen, E; Bieschke, J; Perciavalle, RM; Kelly, JW; Dillin, A. Opposing activities protect against age-onset proteotoxity. *Science*, 2006 313, 1604-1610.

Cohen, J. DNA duplications and deletions help determine health. *Science*, 2007 317, 1315-1317.

Conlon, JM. Evolution of the insulin molecule: insights into structure-activity and phylogenetic relationships. *Peptides*, 2001 22, 1183-1193.

Connor, RC. Dolphin social intelligence: complex alliance relationships in bottlenose dolphin and a consideration of selective environments for extreme brain size evolution in mammals. *Phil. Trans. R. Soc. B.*, 2007 362, 587-602.

Conrad, DF et al., Origins and functional impact of copy number variation in the human genome. *Nature*, 2010 464, 704-712.

Contreras, RJ; Kosten, T. Prenatal and early postnatal sodium chloride intake modifies the solution preferences of adult rats, *J. Nutr.*, 1983 113, 1051-1062.

Contreras, RJ. Differences in perinatal NaCl exposure alters blood pressure levels of adult rats, *Am. J. Physiol. Regul. Integr. Comp. Physiol.*, 1989 256, R70-R77.

Cowley, MA; Pronchuk, N; Fan, W; Dinulescu., DM; Colmers, WF; Cone, RD. Integration of NPY, AGRP, and melanocortin signals in the hypothalamic paraventricular nucleus: evidence of a cellular basis for the adipostat. *Neuron*, 1999 24, 155-163.

Crawford, TN; Alfaro III, DV; Kerrison, JB; Jablon, EP. Diabetic retinopathy and angiogenesis. *Curr. Diabetes Rev.*, 2009 5, 8-13.

Crawford, DL; Oleksiak, MF. The biological importance of measuring individual variation. *J. Exp. Biol.*, 2007 210,1613-1621.

Crosio, C; Heitz, E; Allis, CD; Borrelli, E; Sassone-Corsi, P. Chromatin remodeling and neuronal response: multiple signaling pathways induce specific histone H-3 modifications and early gene expression in hippocampal neurons. *J. Cell Sci.,* 2003 116, 4905-4914.

Crow, JF. The origins, patterns and implications of human spontaneous mutation. *Nature Reviews Genetics*, 2000 1, 40-47.

Csiszar, A; Labinskyy, N; Orosz, Z; Xiangmin, Z; Buffenstein, R; Unguari, Z. Vascular aging in the longest-living rodent, the naked mole rat. *Am. J. Physiol. Heart Circ. Physiol.*, 2007 293, H 919-H927.

Curtis, AM; Cheng, Y; Kapoor, S; Reilly, D; Price, TS.; Fitzgerald, GA. Circadian variation of blood pressure and the vascular response to asynchronous stress. *PNAS*, 2007 104, 3450-3455.

Dantzler, B; Swansdon, EM. Mediation of vertebrate life histories via insulin-like growth factor-1. *Biol. Rev.*, 2012 87, 414-429.

Davidson, AJ; London, B; Block, GD; Menaker, M. Cardiovascular tissues contain independent circadian clocks. *Clin. Exp. Hypertens.*, 2005 2 and 3, 307-311.

Davies, PF. Flow-mediated endothelial mechanotransduction. *Physiol. Rev.*, 1995 75, 519-560.

Davis, MJ; Hill, MA. Signaling mechanisms underlying the vascular myogenic response. *Physiol. Rev.*, 1999 79, 387-423.

Davis, S; Bozon, B; Laroche, S. How necessary is the activation of the immediate early gene zif 268 in synaptic plasticity and learning? *Behavioural Brain Res.*, 2003 142, 17-30.

Davisson, RL; Oliverio, MI; Coffman, TM; Sigmund, CD. Divergent functions of angiotensin II receptor isoforms in the brain. *J. Clin. Invest.*, 2000 106, 103-106.

deMagalhaes, JP; Sanberg, A. Cognitive aging as an extension of brain development: a model linking learning, brain plasticity, and neurodegeneration. *Mech. Ageing Develop.*, 2005 126, 1026-1033.

De Man, SA; Andre, J-L; Bachmann, H; Grobbee, DE; Ibsen, KK; Laaser, U; Lippert, P; Hofman, A. Blood pressure in childhood: pooled findings of six European studies. *J. Hypertens.*, 1991 9, 109-114.

De Mayer, G. et al., Diagnosis- independent Alzheimer's disease biomarker signature in cognitively normal elderly people. *Arch. Neurol.*, 2010 67, 949-956.

Denton, D. et al., The effect of increased salt intake on blood pressure of chimpanzees. *Nature Medicine*, 1995 1, 1009-1016.

De Strooper, B; Voet, T. A protective mutation. *Nature*, 2012 488, 38-39.

Diabetes Control and Complications Trial Research Group. The effect of intensive treatment of diabetes on the development and progression of long-term complications in insulin-dependent diabetes mellitus. *New Eng. J. Med.*, 1993 329, 977-986.

Dibner, C; Schibler, U; Albrecht, U. The mammalian circadian timing system: organization and coordination of central and peripheral clocks. *Annu. Rev. Physiol.*, 2010 72, 517-549.

Dill, KA; MacCallum, JL. The protein-folding problem, 50 years on. *Science*, 2012 338, 1042-1046.

Dobson, CM. Protein folding and misfolding. *Nature*, 2003 426, 884-890.

Doherty, CJ; Kay, SA. Circadian surprise- It's not all about transcription. *Science*, 2012 338, 338-340.

Doidge, ND. The Brain that Changes Itself. New York, USA: Penguin Books; 2007.

Donaldson, ZR; Young, LJ. Oxytocin, vasopressin, and the neurogenetics of sociality. *Science*, 2008 322, 900-904.

Donnelly, P. Progress and challenges in genome-wide association studies in humans. *Nature*, 2008 456, 728-731.

Duffin, J. Lovers and Livers. Toronto, Canada: University of Toronto Press; 2005.

Dunaif, A; Tattersa II, I. Prevalence of glucose intolerance in free-ranging Macaca fascicularis of Mauritius. *Am. J. Primatol.*, 1987 13, 435-442.

Dunbar, RIM; Shultz, S. Evolution in the social brain. *Science*, 2007 317, 1344-1347.

Dunbar, RIM; Shultz, S. Understanding primate brain evolution. *Phil. Trans. R. Soc. B.*, 2007 362, 649-658.

Dupont, HJ; Tesseraud, S; Simon, J. Insulin signaling in chicken liver and muscle. *Gen. Comp. Endocrinol.*, 2009 163, 52-57.

Duran, AC; Rodriguez, C; de Sola, LG; Fernandez, B; Arque, JM; Sans-Coma, V. Intimal thickening of coronary arteries in the rabbitfish, Chimaera monstrosa L. (Chondrichthyes: Holocephali). *J. Fish Dis.*, 2010 33, 675-682.

Duyao, MP; Auerbach, AB; Ryan, A; Persichetti, F; Barnes, GT; McNeil, SM; Ge, P; Vonsattel, J-P; Gusella, JF; Joyner, AL; MacDonald, ME. Inactivation of the mouse Huntington's disease gene homolog Hdh. *Science*, 1995 269, 407-410.

Ecker, JR. Encode explained, *Nature*, 2012 489, 52-53.

Editorial. Evolution and the brain. *Nature*, 2007 447, 753.

Edrey, YH; Park, TJ; Kang, H; Biney, A; Buffenstein, R. Endocrine function and neurobiology of the longest-living rodent, the naked mole-rat. *Exp. Geront.*, 2011 b) 46, 116-123.

Edrey, YH; Hanes, M; Pinto, M; Mele, J; Buffenstein, R. Successful aging and sustained good health in the naked mole rat: a long lived mammalian model for biogerontology and biomedical research. *ILAR J.*, 2011 a), 52, 41-53.

Eisch, AJ; Petrik, D. Depression and hippocampal neurogenesis: a road to remission? *Science*, 2012 338, 72-75.

Eisenberg, DTA; Kuzawa, CW; Hayes, MG. Worldwide allele frequencies of the human apolipoprotein E gene: climate, local adaptations, and evolutionary history. *Am. J. Physical Anthropology*, 2010 143, 100-111.

Eisenstein, M. Finding risk factors, *Nature*, 2011 474, S20-S22.

El-Osta, A; Brasacchio, D; Yao, D; Pocai, A; Jones, PL; Roeder, RG; Cooper, ME; Brownlee, M. Transient high glucose causes persistent epigenetic changes and altered gene expression during subsequent normoglycemia. *J. Exp. Med.*, 2008 205, 2409-2417.

Elton, TS; Martin, MM. Angiotensin II type 1 receptor gene regulation: transcriptional and posttranscriptional mechanisms. *Hypertens*., 2007 49, 953-961.

Emery, NJ; Seed, AM; von Bayern, AMP; Clayton, NS. Cognitive adaptations of social bonding in birds. *Phil. Trans. R. Soc. B.,* 2007a) 362, 489-505.

Emery, NJ; Clayton, NS; Firth. CD. Introduction. Social Intelligence: from brain to culture. *Phil. Trans. R. Soc. B.,* 2007 b) 362, 485-488.

Emmanouilides, GC; Moses, AJ; Duffie Jr, ER; Adams, FH. Pulmonary artery pressure changes in human newborn infants from birth to 3 days of age. *J. Pediat*., 1964 65, 327-333.

ENCODE Project Consortium. Identification and analysis of functional elements in 1% of the human genome by the ENCODE pilot project. *Nature*, 2007 447, 700-816.

Engel, JE; Xie, X-J; Sokolowski, MB; Wu, C-F. cGMP dependent protein kinase gene, Foraging, modifies habituation-like response decrement of the giant fiber escape circuit in Drosophila. *Learn Mem*., 2000 7, 341-352.

Engelgau, MM; Thompson, TJ; Herman, WH; Boyle, JP; Aubert, RE; Kenny, SJ; Badran, A; Sous, ES; Ali, MA. Comparison of fasting and 2-hour glucose and HbA1c levels for diagnosing diabetes. *Diabetes Care*, 1997 20, 785-791.

Ezenwa, VO; Gerardo, NM; Inouye, DW; Medina, M; Xavier, JB. Animal behavior and the microbiome. *Science*, 2012 338, 198-199.

Falush, D; Almqvist, EW; Brinkmann, RR; Iwasa, Y; Hayden, MR. Measurement of mutational flow implies both a high new-mutation rate for Huntington's disease and substantial underascertainment of late-onset cases. *Am. J. Hum. Gen*., 2001 68, 373-385.

Fan, J; May, SJ; Zhou, Y; Barrett-Connor, E. Bimodality of 2-h plasma glucose distributions in whites. *Diabetes Care*, 2005 28, 1451-1456.

Farrell, AP. Coronary arteriosclerosis in salmon: growing old or growing fast? *Comp. Biochem. Physiol. A*, 2002 132, 723-735.

Federoff, NV. Transposable elements, epigenetics, and genome evolution. *Science*, 2012 338, 758-767.

Feinberg, AP; Irizarry, RA. Stochastic epigenetic variation as a driving force of development, evolutionary adaptation, and disease. *PNAS*, 2010 107, 1757-1764.

Fernald, RD. Casting a genetic light on the evolution of eyes. *Science*, 2006 313, 1914-1918.

Ferrara, N; Gerber, H-P; LeCouter, J. The biology of VEGF and its receptors. *Nature Medicine*, 2003 9, 669-676.

Feuk, L; Carson, AR; Scherer, SW. Structural variations in the human genome. *Nature Reviews Genetics*, 2006 7, 85-97.

Filipkowski, RK. Inducing gene expression in barrel cortex-focus on immediate early genes. *Acta Neurobiol. Exp*., 2000 60, 411-418.

Finch, CE. Evolution of the human lifespan and diseases of aging: roles of infection, inflammation, and nutrition. *PNAS*, 2010 107, 1718-1724.

Finkel, T; Serrano, M; Blasco, MA. The common biology of cancer and ageing. *Nature Reviews,* 2007 448, 767-774.

Fisher, SE. Tangled webs: tracing the connections between genes and cognition. *Cognition*, 2006 101, 270-297.

Flickinger, GL. Effect of grouping on adrenals and gonads of chickens. *Gen. Comp. Endocrinol.*, 1061 1, 332-340.

Flint, J; Mackay, TFC. Genetic architecture of quantitative traits in mice, flies, and humans. *Genome Research*, 2009 19, 723-733.

Fokkema, DS; Smit, K; DerGugten, JV; Koolhaas, JM. A coherent pattern among social behavior, blood pressure, corticosterone and catecholamine measures in individual male rats. *Physiol. Behav.*, 1988 42, 485-489.

Ford, LE. Heart size. *Circ. Res.,* 1976 39, 297-303.

Francis, D; Diorio, J; Liu, D; Meaney, MJ. Nongenomic transmission across generations of maternal behavior and stress responses in the rat. *Science*, 1999 286, 1155-1158.

Frigo, DE; tang, Y; Beckman, BS; Scandurro, AB; Alam, J; Burow, ME; McLachlan, JA. Mechanism of AP-1 mediated gene expression by select organochlorines through the p38 MAPK pathway. *Carcinogenesis*, 2004 25, 249-261.

Fukumoto, H; Rosene, DL; Moss, MB; Raju, S; Hyman, BT; Irizarry, MC. B-secretase activity increases with aging in human, monkey, and mouse brain. *Am. J. Pathol.*, 2004 164, 719-725.

Fumagalli, M. et al. Telomeric DNA damage is irreparable and causes persistent DNA-damage –response activation. *Nature Cell Biology*, 2012 14, 355-367.

Funder, J. Mineralocorticoids and cardiac fibrosis: the decade in review. *Clin. Exper. Pharmacol. Physiol.*, 2001 28, 1002-1006.

Gao, V; Raj; JU. Regulation of the pulmonary circulation in the fetus and newborn. *Physiol. Rev.*, 2010 890, 1291-1335.

Garcia-Garrido, L; Munoz-Chapuli, R; de Andres, V. Coronary arteriosclerosis in dogfish (Scyliorhinus canicula). *Arterio Thrombosis*, 1993 13, 876-885.

George, LA; Zhang, L; Tuersunjiang, N; Ma, Y; Long, NM; Uthlaut, AB; Smith, DT; Nathanielsz, PW; Ford, SP. Early maternal under nutrition programs increased food intake, altered glucose metabolism and insulin secretion, and liver function in aged female offspring. *Am. J. Physiol. Regul. Integr. Comp. Physiol.*, 2012 302, R795-R804.

Geraldes, P; Hiraoka-Yamamoto, J; Matsumoto, M; Clermont, A; Leitges, M; Marette, A; Aiello, LP; Kern, TS; King, GL. Activation of PKC-delta and SHP-1 by hyperglycemia causes vascular cell apoptosis and diabetic retinopathy. *Nature Medicine*, 2009 15, 1298-1307.

Gerlinger, M, et al. Intratumor heterogeneity and branched evolution revealed by multiregion sequencing. *New Eng. J. Med.*, 2012 366, 883-892.

Gerstner, JR; Perren, IJ; Pack, AI. The nexus of AB, aging, and sleep. *Science Translational Medicine*, 2012 4, 150fs34.

Gibbons, A; turning back the clock: slowing the pace of prehistory. *Science*, 2012 338, 189-191.

Gidalevitz, T; ben-Zvi, A; Ho, KH; Brignull, HR; Morimoto, RI. Progressive disruption of cellular protein folding in models of polyglutamine diseases. *Science*, 2006 311, 1471-1474.

Gingeras, Tr. The multitasking genome. *Nature Genetics*, 2006 38, 608-609.

Glagov, S; zarins, C; Giddens, DP; Ku, DN. Hemodynamics and atherosclerosis. Insights and perspectives gained from studies of human arteries. *Arch. pathol. Lab. Med.*, 1988 112, 1018-1031.

Glickman. D; Parker, L; Sim, LJ; Cook, HDV; Miller, EA. Accelerating progress in obesity prevention: solving the weight of the nation. *National Academy of Sciences* (USA); 2012.

Goetz, RH; Keen, N. Some aspects of the cardiovascular system in the giraffe. *Angiology*, 1957 8, 542-564.

Goldberg, TE; Weinberger, DR. Genes and the parsing of cognitive processes. *Trends in Cognitive Sciences*, 2004 6, 325-335.

Goldstein, DB. Common genetic variation and human traits. *New Eng. J. Med.*, 2009 360, 1696-1698.

Gordus, A; Krall, JA; Beyer, EM; Kaushansky, A; Wolf-Yadlin, A; Sevecka, M; Chang, BH; Rush, J; MacBeath, G. Linear combinations of docking affinities explain quantitative differences in RTK signaling. *Molec. Syst. Biol.*, 2009 5, 1-10.

Gould, SJ. *The Panda's Thumb*. New York, USA: W.W. Norton and Company, 1980.

Gould, SJ. *Full House*. New York, USA: Three Rivers Press; 1996.

Gould, SJ. *Wonderful Life*. New York: USA: W.W. Norton and Company; 1989.

Graff, J. et al. An epigenetic blockade of cognitive functions in the neurodegenerating brain. *Nature*, 2012 483, 222-228.

Grainger, J; dufau, S; Montant, M; Ziegler, JC; Fagot, J. Orthographic processing in baboons (Papio papio). *Science*, 2012 336, 245-248.

Greally, JM. Encyclopaedia of humble DNA. *Nature*, 2007 447, 782-783.

Greenwood, AK; Butler, PC; White, RB; DeMarco, U; Pearce, D; Fernald, RD. Multiple corticosteroid receptors in the teleost fish: distinct sequences, expression patterns, and transcriptional activities. *Endocrinol.*, 2003 144, 4226-4236.

Grossmann, C; Krug, AW; Freudinger, R; Mildenberger, S; Voelker, K; Gekle, M. Aldosterone-induced EGFR expression: interaction between the human mineralocorticoid receptor and the human EGFR promoter. *Am. J. Physiol. Endocrinol. Metab.*, 2007 292, E1790-E1800.

Grossman, W. Cardiac hypertrophy: useful adaptation or pathologic process? *Am. J. Med.*, 1980 69, 576-584.

Grubb, BR. Allometric relations of cardiovascular functions in birds. *Am. J. Physiol. Heart Circ. Physiol.*, 1983 245, H567-H572.

Grueter, CE; Van Rooij. E; Johnson, BA; DeLeon, SM; Sutherland, LB; Qi, X: Gautron, L; Elmquist, JK; Bassel-Duby, R; Olson, EN. A cardiac microRNA governs systemic energy homeostasis by regulation of MED13. *Cell*, 2012 149, 671-683.

Guerriero, CJ; Brodsky, JL. The delicate balance between secreted protein folding and endoplasmic reticulum associated degradation in human physiology. *Physiol. Rev.*, 2012 92, 537-576.

Gunther, S; Grossman, W. Determinants of ventricular function in pressure-overload hypertrophy in man. *Circ.*, 1979 59, 679-688.

Guo, D-F; Uno, S; Ishihata, A; nakamura, N; Inagami, T. Identification of a cis-acting glucocorticoid responsive element in the rat angiotensin II type 1 A promoter. *Circ. Res.*, 1995 77, 249-257.

Guyenet, PG. The sympathetic control of blood pressure. *Nature Reviews Neuroscience*, 2006 7, 335-346.

Guyton, AC. Renal function curve-a key to understanding the pathogenesis of hypertension. *Hypertens.*, 1987 10, 1-6.

Guzowski, JF; Lyford, GL; Stevenson, GD; Houston, FP; McGaugh, JL; Worley, PF; Barnes, CA. Inhibition of activity-dependent Arc protein expression in the rat hippocampus impairs the maintenance of long-term potentiation and the consolidation of long-term memory. *J. Neurosci.*, 2000 20, 3993-4001.

Haass, C; Selkoe, DJ. Soluble protein oligomers in neurodegeneration: lessons from the Alzheimer's amyloid B-peptide. *Nature Reviews Molecular Cell Biology*, 2007 8, 101-112.

Haesler, S; Wada, K; Nshdejan, A; Morrisey, EE; Lints, T; Jarvis, ED; Scharff, C. FoxP2 expression in avian vocal learners and non-learners. *J. Neurosci.*, 2004 24, 3164-3175.

Hahn, C; Schwartz, MA. Mechanotransduction in vascular physiology and atherogenesis. *Nature Reviews Molecular Cell Biology*, 2009 10, 53-62.

Hamylyn JM; Manunta, P. Endogenous oubain; a link between sodium intake and hypertension. *Curr. Hypertens. Rep.*, 2011 13, 14-20.

Hargens, AR; Danzig, LA; Gershuni, DH; Millard, RW. Tissue adaptations to gravitational stress: newborn versus adult giraffes. *Physiologist*, 1988 31 (suppl) S110-S113.

Hargens, AR; Millard, RW; Pettersson, K; Johansen, K. Gravitational haemodynamics and oedema prevention in the giraffe. *Nature*, 1987 329, 59-60.

Harold, D. et al. Genome-wide association study identifies variants at CLU and PICALM associated with Alzheimer's disease. *Nature Genetics*, 2009 41, 1088-1095.

Harris, P. Evolution and the cardiac patient. *Cardiovasc. Res.*, 1983 17, 373-378.

Haworth, SG; Hall, SM; Chew, M; Allen, K. Thinning of fetal pulmonary arterial wall and postnatal remodeling: ultrastructural studies on the respiratory unit arteries of the pig. *Virchows Arch.*, 1987 A 4511, 161-171.

Haygood, R; Fedrigo, O; Hanson, B; Yokoyama, K-D; Wray, GA. Promoter regions of many neural-and nutrition-related genes have experienced positive selection during human evolution. *Nature Genetics*, 2007 39, 1140-1144.

Henderson, J; Hurly, TA; Bateson, M; Healy, SD. Timing in free-living Rufous hummingbirds, Selasphorus rufus. *Curr. Biol.*, 2006 16, 512-515.

Herbig, U; Ferreuira, M; Condel, L; Carey, D; Sedivy, JM. Cellular senescence in aging primates. *Science*, 2006 311, 1257.

Herman, MA; Kahn, BB. Glucose transport and sensing in the maintenance of glucose homeostasis and metabolic harmony. *J. Clin. Invest.*, 2006 116, 1767-1775.

Hernadez-Sanchez, C; Mansilla, A; dePablo, F; Zardoya, R. Evolution of the insulin receptor family and receptor isoform expression in vertebrates. *Molec. Biol. Evol.*, 2008 25, 1043-1053.

Herndon, JG; Moss, MB; Rosene, DL; Killiany, RJ. Patterns of cognitive decline in aged rhesus monkeys. *Behav. Brain Res.*, 1997 87, 25-34.

Herskiovits AZ; Growdon, JH. Sharpen that needle. *Arch. Neurol.*, 2010 67, 918-920.

Herzog, ED. Neurons and networks in daily rhythms. *Nature Reviews*, 2007 8, 790-802.

High, FA; Epstein, JA. The multifaceted role of Notch in cardiac development and disease. *Nature Reviews Genetics*, 2008 9, 44-61.

Higuchi, A; Ohashi, K; Kihara, S; Walsh, K; Ouchi, N. Adiponectin suppresses pathological microvessel formation in retina through modulation of tumor necrosis factor alpha expression. *Circ. Res.*, 2009 104, 1058-1065.

Ho, M; Oliverio, MI; Mannon, PJ; Best, CF; Maeda, N; Smithies, O; Coffman, TM. Regulation of blood pressure by the type 1 A angiotensin II receptor gene. *PNAS*, 1995 92, 3521-3525.

Hocht, C; Mayer, M; Taira, CA. Therapeutic perspectives of angiotensin-(1-7) in the treatment of cardiovascular disease. *The Open Pharmacology Journal*, 2008 3, 21-31.

Hof. PR; Gilissen, EP; Sherwood, CC; Duan, H; Lee, PWH; Delman, BN; Naidich, TP; Gannon, PJ; Perl, DP; Erwin, JM. Comparative neuropathology of brain aging in primates. In : Erwin,JM; Hof, PR. Editors. *Aging in nonhuman primates*. Basel, Karger, 2002 vol 31 pp 130-154.

Hofman, JJ; Iruela-Arispe, ML. Notch signaling in blood vessels: who is talking to whom about what? *Circ. Res.*, 2007 100, 1556-1568.

Hohlfeld, R; Wekerle, H. B-amyloid: enemy or remedy. *Science Translational Medicine*, 2012 4, 1-2.

Holmes, DJ; Austad, SN. The evolution of avian senescence patterns: implications for understanding primary aging processes. *Am. Zool.*, 1995 35, 307-317.

Holtmaat, Al; Svoboda, K. Experience-dependent structural synaptic plasticity in the mammalian brain. *Nature Reviews Neuroscience*, 2009 10, 647-658.

Holtmaat, AJGD; Trachtenberg, TT; Wilbrecht, L; Shepherd, GM; Zhang, X; Knott, GW; Svoboda, K. Transient and persistent dendritic spines in the neocortex in vivo. *Neuron*, 2005 45, 279-291.

Hooper, SL. Multiple routes to similar network output. *Nature Neuroscience*, 2004 7, 1287-1288.

Horuk, R; Goodwin, P; O'Connor, K; Nevelle, RWJ; Lazarus. NR. Evolutionary change in the insulin receptors of hystricomorph rodentsd. *Nature*, 1979 279, 439-440.

Horuk, R; Blundell, TL; Lazarus, NR; Neville, RWJ; Stone, D; Wollmer, A. A monomeric insulin from the porcupine (Hystrix cristata), an old world hystricomorph. *Nature*, 1980 286, 822-824.

Hosking, R. mTOR the master regulator. *Cell*, 2012 149, 955, 957.

Howard, Jr. CF; Kessler, MJ; Schwartz, S. Carbohydrate impairment and insulin secretory abnormalities among Macaca mulatta from Cayo Santiago. *Am. J. Primatol.*, 1986, 11, 147-162.

Howard, Jr. CF; Kessler, MJ; Schwartz, S. Metabolic abnormalities among free-ranging Macaca mulatta on Cayo Santiago: comparisons with Macaca mulatta at Sabana Seca. *Am. J. Primatol.,* 1990 21, 189-200.

Huhtala, M; Heino, J; Casciari, D; deLuise, A; Johnson, MS. Integrin evolution: insights from ascidian and teleost fish genomes. *Matrix Biol.*, 2005 24, 83-95.

Imarisio, S. et al. Huntington's disease: from pathology and genetics to potential therapies. *Biochem. J.,* 2008 412, 191-209.

Ingber, DE. Cellular mechanotransduction: putting all the pieces together again. *The FASEB J.*, 2006 20, 811-827.

Irwin, DM. Molecular evolution of mammalian incretin hormone genes. *Regulatory Peptides*, 2009 155, 121-130.

Irwin, DM; Wong, K. Evolution of new hormone function: loss and gain of a receptor. *J. Heredit.,* 2005 96, 205-211.

Ittner, LM; Gotz, J. Amyloid-B and tau- a toxic pas de deux in Alzheimer's disease. *Nature Reviews Neuroscience*, 2011 12, 67-72.

Jain, R; Rentschler, S; Epstein, JA. Notch and cardiac outflow tract development. *Ann. N. Y. Acad. Sci.*, 2010 1188, 184-190.

Jeyapalan, JC; Ferreira, M; Sedivy, JM; Herbig, U. Accumulation of senescent cells in mitotic tissue of aging primates. *Mech. Ageing Develop.*, 2007 128, 36-44.

Jiang, B-H; Zheng, JZ; Aoki, M; Vogt, PK. Phosphatidyl inositol 3-kinase signaling mediates angiogenesis and expression of vascular endothelial growth factor in endothelial cells. *PNAS*, 2000 97, 1749-1753.

Jiang, G; Zhang, BB. Glucagon and regulation of glucose metabolism. *Am. J. Physiol. Endocrinol. Metab.*, 2003 284, E671-E678.

Johansen, IB; Lunde, IG; Rosjo, H; Christensen, G; Nilsson, GE; Bakken, M; Overli, O. Cortisol response to stress is associated with myocardial remodeling in salmonid fishes. *J. Exp. Biol.*, 2011 214, 1313-1321.

Jones, R; Two sides to B-amyloid. *Nature Reviews Neuroscience*, 2012 13, 666.

Jonker, JW, et al. A PPAR gamma-FGF1 axis is required for adaptive adipose remodeling and metabolic homeostasis. *Nature*, 2012 485, 391-395.

Jonsson, T. et al. A mutation in APP protects against Alzheimer's disease and age-related cognitive decline. *Nature*, 2012 488, 96-99.

Kadowaki, T; Yamauchi, T. Adiponectin and adiponectin receptors. *Endocrinol. Rev.*, 2005 26, 439-451.

Kamakura, M. Royalactin induces queen differentiation in honeybees. *Nature*, 2011 473, 478-483.

Kaplan, G. Pointing gesture in a bird- merely instrumental or a cognitively complex behavior? *Curr. Zool.*, 2011 57, 453-467.

Karin, M; Liu, Z; Zandi, E. AP-1 function and regulation. *Curr. Opin. Cell Biol.*, 1997 9, 240-246.

Karran, E; Mercken, M; DeStrooper, B. The amyloid cascade hypothesis for Alzheimer's disease: an appraisal for the development of therapeutics. *Nature Reviews*, 2011 10, 698-712.

Kazda, A; Zellinger, B; Rossler, M; Derboven, E; Kusenda, B; Riha, K. Chromosome end protection by blunt-ended telomeres. *Genes Dev.*, 2012 26, 1703-1713.

Kean, BH; Hammill, JF. Anthropathology of arterial tension. *Arch. Int. Med.*, 1949 83, 355-362.

Keller, L; genoud, M. Extraordinary lifespans in ants: a test of evolutionary theories of ageing. *Nature*, 1997 389, 958-960.

Keller, A. et al. New insights into the Tyrolean Iceman's origin and phenotype as inferred by whole-genome sequencing. *Nature Communications*, 2012 3: 698/DOI: 10, 1038/ ncommsw 1701 (Feb, 28, 2012).

Kelly, SA; Panhuis, TM; Stoehr, AM. Phenotypic plasticity: molecular mechanisms and adaptive significance. *Compr. Physiol.*, 2012 2, 1417-1439.

Kershaw, EE; Flier, JS. Adipose tissue as an endocrine organ. *J. Clin. Endocrinol. Metab.*, 2004 89, 2548-2556.

Kim, J; Basak, JM; Holtzman, DM. The role of apolipoprotein E in Alzheimer's disease. *Neuron*, 2009 63, 287-303.

Klunk, WE. et al., Imaging brain amyloid in Alzheimer's disease with Pittsburgh Compound-B. *Ann. Neurol.*, 2004 55, 306-319.

Koike, N; Yoo, S-H; Huang, H-C; Kumar, V; Lee, C; Kim, T-K; Takahashi, JS. Transcriptional architecture and chromatin landscape of the core circadian clock in mammals. *Science*, 2012 338, 349-354.

Kondo, T; Vicent, D; Suzama, K; Yanagisawa, M; King, GL; Holzenberger, M; Kahn, CR. Knockout of insulin and IGF-1 receptors on vascular endothelial cells protects against retinal neovascularization. *J. Clin. Invest.*, 2003 111, 1835-1842.

Kondrashov, A. The rate of human mutation. *Nature*, 2012 488, 467-468.

Kong, A. et al. Rate of de novo mutations and the importance of father's age to disease risk. *Nature*, 2012 488, 471-475.

Kong, A, et al. Parental origin of sequence variants associated with complex diseases. *Nature*, 2009 462, 868-875.

Konopka, G, et al. Human-specific transcriptional networks in the brain. *Nature*, 2012 75, 601-617.

Konopka, G; Bomar, JM; Winden, K; Coppola, G; Jonsson, ZO; gao, F; Peng, S; Preuss, TM; Wohlschlegel, JA; Geschwind, DH. Human-specific transcriptional regulation of CNS development genes by FOXP2. *Nature*, 2009 462, 213-218.

Koppang, EO; Fischer, U; Satoh, M; Jirillo, E. Inflammation in fish as seen from a morphological point of view with special reference to the vascular compartment. *Curr. Pharmaceutical Design*, 2007 13, 3649-3655.

Korbel, JO, et al. Paired-end mapping reveals extensive structural variation in the human genome. *Science*, 2007 318, 420-426.

Kornel, L. the role of vascular steroid receptors in the control of vascular contractility and peripheral vascular resistance. *J. Steroid Biochem. Molec. Biol.*, 1993 45, 195-203.

Koudinov, AR; Berezov, TT. Alzheimer's amyloid-beta (AB) is an essential synaptic protein, not neurotoxic junk. *Acta Neurobiol. Exp.*, 2004, 64, 71-79.

Kubota, H. Quality control against misfolded proteins in the cytosol: a network for cell survival. *J. Biochem.*, 2009 146, 609-616.

Kubota, N. et al. Disruption of adiponectin causes insulin resistance and neointimal formation. *J. Biol. Chem.*, 2002 277, 25863-25866.

Kucharski, R; Maleszka, J; Foret, S; Maleszka, R. Nutritional control of reproductive status in honeybees via DNA methylation. *Science*, 2008 319, 1827-1830.

Kuo, LE, et al. Neuropeptide Y acts directly in the periphery on fat tissue and mediates stress-induced obesity and metabolic syndrome. *Nature Medicine*, 2007 13, 803-811.

Lammers, R; Gray, A; Schlessinger, J; Ullrich, A. Differential signaling potential of insulin- and IGF-1-receptor cytoplasmic domains. *The EMBO J.*, 1089 3, 1369-1375.

Lamming, DW, et al. Rapamycin-induced insulin resistance is mediated by mTORC2 loss and uncoupled from longevity. *Science*, 20-12 335, 1638-1643.

Lahiri, DK; Maloney, B. Beyond the signaling effect role of amyloid-B42 on the processing of ABPP, and its clinical implications. *Exp. Neurol.*, 2010 225, 51-54.

Lahti, DC; Johnson, NA; Ajie, BC; Otto, SP; Hendry, AP; Blumstein, DT; Coss, RG; Donohue, K; Foster, SA. Relaxed selection in the wild. *Trends Ecol. Evol.*, 2009 24, 487-496.

Lander, ES. Initial impact of the sequencing of the human genome. *Nature*, 2011 470, 187-197.

Lang, F; Bohmer, C; Palmada, M; Seebohm, G; Strutz-Seebohm, N; Vallon, V. (Patho)physiological significance of the serum- and glucocorticoid- inducible kinase isoforms. *Physiol. Rev.*, 2006 86, 1151-1178.

Laurent, P; Marenco, P; Castagna, O; Smulyan, H; Blacher, J; Safar, ME. Differences in central systolic blood pressure and aortic stiffness between aerobically trained and sedentary individuals. *J. Am. Soc. Hypertens.*, 2011 5, 85-93.

Learoyd, BM; Taylor, MG. Alterations with age in the viscoelastic properties of human arterial walls. *Circ. Res.*, 1966 18, 278-292.

Lecomte, VJ, et al. Patterns of aging in the long-lived wandering albatross. *PNAS*, 2010 107, 6370-6375.

Leenen, FHH. The central role of the brain- "oubain" pathway in salt-sensitive hypertension. *Biochim. Biophys. Acta*, 2010 1802, 1132-1139.

Lehoux, S; Esposito, B; Merval, R; Tedgui, A. Differential regulation of vascular focal adhesion kinase by steady stretch and pulsatility. *Circ*, 2005 111, 643-649.

Lehoux, S; Tedgui, A. Cellular mechanics and gene expression in blood vessels. *J. Biomech.*, 2003 36, 631-643.

Lehoux, S; castier, Y; Tedgui, A. Molecular mechanisms of the vascular responses to haemodynamic forces. *J. Int. Med.*, 2006 259, 381-392.

Lemons, D; McGinnis, W. Genomic evolution of HOX gene clusters. *Science*, 2006 313, 1918-1922.

Leung, DY; Glagov, S; Mathews, MB. Elastin and collagen accumulation in rabbit ascending aorta and pulmonary trunk during postnatal growth. Correlation of cellular synthetic response with medial tension. *Circ. Res.*, 1077 41, 316-323.

Levin, BE; Sullivan, AC. Glucose, insulin and sympathoadrenal activation. *J. Autonomic Nerv. Sys.*, 1987 20, 233-242.

Levin, BE. Neuronal glucose sensing: still a physiological orphan? *Cell Metab.*, 2007 6, 252-254.

Levin, BE; Routh, VH; Kang, L; Sanders, NNM; Dunn-Meynell, AA. Neuronal glucosensing. What do we know after 50 years? *Diabetes*, 2004 53, 2521-2528.

Lewington, S; Clarke, R; Qizilbash, N; Peto, R; Collins, R. Age-specific relevance of usual blood pressure to vascular mortality: a meta-analysis of individual data for one million adults in 61 prospective studies. *Lancet*, 2002 360, 1903-1913.

Li, J, et al. Genomic hypomethylation in the human germline associates with selective structural mutability in the human genome. *PLoS Genetics*, 2012 vol 8 (issue 5) 1-17.

Lifton, RP; Gharavi, AG; Geller, DS. Molecular mechanisms of human hypertension. *Cell*, 2001 104, 545-556.

Lillywhite, HB. Gravity, blood circulation, and the adaptation of form and function in lower vertebrates. *J. Exp. Zool.*, 1996 275, 217-225.

Lim. T-O; Bakri, R; Morad, Z; Hamid, MA. Bimodality in blood glucose distribution. *Diabetes Care*, 2002 25, 2212-2217.

Lindner, V; Booth, C; Prudovsky< I; Small, D; Maciag,, T; Liaw, L. Members of the Jagged/Notch gene families are expressed in injured arteries and regulate cell phenotype via alteration in cell matrix and cell-cell interaction. *Am. J. Pathol.*, 2001 159, 875-883.

Lister, R,et al. Human DNA methylomes at base resolution show widespread epigenomic differences. *Nature*, 2009 462, 315-322.

Liu, D; Diorio, J; Tannenbaum, B; Caldji, C; Francis, D; Freedman, A; Sharma, S; Pearson, D Plotsky, PM; Meaney, MJ. Maternal care, hippocampal glucocorticoid receptors, and hypothalamic-pituitary-adrenal responses to stress. *Science*, 1997 277, 1659-1662.

Liu, N; Landreh, M; Cao, K; Abe, M; Hendriks, G-J; Kennerdell, JR; Zhu, Y. The microRNA miR-34 modulates ageing and neurodegeneration in Drosophila. *Nature*, 2012 482, 519-525.

Longo, DL. Tumor heterogeneity and personalized medicine. *New Eng. J. Med.*, 2012 366, 956-957.

Loo, SG; Dowse, GK; Finch, C; Zimmet, P. Bimodality analysis of frequency distributions of 2-hour plasma glucose concentrations in the urban Micronesia population of Kiribati. *J. Diab. Comp.*, 1993 7, 73-80.

Lynch, M. Rate, molecular-spectrum, and consequences of human mutation. *PNAS*, 2010 107, 961-968.

Lucas, L-R; Pompei, P; McEwen, BS. Salt appetite in salt-replete rats: involvement of mesolimbic structures in deoxycorticosterone- induced salt craving behavior. *Neuroendocrinol.*, 2000 71, 386-395.

Luk, KC; Kehm, V; Carroll, J; Zhang, B; O'Brien, P; Trojanowski, JQ; Lee, VM-Y. Pathological alpha-synuclein transmission initiates Parkinson-like neurodegeneration in non transgenic mice. *Science*, 2012 338, 949-953.

Lunau, K. In the company of whales. *Macleans's Magazine*, August 8, 2011 pages 57-59.

MacArthur, DG, et al. A systematic survey of loss-of –function variants in human protein-coding genes. *Science*, 2012 335, 823-828.

Maher, B; The case of the missing heritability. *Nature*, 2008 456, 18-21.

Makinodan, M; Rosen, KM; Ho, S; Corfas, G. A critical period for social experience-dependent oligodendrocyte maturation and myelination. *Science*, 2012 337, 1357-1360.

Maldonado, TA; Jones, RE; Norris, DO. Distribution of B-amyloid and amyloid precursor protein in the brain of spawning (senescent) salmon: a natural, brain-aging model. *Brain Res.*, 2000 858, 237-251.

Maldonado, TA; Jones, RE; Norris, DO. Timing of neurodegeneration and beta-amyloid (AB) peptide deposition in the brain of aging kokanee salmon. *J. Neurobiol.*, 2002 53, 21-35.

Maluf, NSR. Kidney of giraffes. *Anat. Rec.*, 2002 267, 94-111.

Mandrioli, M. Epigenetic tinkering and evolution: is there any continuity in the role of cytosine methylation from invertebrates to vertebrates? *Cellular Molec. Life Sciences*, 2004 61, 2425-2427.

Manning, BD; Cantley, LC. AKT/PKB signaling: navigating downstream. *Cell*, 2007 129, 1261-1274.

Manunta, P; Hamilton, BP; Hamlyn, JM. Salt intake and depletion increase circulating levels of endogenous oubain in normal men. *Am. J. Physiol. Regul. Integr. Comp. Physiol.*, 2006 290, R553-R559.

Marcheva, B, et al. Disruption of the clock components CLOCK and BMAL 1 leads to hypoinsulinemia and diabetes. *Nature*, 2010 466, 627-631.

Marino, L, et al. Cetaceans have complex brains for complex cognition. *PLoS Biology*, 2007 5, issue 5.

Marques-Bonet, T; Ryder, OA; Eichler, EE. Sequencing primate genomes: what have we learned? *Annu. Rev. Genomics Hum. Genetics*, 2009 10, 355-386.

Martinez, DE. Mortality patterns suggest lack of senescence in hydra. *Exper. Geront.*, 1998 33, 217-225.

Marx, J. Huntington's research points to possible new therapies. *Science*, 2005 310, 43-45.

Mattick, JS. Challenging the dogma: the hidden layer of non-protein coding RNAs in complex organisms. *BioEssays*, 2003 25, 930-939.

Mattick, JS. The genomic foundation is shifting. *Science*, 2011 331, 874.

Mattison, JA, et al. Impact of caloric restriction on health and survival in rhesus monkeys from the NIA study. *Nature*, 2012 489, 318-323.

Maurano, MT, et al. Systematic localization of common disease-associated variation in regulator DNA. *Science*, 2012 337, 1190-1195.

McCance, DR; Hanson, RL; Charles, M-A; Jacobsson, LTH; Pettitt, DJ; Bennett, PH; Knowler, WC. Comparison tests for glycated haemoglobin and fasting and two hour plasma glucose concentrations as diagnostic methods for diabetes,. *Brit. Med. J.*, 1994 308, 1323-1328.

McCullagh, KG. Arterosclerosis in the African elephant. Part 1. Intimal atherosclerosis and its possible causes. *Atherosclerosis*, 1972 16, 307-335.

McEwen, BS. Protective and damaging effects of stress mediators. *New Eng. J. Med.*, 1998 338, 171-179.

McEwen, BS. From molecules to mind. Stress, individual differences, and the social environment. *Ann. N. Y. Acad. Sci.*, 2001 935, 42-49.

McGonnell, IM; Fowkes, RC. Fishing for gene function-endocrine modelling in the zebra fish. *J. Endocrinol.*, 2006 189, 425-439.

McLean, CY, et al. Human- specific loss of regulatory DNA and the evolution of human-specific traits. *Nature*, 2011 471, 216-219.

Mettke-Hofmann, C; Gwinner, E. Long-term memory for a life on the move. *PNAS*, 2003 100, 5863-5866.

Micali, A; Pisani, A; Ventrici, C; Puzzolo, D; Roszkowska, AM; Spinella, R; Aragona, P. Morphological and morphometric study of the pectin oculi in the Budgerigar (Melopsittacus undulates). *Anat. Rec.*, 2012 295, 540-550.

Michel, RP; Gordon, JB; Chu, K. Development of the pulmonary vasculature in newborn lambs: structure- function relationships. *J. Appl. Physiol.*, 1001 70, 1255-1264.

Mick, GJ; Wang, X; McCormick, K. White adipocyte vascular endothelial growth factor: regulation by insulin. *Endocrinol.*, 2002 143, 948-953.

Miller, CA; Sweatt, JD. Covalent modification of DNA regulates memory formation. *Neuron*, 2007 53, 857-869.

Miller, G. Why are you and your brain unique? *Science*, 2012 338, 35-36.

Miller, G. Stopping Alzheimer's before it starts. *Science*, 2012 337, 790-792.

Miller-Jensen, K; Janes, KA; Brugge, JS; Lauffenburger, DA. Common effector processing mediates cell- specific responses to stimuli. *Nature*, 2007 448, 604-609.

Mills, Re, et al. Mapping copy number variation by population- scale genome sequencing. *Nature*, 2011 470, 59-65.

Mitchell, G; Skinner, JD. An allometric analysis of the giraffe cardiovascular system. *Comp. Biochem. Physiol.* Part A, 2009 154, 523-529.

Moon., TW. Glucose intolerance in teleost fish: fact or fiction? *Comp. Biochem. Physiol.*, 2001 Part B 129, 243-249.

Morley, JE; Farr, SA; banks, WA; Johnson, SN; Yamada, KA; Xu,L. A physiological role for amyloid-B protein: enhancement of learning and memory. *J. Alzheimer's Disease*, 2010 19, 441-449.

Morris, MJ; Na, ES; Johnson, AK. Salt craving: the psychobiology of pathogenic sodium intake. *Physiol. Behav.*, 2008 94, 709-721.

Muller, C; Zheng, H. Physiological functions of APP family proteins. *Cold Spring Harb. Perspect. Med.*, 2012 4: a 006288.

Munoz-Sanjuan, I; Bates, GP. The importance of integrating basic and clinical research toward the development of new therapies for Huntington Disease. *J. Clin. Invest.*, 2011 121, 476-483.

Musson, MC; jepeal, LI; Mabray, PD; Zhdanova, IV; Cardoso, WV; Wolfe, MM. Expression of glucose- dependent insulintropic polypeptide in the zebra fish. *Am. J. Physiol. Regul. Integr. Comp. Physiol.*, 2009 297, R1803-R1812.

Nakayama, H; Katayama, K-I; Ikawa, A; Miyawaki, K; Shinozuka, J; Uetsuka, K; Nakamura, S-I; Kimura, N; Yoshikawa, Y; Doi, K. Cerebral amyloid angiopathy in an aged great spotted wood pecker (Picoides major). *Neurobiol. Aging*, 1999 20, 53-56.

Nakamura, Y, et al. NDM2: a novel mineralocorticoid-responsive gene involved in aldosterone- induced human vascular structural remodeling. *Amer. J. Pathol.*, 2006 169, 362-371.

Nathwani, AC, et al. Adenovirus-associated virus vector- mediated gene transfer in Hemophilia B. *New Eng. J. Med.*, 2011 365, 2357-2365.

Nathan, DM. International expert committee report on the role of the A1C assay in the diagnosis of diabetes. *Diabetes ,Care*, 2009 32, 1327-1334.

National Research Council; Toward Precision Medicine, Building a Knowledge Network for Biomedical Research and a new Taxonomy of Disease. National Academy Press, Washington, D.C., 2011.

Nawata, H; Takayanagi, R; Ohnaka, K; Sakai, Y; Imasaki, K; Yanase, T; Ikuyama, S; Tanaka, S; Ohe, K. Type 1 angiotensin II receptors of adrenal tumors. *Steroids*, 1995 60, 28-34.

Nelson, ADL; Shippen,DE. Blunt-ended telomeres: an alternative ending to the replication and end protection stories. *Genes Dev.*, 2012 26, 1648-1652.

Nestler, EJ. Stress makes its molecular mark. *Nature*, 2012 490, 171-172.

Neufeld, HN; Wagenvoort, Edwards,, JE. Coronary arteries in fetuses, infants, juveniles, and young adults. *Lab. Invest.*, 1962 11, 837-844.

Nicholson, JK; Holmes, E; Kincross, J; Burcelin, R; Gibson, G; Jia, W; Pettersson, S. Host-gut microbiota metabolic interactions. *Science*, 2012 336, 1262-1267.

Nicolucci, A. Epidemiological aspects of neoplasms in diabetes. *Acta Diabetol.*, 2010 47, 87-95.

O'Donnell, CJ, et al. Genome wide association study for subclinical atherosclerosis in major arterial territories in the NHLBI's Framingham Heart Study. *BMC Medical Genetics*, 2007 B (suppl 1): S4.

Oliver, WJ; Cohen, EL; Neel, JV. Blood pressure, sodium intake, and sodium related hormones in the Yanomamo Indians, a "no-salt" culture. *Circ.*, 1975, 52, 146-151.

Olson, MV; Varki, A. Sequencing the chimpanzee genome: insights into human evolution and disease. *Nature Reviews Genetics*, 2003 4, 20-28.

Olson, MV. What does a "normal" human genome look like? *Science*, 2011 331, 872.

Osborn, JW; Jacob, F; Guzman, P. A neural set point for the long-term control of arterial pressure: beyond the arterial baroreceptor reflex. *Am. J. Physiol. Regul. integr. Comp. Physiol.*, 2005 288, R846-R855.

Osika, W; Dangardt, F; Gronros, J; Lundstram, U; Myredal, A; Johansson, M; Volkmann, R; Gustavsson, T; Gan, LM; Friberg, P. Increasing peripheral artery intimal thickness from childhood to seniority. *Arteriosclerosi. Thromb. Vasc. Biol.*, 2007 27, 671-676.

Ozaki, T; Iizuka, K; Suzuki, M; Murakami, T; Kitabatake, A; Kawaguchi, H. Threshold-dependent DNA synthesis by pure pressure in human aortic smooth muscle cells: Gi alpha- dependent and- independent pathways. *Biochem. Biophys. Res. Comm.*, 1999 256, 212-217.

Page, LB; Damon, A; Moellering, Jr, RC. Antecedents of cardiovascular disease in six Solomon Islands Societies. *Circ.*, 1974, 49, 1132-1146.

Page, Jr, RE; Peng, CY-S. Aging and development in social insects with emphasis on the honey bee, Apis mellifera L. *Exp. Geront.*, 2001 36, 695-711.

Pani, LN; Kovenda, L; Meigs, JB; Driver, C; Chamany, S; Fox, C; Sullivan, L; D'Agostino, RB; Nathan, DM. Effect of aging on A1C levels in individuals without diabetes. *Diabetes Care*, 2008 31, 1991-1996.

Pape, LA; Price, JM; Alpert, JS; Rippe, JM. Hemodynamics and left ventricular function: a comparison between adult racing greyhounds and greyhounds completely untrained from birth. *Basic Res. Cardiol.*, 1986 81, 417-424.

Parton, LE, et al. Glucose sensing by POMC neurons regulates glucose homeostasis and is impaired in obesity. *Nature*, 2007 449, 228-233.

Paton, JFR; Dickinson, CJ; Mitchell, G. Harvey Cushing and the regulation of blood pressure in giraffe, rat and man: introducing "Cushing's mechanism". *Exp. Physiol.*, 2009 94, 11-17.

Pava, L; Casiglia, E; Braga, LMC; Winnicki, M; Puato, M; Pauletto, P; Pessina, AC. Effects of a traditional lifestyle on the cardiovascular risk profile: the Amondava population of the Brazilian Amazon. Comparisons with matched African, Italian and Polish populations. *J. Hypertens.,* 1999 17, 749-756.

Pearson, TA; Manolio, TA. How to interpret a genome wide association study. *JAMA*, 2008 299, 1335-1344.

Pelkmans, L. Using cell-to-cell variability-a new era in molecular biology. *Science*, 2012 336, 425-426.

Pennisi, E,. Gene duplication's role in evolution gets richer, more complex. *Science*, 2012 a) 338, 316-317.

Pennisi, E. ENCODE project writes eulogy for junk DNA. *Science*, 2012 b) 337, 1159-1161.

Pennisi. E. DNA study forces rethink of what it means to be a gene. *Science*, 2007 316, 1556-1557.

Perez, W; Lima, M; Pedrana, G; Cirillo, F. Heart anatomy of Giraffa camelopardalis rothschildi: a case report. *Veterinarni Medicina*, 2008 53, 165-168.

Pessin, JE; Saltiel, AR. Signaling pathways of insulin action: molecular targets of insulin resistance. *J. Clin. Invest.*, 2000 106, 165-169.

Phillips, MI; deOliveira, EM. Brain renin angiotensin in disease. *J. Molec. Med.*, 2008 86, 715-722.

Pinheiro, SVB; eSilva, ACS. Angiotensinn converting enzyme 2, angiotensin- (1-7), and receptor Mas axis in the kidney. *Int. J. Hypertens.*, 2012 vol 2012, article ID 414128, 8 pages.

Pilny, AA; Luong, R. Diabetes mellitus in a chestnut-fronted macaw (Ara severa). *J. Avian Med. Surg.*, 2005 19, 297-302.

Polakof, S; Miguez, JM; Moon, TW; Soengas, JL, Evidence for the presence of a glucosensor in hypothalamus, hindbrain, and Brockmann bodies of rainbow trout. *Am. J. Physiol. Regul. Integr. Comp. Physiol.*, 2007 292, R1657-R1666.

Polakof, S; Mommsen, TP; Soengas, JL. Glucosensing and glucose homeostasis: from fish to mammals. *Comp. Biochem. Physiol.*, 2011 Par B 160, 123-149.

Pollack, A. DNA sequencing is caught in a deluge of data. New York Times, December 18, 2011, page 7.

Pollak, M. Insulin and insulin-like growth factor signaling in neoplasia. *Nature Reviews Cancer*, 2008 8, 915-928.

Pollard, KS, et al. An RNA gene expressed during cortical development evolved rapidly in humans. *Nature*, 2006 443, 167-172.

Pollock, ML; Mengelkoch, LJ; Graves, JE; Lowenthal, DT; Limacher, MC; Foster, C; Wimore, JH. Twenty- year follow-up of aerobic power and body composition of older track athletes. *J. Appl. Physiol.*, 1997 82, 1508-1516.

Ponder, KP. Merry Christmas for patients with Hemophilia B. *New Eng. J. Med.*, 2011 365, 2424-2425.

Portier, H; Louisy, F; Laude, D; Berthelot, M; Guezennec, C-Y. Intense endurance training on heart rate and blood pressure variability in runners. *Med. Sci. Sports Exerc.*, 2001 33, 1120-1125.

Post, RH. Possible cases of relaxed selection in civilized populations. Humangenetik, 1971 13, 253-284.

Poulter, N; Khaw, KT; Hopwood, BEC; Mugambi, M; Peart, WS; Rose, G; Sever, PS. Blood pressure and its correlates in an African tribe in urban and rural environments. *J. Epidem. Community Health*, 1984, 38, 181-186.

Poupa, O; Lindstrom, L. Comparative and scaling aspects of heart and body weights with reference to blood supply of cardiac fibers. *Comp. Biochem. Physiol.*, 1983 76A, 413-421.

Poupa, O; Ostadal, B. Experimental cardiomegalies and "cardiomegalies" in free-living animals. *Ann. N. Y. Acad. Sci.*, 1969 156, 445-468.

Pravosudov, V; Kitaysky, AS; Omanska, A. The relationship between migratory behavior, memory and the hippocampus: an intraspecific comparison. *Proc. R. Soc. B.*, 2006 273, 2641-2649.

Prinz, AA; Bucher, D; Marder, E. Similar network activity from disparate circuit parameters. *Nature Neurosciences*, 2004 7, 1345-1352.

Pyorala, K; Karronen, MJ; Taskinen, P; Takkunen, J; Kyronseppa, H; Peltokallio, P. cardiovascular studies on former endurance athletes. *Am. J. Cardiol.*, 1967 20, 191-205.

Raichlen, DA; Foster, AD; Gerdeman, GL; Seillier, A; Giuffrida, A. Wired to run: exercise-induced endocannabinoid signaling in humans and cursorial mammals with implications for the " runner's high". *J. Exp. Biol.*, 2012 215, 1331-1336.

Ramus, F. Genes, brain, and cognition: a road map for the cognitive scientist. *Cognition*, 2006 101, 247-269.

Rando, OJ. Daddy issues: paternal effects on phenotype. *Cell*, 2012 151, 702-708.

Ratcliffe, HL; Snyder, RL. Myocardial infarction: a response to social interactions among chickens. *Science*, 1964 144, 425-426.

Ratcliffe, HL; Yerasimides, TG; Elliott, GA. Changes in the character and location of arterial lesions in mammals and birds in the Philadelphia Zoological Garden. *Circ.*, 1960 21, 730-738.

Ratcliffe, HL. Age and environment as factors in the nature and frequency of cardiovascular lesions in mammals and birds in the Philadelphia Zoological Garden. *Ann. N. Y. Acad. Sci.*, 1965 127, 715-735.

Ratcliffe, HL; Cronon, MTI. Changing frequency of arteriosclerosis in mammals and birds in the Philadelphia Zoological Garden. *Circ.*, 1958, 18, 41-52.

Ravichand, KS. Signaling via Shc family adapter proteins. Oncogene, 2001 20, 6322-6330.

Ravioli, E; Raviola, G. A light and electron microscopic study of the pectin of the pigeon eye. *Am. J. Anat.,* 1967 120, 427-462.

Reilly, DF; Westgate, EJ; FitzGerald, GA. Peripheral circadian clocks in the vasculature. *Arteriosclerosis Thromb. Vasc. Biol.*, 2007 27, 1694-1705.

Rendell, M; Srephen, PM; Paulsen, R; Valentine, JL; Rasbold, K; Hestorff, T; Eastberg, S; Shint, DC. An interspecies comparison of normal levels of glycosylated hemoglobin and glycosylated albumin. *Comp. Biochem. Physiol.* 1985 81B, 819-822.

Riccio, AP; Goldman, BD. Circadian rhythms of body temperature and metabolic rate in naked mole-rats. *Physiol. Behav.*, 2000 a) 71, 15-22.

Riccio, AP; Goldman, BD. Circadian rhythms of locomotor activity in naked mole-rats. *Physiol. Behav.*, 2000 b) 71, 1-13.

Richards, MP; McMurtry, JP. The avian proglucagon system. *Gen. Comp. Endocrinol.*, 2009 163, 39-46.

Richards, EJ. Inherited epigenetic variation- revisiting soft inheritance. *Nature Reviews Genetics*, 2006 7, 395-401.

Ridker, PM, et al. Rosuvastatin to prevent vascular events in men and women with elevated c-reactive protein. *New Eng. J. Med.*, 2008 359, 2195-2207.

Robertson, OH; Krupp, MA; Thomas, SF; Favour, CB; Hane, S; Wexler, BC. Hyperadrenocorticism in spawning migratory and nonmigratory Rainbow trout (Salmo gairdnerii); comparison with Pacific salmon (Genus Oncorhynchus). *Gen. Comp. Endocrinol.*, 1961 1, 473-484.

Robinson, GE; Fernald, RD; Clayton, DF. Genes and social behavior. *Science*, 2008 322, 896-900.

Rockman, MV; Kruglyak, L. Genetics of global gene expression. *Nature Reviews Genetics*, 2006 7, 862-872.

Rogers, KM; Bonar, CA; Estrella, JL; Yang, S. Inhibitory effect of glucocorticoid on coronary artery endothelial function. *Am. J. Physiol. Heart Circ. Physiol.*, 2002 283, H1922-H1928.

Roh, JH; Huang, Y; Bero, AW; Kasten, T; Stewart, FR; Bateman, RJ; Holtzman, DM. Disruption of the sleep-wake cycle and diurnal fluctuation of amyloid-B in mice with Alzheimer's disease pathology. *Science Translational Medicine*, 2012 4, 150ra122.

Ron, D; Walter, P. Signal integration in the endoplasmic reticulum unfolded protein response. *Nature Reviews Molecular Cell Biology*, 2007 8, 519-529.

Rose, MR. Adaptation, aging and genomic information. *Aging*, 2009 1, 444-451.

Routh, VH. Glucosensing neurons in the ventromedial hypothalamic nucleus (VMN) and hypoglycema- associated autonomic failure (HAAF). *Diabetes Metab. Res. Dev.*, 2003 19, 348-356.

Rudic, RD; McNamara. P; Reilly, D; Grosser, T; Curtis, A-M; Price, TS; Panda, S; Hogenesch, JB; FitzGerald, GA. Bioinformatic analysis of circadian gene oscillation in mouse aorta. *Circ.*, 2005 112, 2716-2724.

Russell, SJ; Kahn, CR. Endocrine regulation of ageing. *Nature Reviews Molecular Cell Biology*, 2007 8, 681-691.

Saltiel, AR; Kahn, CR. Insulin signaling and the regulation of glucose and lipid metabolism. *Nature*, 2001 414, 799-806.

Samuel, VT; Shulman, GI. Mechanisms for insulin resistance: common threads and missing links. *Cell*, 2012 148, 852-871.

Sanyal, S; Sandstrom, DJ; Hoeffer, CA; Ramaswami, M. AP-1 functions upstream of CREB to control synaptic plasticity in Drosophila, *Nature*, 2002 416, 870-874.

Scally, A; Durbin, R. Revising the human mutation rate: implications for understanding human evolution. *Nature Reviews Genetics*, 2012 13, 745-753.

Scarf, D; Hayne, H; Colombo, M. Pigeons on par with primates in numerical competence. *Science*, 2011 334, 1664.

Schafer, WR. PKG and the neural basis for behavioral phenotypes. *Neuron*, 2002 36, 991-993.

Scharff, C; Petri, J. Evo-devo, deep homology, and FoxP2: implications for the evolution of speech and language. *Phil. Trans. R. Soc. B.*, 2011 366, 2124-2140.

Schlegel, A; Stainier, DYR. Lessons from "lower" organisms: what worms, flies, and zebra fish teach us about human energy metabolism. *PLoS Genetics*, 2007 3, issue 11.

Schlessinger, J; Lemmon, MA. Nuclear signaling by receptor tyrosine kinases: the first robin of spring. *Cell*, 2006 127, 45-48.

Schmidt, DA; Koutsos, EA; Ellersieck, MR; Griffin, ME. Serum concentration comparisons of amino acids, fatty acids, lipoproteins, vitamins A and E, and minerals between Zoo and free-ranging giraffes (Giraffa camelopardalis), *J. Zoo Wildlife Med.*, 2009 40,29-38.

Schnabel, J. Little proteins, big clues. *Nature*, 2011 475, S12-S14.

Schoenenberger, P; Gerosa, D; Oertner, TG. Temporal control of immediate early gene induction by light. *PLoS ONE*, 2009 4, issue 12.

Schreihofer, AM; Ho, S; Sved, AF. Brain stem control of arterial pressure in chronic arterial baroreceptor- denervated rats. *Am. J. Physiol. Regul. Integr. Comp. Physiol.*, 2005 289, R1746-R1755.

Schrufner, TL; Antoneth, DA; Sonenberg, N; Kimball, SR; Gardner, TW; Jefferson, LS. Ablation of 4E-BP1/2 prevents hyperglycemia- mediated induction of VEGF expression in the rodent retina and in Muller cells in culture. *Diabetes*, 2010 59, 2107-2116.

Schwartz, MW. Brain pathways controlling food intake and body weight. *Exp. Biol. Med.*, 2001 226, 978-981.

Schuit, FC; Huypens, P; Heimberg, H; Pipeleers, DG. Glucose sensing in pancreatic B –cells. A model for the study of other glucose- regulated cells in gut, pancreas, and hypothalamus. *Diabetes*, 2001 50, 1-11.

Schulz, LO; Bennett, PH; Ravussin, E; Kidd, JR; Kidd, KK; Esparza, J; Valencia, ME. Effects of traditional and western environments on prevalence of type 2 diabetes in Pima Indians in Mexico and the US. *Diabetes Care*, 2006 29, 1866-1871.

Seirstad, SL; Svindland, A; Larsen, S; Rosenlund, G; Torstensen, BE; Evensen, O. Development of intimal thickening of coronary arteries over the lifetime of Atlantic salmon, Salmo salar L., fed different lipid sources. *J. Fish Dis.*, 2008 31, 401-413.

Selkoe, DJ. Preventing Alzheimer's Disease. *Science*, 2012 a) 337, 1488-1492.

Selkoe, DJ. Alzheimer's Disease is a synaptic failure. *Science*, 2002 298,789-791.

Selkoe, D; Mandelkow, E; Holtzman, D. Deciphering Alzheimer Disease. *Cold Spring Harb. Perspect Med.*, 2012 b) 2:a011460.

Selkoe, DJ. Cell biology of protein misfolding: the examples of Alzheimer's and Parkinson's diseases. *Nature Cell Biology*, 2004 6, 1054-1061.

Seymour, RS; Lillywhite, HB. Blood pressure in snakes from different habitats. *Nature*, 1976 264, 664-666.

Seymour, RS; Blaylock, AJ. The principle of Laplace and scaling of ventricular wall stress and blood pressure in mammals and birds. *Physiol. Biochem. Zool.*, 2000 73, 389-405.

Shabalina, SA; Yampolsky, LY; Kondrashov, A. rapid decline of fitness in panmictic populations of Drosophila melanogaster maintained under relaxed natural selection. *PNAS*, 1997 94, 13034-13039.

Shadwick, RE. mechanical design in arteries. *J. Exp. Biol.*, 1999 202, 3305-3313.

Sharif-Naeini, R; Folgering, JHA; Bichet, D; Duprat, F; Delmas, P; Patel, A; Honore, E. Sensing pressure in the cardiovascular system: Gq- coupled mechanoreceptors and TRP channels. *J. Molec. Cell Cardiol.*, 2010 48, 83-89.

Shibata, D. Heterogeneity and tumor history. *Science*, 2012 336, 304-305.

Shively, CA; Register, TC; Clarkson, TB. Social stress, visceral obesity, and coronary artery atherosclerosis: product of a primate adaptation. *Am. J. Primatol.*, 2009 71, 742-751.

Siegel, JM. Suppression of sleep for mating. *Science*, 2012 337, 1610-1611.

Sikes, SK. The disturbed habitat and its effects on the health of animal populations, with special reference to cardiovascular disease in elephants. *Proc. R. Soc. Med.*, 1968 61, 160-161.

Singer, MA. Comparative Physiology, Natural Animal Models and Clinical Medicine. London, UK: Imperial College Press; 2007.

Singer, MA. Insights into biomedicine from animal adaptations. *Compr. Physiol.*, 2011 1, 2063-2081.

Snodgrass, JJ; Leonard, WR; Sorensen, MV; Tarskaia, LA; Mosher, MJ. The influence of basal metabolic rate on blood pressure among indigenous Siberians. *Am. J. Phys. Anthropology*, 2008 137, 145-155.

Soivio, A; Nynolm, K; Westman, K. A technique for repeated sampling of the blood of individual fish. *J. Exp. Biol.*, 1975 62, 207-217.

Soto, C; Estrada, KL; Castilla, J. Amyloids, prions and the inherent infectious nature of misfolded protein aggregates. *Trends Biochem. Sci.*, 2006 31, 150-155.

Spassova, MA; Hewavitharana, T; Xu, W; Soboloff, J; Gill, DL. A common mechanism underlies stretch activation and receptor activation of TRPC 6 channels. *PNAS*, 2006 103 16586-16591.

Staessen, JA, et al. Randomized double- blind comparison of placebo and active treatment for older patients with isolated systolic hypertension. *Lancet*, 1997 350, 757-764.

Stamler, J. The INTERSALT study: background, methods, findings, and implications. *Am. J. Clin. Nutr.*, 1997 65 (suppl), 626S-642S.

Stanfel, MN; Shamieh, LS; Kaeberlein, M; Kennedy, BK. The TOR pathway comes of age. *Biochim. Biophys. Acta*, 2009 1790, 1067-1074.

Stehbens, WE. Structural and architectural changes during arterial development and the role of hemodynamics. *Acta Anat.*, 1996 157, 261-274.

Stewart, CE; Rotwein, P. Growth, differentiation, and survival: multiple physiological functions for insulin-like growth factors. *Physiol. Rev.*, 1996 76, 1005-1026.

Sugii, S, et al. PPAR gamma activation in adipocytes is sufficient for systemic insulin sensitization. *PNAS*, 2009 106, 22504-22509.

Sugiyama, T; Yoshimoto, T; Tsuchiya, K; Gochou, N; Hirono, Y; Tateno, T; Fukai, N; Shichiri, M; Hirata, Y. Aldosterone induces angiotensin converting enzyme gene expression via JAK 2-dependent pathway in rat endothelial cells. *Endocrinol.*, 2005 146, 3900-3906.

Suter, M; Ma, J; Harris, A; Patterson, L; Brown, KA; Shope, C; Showalter, L; Abramovici, A; Aagaard,-Tillery, KM. Maternal tobacco use modestly alters correlated epigenome-wide placental DNA methylation and gene expression. *Epigenetics*, 2011 6, 1284-1294.

Taft, RJ; Pheasant, M; Mattick, JS. The relationship between non-protein coding DNA and eukaryotic complexity. *BioEssays*, 2007 29, 288-299.

Talchai, C; Xuan, S; Lin, HV; Sussel, L; Accili, D. Pancreatic B cell dedifferentiation as a mechanism of diabetic B cell failure. *Cell*, 2012 150, 1223-1234.

Tallec, LP; Lombes. M. The mineralocorticoid receptor: a journey exploring its diversity and specificity of action, *Molec. Endocrinol.*, 2005 19, 2211-2221.

Taniguchi, CM; Emanuelli, B; Kahn, CR. Critical nodes in signaling pathways: insights into insulin action. Nature Reviews Molecular *Cell Biology*, 2006 7, 85-96.

Thomson, CA; Geraci, JR. Cortisol, aldosterone, and leukocytes in the stress response of bottlenose dolphins, Tursiops truncatus. *Can. J. Fish. Aquat. Sci.*, 1986 43, 1010-1016.

Toma, DP; Bloch, G; Moore, D; Robinson, GE. Changes in Period mRNA levels in the brain and division of labor in honey bee colonies. *PNAS*, 2000 97, 6914-6919.

Toth, AL; Robinson, GE. Evo-devo and the evolution of social behavior. *Trends Genetics*, 2007 23, 334-341.

Tran, V; Lim, C; Xie, J; Chen, X. Asymmetric division of Drosophila male germline stem cell shows asymmetric histone distribution. *Science*, 2012 338, 679-682.

Trenzado, CE; Carrick, TR; Pottinger, TG. Divergence of endocrine and metabolic responses to stress in rainbow trout lines selected for differing cortisol responsiveness to stress. *Gen. Comp. Endocrinol.*, 2003 133, 3322-340.

Tzima, E; Irabni-Tehrani, M; Kiosses, WB; Dejanna, E; Schultz, DA; Engelhardt, B; Cao, G; DeLisser, H; Schwartz, MA. A mechanosensory complex that mediates the endothelial cell response to fluid shear stress. *Nature*, 2005 437, 426-431.

Tzingounis, AV; Nicoll, RA. Arc/Arg3.1: linking gene expression to synaptic plasticity and memory. *Neuron*, 2006 52, 403-407.

Ullian, ME; Walsh, LG; Morinelli, TA. Potentiation of angiotensin II action by corticosteroids in vascular tissue. *Cardiovascular Res*., 1996 32, 266-273.

Ullrich, A, et al. Insulin-like growth factor 1 receptor primary structure: comparison with insulin receptor suggests structural determinants that define functional specificity. *The EMBRO J.*, 1986 5, 2503-2512.

Underwood, E. Early isolation impairs brain connections. *Science Now*., Sept 13, 2012.

Unoki, H, et al. SNPs in KCNQ1 are associated with susceptibility to type 2 diabetes in East Asian and European populations. *Nature Genetics*, 2008 40, 1098-1102.

Urban, N; Tripathy, S. Circuits drive cell diversity. *Nature*, 2012 488, 289-290.

Vabulas, RM; Raychaudhuri, S; Hayer-Hartl, M; Hartl, FU. Protein folding in the cytoplasm and the heat shock response. *Cold Spring Harb. Perspect Biol*., 2010; 2: a004390.

VanCraenenbroeck, K; De Bosscher, K; Berghe, WV; Vanhoenacker, P; Haegeman, G. Role of glucocorticoids in dopamine-related neuropsychiatric disorders. *Molec. Cell Endocrinol*., 2005 245, 10-22.

Van ES, M; van den Berg, LH. Alzheimer's disease beyond APOE. *Nature Genetics*, 2009 41, 1047-1048.

VanSittert, SJ; Skinner, JD; Mitchell, G. From fetus to adult- an allometric analysis of the giraffe vertebral column. *J. Exp. Zool*.,(Mol Dev Evol) 2010 314 B, 469-479.

Vaquerizas, JM; Kummerfeld, SK; Teichmann, SA; Luscombe, NM. A census of human transcription factors: function, expression and evolution. *Nature Reviews Genetics*, 2009 10, 252-263.

Vastesaeger, MW. Coronary arterial lesions in exotic vertebrates. *Ann. N. Y. Acad. Sci*., 1965 127, 709-714.

Vastesaeger, MW; Delcourt, R. The natural history of atherosclerosis. *Circ*., 1962 26, 841-855.

Velican, C; Velican, D. Some particular aspects of the microarchitecture of human coronary arteries. *Atherosclerosis*, 1979 a), 33, 191-200.

Velican, D; Velican, C. Study of fibrous plaques occurring in the coronary arteries of children. *Atherosclerosis*, 1979 b) 33, 201-215.

Velican, C; Velican, D. Intimal thickening in developing coronary arteries and its relevance to atherosclerotic involvement. *Atherosclerosis*, 1976 23, 345-355.

Veraksa, ; DelCampo, M; McGinnis, W. Developmental patterning genes and their conserved functions: from model organisms to humans. *Molec. Genetics Metab*., 2000 69, 85-100.

Viengchareun, S; LeMenuet, D; Martinerie, L; Munier, M; Tallec, LP; Lombes, M. The mineralocorticoid receptor: insights into its molecular and (patho)physiological biology. *Nuclear Receptor Signaling*, 2007 5, e012.

Vijay-Kumar, M; Aitken, JD; Carvalho, FA; Cullender, TC; Mwangi, S; Srinivasan, S; Sitaraman, SV; Knight, R; Ley, RE; Gerwitz, AT. Metabolic syndrome and altered gut microbiota in mice lacking Toll-like receptor 5. *Science*, 2010 328, 228-231.

Wagensteil, JE; Mecham, RP. Vascular extracellular matrix and arterial mechanics. *Physiol. Rev.,* 2009 89, 957-989.

Wagner, JD; Cline, JM; Shadoan, MK; Bullock, BC; Rankin, SE; Cefalu, WT. Naturally occurring and experimental diabetes in cynomolgus monkeys: a comparison of carbohydrate and lipid metabolism and islet pathology. *Toxicol. Pathol*., 2001, 29, 142-148.

Wagner, JD; Kavanagh, K; Ward, GM; Auerbach, GJ; Harwood Jr, HJ; Kaplan, JR. Old world nonhuman primate models of type 2 diabetes mellitus. *ILAR J.*, 2006 47, 259-271.

Wang, X; Ishimori, N; Korstanje, R; Rollins, J; Paigen, B. Identifying novel genes for atherosclerosis through mouse-human comparative genetics. *Am. J. Hum. Genet.*, 2005 77, 1-16.

Wang, B, et al. Gamma- secretase gene mutations in familial acne inversa. *Science*, 2010 330, 1065.

Wagner, GP. The inner life of proteins. *Nature*, 2012 490, 493-494.

Wagner, GP; Lynch, VJ. Evolutionary novelties. *Curr. Biol.*, 2010 20, R48-R52.

Watanabe, H; Hoang, VT; Mattner, R; Holstein, TW. Immortality and the base of multicellular life: lessons from cnidarian stem cells. *Semin. Cell Develop. Biol.* 2009 20, 1114-1125.

Watkins-Chow, DE; Pavan WJ. Genomic copy number and expression variation within the C57BL/6J inbred mouse strain. *Genome Res.*, 2008 18, 60-66.

Weaver, ICG; Diorio, J; Seckl, JR; Szyf, M; Meaney, MJ. Early environmental regulation of hippocampal glucocorticoid receptor gene expression. *Ann. N. Y. Acad. Sci.*, 2004 1024, 182-212.

Weaver, ICG; D'Alessio, AC; Brown, SE; Hellstrom, IC; Dymov, S; Sharma, S; Syzf, M; Meaney, MJ. The transcription factor nerve growth factor-inducible protein A mediates epigenetic programming: altering epigenetic marks by immediate early genes. *J. Neurosci.*, 2007 27, 1756-1768.

Weaver, ICG; Cervoni, N; Champagne, FA; D'Alessio, AC; Sharma, S; Seckl, JR; Dymov, S; Szyf, M; Meaney, MJ. Epigenetic programming by maternal behavior. *Nature Neuroscience*, 2004 7, 847-854.

Webb, DM; Zhang, J. FoxP2 in song-learning birds and vocal learning mammals. *J. Heredity*, 2005 96, 212-216.

Wehrwein, P. Repeat to fade. *Nature*, 2012 492, S12-S13.

Wellcome Trust Case Control consortium. Genome-wide association study of 14,000 cases of seven common diseases and 3,000 shared controls. *Nature*, 2007 447, 661—683.

Wellcome Trust Case Control Consortium. Genome-wide association study of CNVs in 16,000 cases of eight common diseases and 3,000 shared controls. *Nature*, 2010 464, 713-722.

Welsh, DG; Morielli, AD; nelson, MT; Brayden, JE. Transient receptor potential channels regulate myogenic tone of resistance arteries. *Circ. Res.*, 2002 90, 248-250.

Weninger, WJ; Muller, GB; Reiter, C; Meng, S; Rabl, SU. Intimal hyperplasia of the infant parasellar carotid artery. *Circ. Res.*, 1999 85, 970-975.

West, JB. Comparative physiology of the pulmonary circulation. *Compr. Physiol.*, 2011 1, 1525-1539.

Wexler, NS, et al. Venezuelan kindreds reveal that genetic and environmental factors modulate Huntington's disease age of onset. *PNAS*, 2004 101, 3498-3503.

White, CR; Frangos, JA. The shear stress of it all: the cell membrane and mechanochemical transduction. *Phil. Trans. R. Soc. B.*, 2007 362, 1459-1467.

Whitfield, CW; Ben-Shahar, Y; Brillet, C; Leoncini, I; Crauser, D; LeConte, Y; Rodriguez-Zas, S; Robinson, GE. Genomic dissection of behavioral maturation in the honey bee. *PNAS*, 2006 103, 16068-16075.

Whitfield, CW; Cziko, A-M; Robinson, GE. Gene expression profiles in the brain predict behavior in individual honey bees. *Science*, 2003 302, 296-299.

Whitehead, A; Galvez, F; Zhang, S; Williams, LM; Oleksiak, MF. Functional genomics of physiological plasticity and local adaptation in killifish. *J. Heredity*, 2011 102, 499-511.

Whithers, DJ, et al. Disruption of IRS-2 causes type 2 diabetes in mice. *Nature*, 1998 391, 900-904.

Whitehouse, PJ. Classification of the dementias. *Lancet*, 2003 361, 1227.

Wilkins, BJ; Dai, Y-S; Bueno, OF; Parsons, SA; Xu, J; Plank, DM; Jones, F; Kimball, TR; Molkentin, JD. Calcineurin/NFAT coupling participates in pathological, but not physiological, cardiac hypertrophy. *Circ. Res*., 2004 94, 110-118.

Williams, JT. Promiscuous vesicles. *Nature*, 2012, 490, 178-179.

Wilson, M, et al. Cardiovascular function and the veteran athlete. *Eur. J. Appl. Physiol*., 2010 110, 459-478.

Wolinsky, H; Glagov, S. Comparison of abdominal and thoracic aortic medial structure in mammals. *Circ. Res*., 1969 25, 672-686.

Woodfin, A; Voisin, M-B; Nourshargh, S. PECAM-1: a multi-functional molecule in inflammation and vascular biology. *Arterioscler. Thromb. Vasc. Biol*., 2007 27, 2514-2523.

Wright Jr, JT; Davis, BR. Major outcomes in high- risk hypertensive patients randomized to angiotensin –converting enzyme inhibitor or calcium channel blocker vs diuretic. *JAMA*, 2002 288, 2981-2997.

Wu, H; Peisley, A; Graef, IA; Crabtree, GR. NFAT signaling and the invention of vertebrates. *Trends Cell Biol*., 2007 17, 251-260.

Wu, Q; Brown, MR. Signaling and function of insulin-like peptides in insects. *Annu. Rev. Entolmol*., 2006 51, 1-24.

Wu, Q; Clark, MS; Palmiter, RD. Deciphering a neuronal circuit that mediates appetite. *Nature*, 2012 483, 594-598.

Xiao, D; Huang, X; Bae, S; Ducsay, CA; Zhang, L. Cortisol-mediated potentiation of uterine artery contractility: effect of pregnancy. *Am. J. Physiol. Heart Circ. Physiol*., 2002 283, H238-H246.

Xu, T; Yu, X; Perlik, AJ; Tobin, WF; Zweig, JA; Tennant, K; Jones, T; Zuo, Y. Rapid formation and selective stabilization of synapses for enduring motor memories. *Nature*, 2009 462, 915-920.

Yamamoto, T; Nakahata, Y; Tanaka, M; Yoshida, M; Soma, H; Shinohara, K; Yasuda, A; Mamine. T; Takumi, T. Acute physical stress elevates mouse Period 1 mRNA expression in mouse peripheral tissues via a glucocorticoid-responsive element. *J. Biol. Chem*., 2005 280, 42036-42043.

Yamazaki, Y; Matsunaga, Y; Tokunaga, Y; Obayashi, S; Saito, M; Morita, T. Snake venom vascular endothelial growth factors (VEGF-Fs) exclusively vary their structures and functions among species. *J. Biol. Chem*., 2009 284, 9885-9891.

Yang, S; Zhang, L. Glucocorticoids and vascular reactivity. *Curr. Vasc. Pharmacol*., 2004 2, 1-12.

Yang, G; Pan, F; Gan, W-B. Stably maintained dendritic spines are associated with lifelong memories. *Nature*, 2009 462, 920-935.

Yoshida, H. ER stress and diseases. *The FEBS J*., 2007 274, 630-658.

Yoshida, K; Fujsawa, T; Hwang, JS; Ikeo, K; Gojobori, T. Degeneration after sexual differentiation in hydra and its relevance to the evolution of aging. *Gene*, 2006 385, 64-70.

Youngson, NA; Whitelaw, E. Transgenerational epigenetic effects. *Annu. Rev. Genomics Hum. Genet.*, 2008 9, 233-257.

Yu, L.; Tucci, V; Kishi, S; Zhdanova, IV. Cognitive aging in zebrafish. *PLoS ONE*, 2006 issue 1, (December) 1-13.

Zeng, C; Jose, PA. Dopamine receptors: important antihypertensive counterbalance against hypertensive factors. *Hypertens.*, 2011 57, 11-17.

Zeng, C: Armando, I; Luo, Y; Eisner, GM; Felder, RA; Jose, PA. Dysregulation of dopamine-dependent mechanisms as a determinant of hypertension: studies in dopamine receptor knockout mice. *Am. J. Physiol. Heart Circ. Physiol.*, 2008 294, H551- H569.

Zheng, H, et al. B-amyloid precursor protein-deficient mice show reactive gliosis and decreased locomotor activity. *Cell*, 1995 81, 525-531.

Zhou, Q-Y; Li, C; Cirelli, O. Characterization of gene organization and promoter region of the rat dopamine D1 receptor gene. *J. Neurochem.*, 1992 59, 1875-1883.

Zimmerman, AE; Moule, ML; Yip, CC. Guinea pig insulin II biological activity. *J. Biol. Chem.*, 1974 249, 4026-4029.

Zinzalla, V; Stracka, D; Oppliger, W; Hall, MN. Activation of mTORC2 by association with the ribosome. *Cell*, 2011 144, 757-768.

Ziv, NE; Ahissar, E. New tricks and old spines. *Nature*, 2009 462, 859-861.

Zuccato, C; Valenza, M; Cattaneo, E. Molecular mechanisms and potential therapeutic targets in Huntington's disease. *Physiol. Rev.*, 2010 90, 905-981.

Index

A

B

D

E

F

G

H

I

J

K

L

M

N

O

P

Q

R

S

T

U

V

W

X

Y

Z